Yoga for Positive Embodiment in Eating Disorder Prevention and Treatment

There is a growing body of research exploring the effectiveness of yoga as a pathway to positive embodiment for those at-risk for and struggling with eating disorders. This book provides a comprehensive look at the state of the field.

This book begins with an introduction to positive embodiment, eating disorders, and yoga. It also offers insights into the personal journey of each of the editors as they share what brought them to this work. The first section of this book explores the empirical and conceptual rationale for approaching eating disorder prevention and treatment through the lens of embodiment and yoga. The next section of the text integrates the history of embodiment theory as related to yoga and eating disorders, provides the logic model for change and guidance for researchers, and offers a critical social justice perceptive of the work to date. The third section addresses the efficacy of yoga in the prevention and treatment of eating disorders including a comprehensive review and meta-analysis as well as five research studies demonstrating the various approaches to exploring the preventative and therapeutic effects of yoga for disordered eating. The final section of this book closes with a chapter on future directions and offers guidance for what is next in both practice and research.

The chapters in this book were originally published as a special edition of *Eating Disorders: The Journal of Treatment & Prevention*.

Catherine Cook-Cottone, PhD, is a psychologist, certified yoga therapist, and Professor in the Department of Counseling, School, and Educational Psychology at the University at Buffalo, SUNY, USA. She has written 8 books and over 80 research articles and chapters specializing in embodiment, mindful self-regulation, eating disorders, and trauma. Passionate about service, she is co-founder and President of Yogis in Service, Inc.

Anne E. Cox is a yoga teacher and Professor of Sport and Exercise Psychology in the kinesiology program at Washington State University, Pullman, USA, where she co-directs the Psychology of Physical Activity Lab. Her research is focused on understanding key determinants of physical activity behaviors and seeks to apply knowledge about motivational processes and body image to create positive physical activity experiences.

Dianne Neumark-Sztainer, PhD, MPH, RD, RYT-500 is McKnight Presidential and Mayo Professor and serves as Head of the Division of Epidemiology and Community Health at the School of Public Health at the University of Minnesota, Minneapolis, USA. Her research focuses on a broad spectrum of eating and weight-related outcomes including eating disorders, unhealthy weight control behaviors, body image, dietary intake, weight stigmatization, and obesity. A certified yoga instructor, she has published approximately 550 articles, and her current research interests include investigating the potential for the practice of yoga to help with body image concerns and eating disorders.

Tracy L. Tylka, PhD, is Professor of Psychology at The Ohio State University, USA. Her research focuses on both positive and negative body image and adaptive and maladaptive eating. To date, she has published 87 journal articles and has written three books and 20 book chapters. She is Editor-in-Chief for *Body Image: An International Journal of Research* and on the editorial board for *Eating Disorders: The Journal of Treatment & Prevention*. She is Fellow of the Academy of Eating Disorders.

Yoga for Positive Embodiment in Eating Disorder Prevention and Treatment

Edited by
Catherine Cook-Cottone, Anne E. Cox,
Dianne Neumark-Sztainer and Tracy L. Tylka

Routledge
Taylor & Francis Group
LONDON AND NEW YORK

First published 2023
by Routledge
4 Park Square, Milton Park, Abingdon, Oxon, OX14 4RN

and by Routledge
605 Third Avenue, New York, NY 10158

Routledge is an imprint of the Taylor & Francis Group, an informa business

British Library Cataloguing-in-Publication Data
A catalogue record for this book is available from the British Library

ISBN13: 978-1-032-06323-2 (hbk)
ISBN13: 978-1-032-06324-9 (pbk)
ISBN13: 978-1-003-20173-1 (ebk)

DOI: 10.4324/9781003201731

Typeset in Minion Pro
by codeMantra

Publisher's Note
The publisher accepts responsibility for any inconsistencies that may have arisen during the conversion of this book from journal articles to book chapters, namely the inclusion of journal terminology.

Disclaimer
Every effort has been made to contact copyright holders for their permission to reprint material in this book. The publishers would be grateful to hear from any copyright holder who is not here acknowledged and will undertake to rectify any errors or omissions in future editions of this book.

Contents

Citation Information   vii
Notes on Contributors   ix

1 Introduction   1
  Dianne Neumark-Sztainer, Catherine Cook-Cottone, Tracy L. Tylka,
  and Anne E. Cox

Theoretical and empirical considerations   **7**

2 Eating disorders, embodiment, and yoga: a conceptual overview   9
  Iris Perey and Catherine Cook-Cottone

3 Yoga and the experience of embodiment: a discussion of possible links 24
  Niva Piran and Dianne Neumark-Sztainer

4 Realizing Yoga's all-access pass: a social justice critique of westernized yoga and
  inclusive embodiment   43
  Jennifer B. Webb, Courtney B. Rogers, and Erin Vinoski Thomas

5 A conceptual model describing mechanisms for how yoga practice may support
  positive embodiment   70
  Anne E. Cox and Tracy L. Tylka

Research update   **95**

6 Yoga and eating disorder prevention and treatment: a comprehensive review
  and meta-analysis   97
  Ashlye Borden and Catherine Cook-Cottone

7 Benefits of yoga in the treatment of eating disorders: results of a randomized
  controlled trial   135
  Margaret A. Brennan, William J. Whelton, and Donald Sharpe

8 Examining the effects of mindfulness-based yoga instruction on positive embodiment and affective responses 155
Anne E. Cox, Sarah Ullrich-French, Catherine Cook-Cottone, Tracy L. Tylka, and Dianne Neumark-Sztainer

9 A yoga-based therapy program designed to improve body image among an outpatient eating disordered population: program description and results from a mixed-methods pilot study 173
Lisa Diers, Sarah A. Rydell, Allison Watts, and Dianne Neumark-Sztainer

10 Yoga practice in a college sample: associated changes in eating disorder, body image, and related factors over time 191
Rachel Kramer and Kelly Cuccolo

11 Yoga's impact on risk and protective factors for disordered eating: a pilot prevention trial 210
CR Pacanowski, L Diers, RD Crosby, M Mackenzie, and D. Neumark-Sztainer

Future directions **239**

12 Future directions for research on yoga and positive embodiment 241
Catherine Cook-Cottone, Anne Elizabeth Cox, Dianne Neumark-Sztainer, and Tracy L. Tylka

Index 247

Citation Information

The chapters in this book were originally published in *Eating Disorders: The Journal of Treatment and Prevention*, volume 28, issue 4 (2020). When citing this material, please use the original page numbering for each article, as follows:

Chapter 1
Introduction to the special issue on yoga and positive embodiment: a note from the editors on how we got here
Dianne Neumark-Sztainer, Catherine Cook-Cottone, Tracy L. Tylka, and Anne Elizabeth Cox
Eating Disorders, volume 28, issue 4 (2020) pp. 309–314

Chapter 2
Eating disorders, embodiment, and yoga: a conceptual overview
Iris Perey and Catherine Cook-Cottone
Eating Disorders, volume 28, issue 4 (2020) pp. 315–329

Chapter 3
Yoga and the experience of embodiment: a discussion of possible links
Niva Piran and Dianne Neumark-Sztainer
Eating Disorders, volume 28, issue 4 (2020) pp. 330–348

Chapter 4
Realizing Yoga's all-access pass: a social justice critique of westernized yoga and inclusive embodiment
Jennifer B. Webb, Courtney B. Rogers, and Erin Vinoski Thomas
Eating Disorders, volume 28, issue 4 (2020) pp. 349–375

Chapter 5
A conceptual model describing mechanisms for how yoga practice may support positive embodiment
Anne E. Cox and Tracy L. Tylka
Eating Disorders, volume 28, issue 4 (2020) pp. 376–399

Chapter 6
Yoga and eating disorder prevention and treatment: A comprehensive review and meta-analysis
Ashlye Borden and Catherine Cook-Cottone
Eating Disorders, volume 28, issue 4 (2020) pp. 400–437

Chapter 7
Benefits of yoga in the treatment of eating disorders: Results of a randomized controlled trial
Margaret A. Brennan, William J. Whelton, and Donald Sharpe
Eating Disorders, volume 28, issue 4 (2020) pp. 438–457

Chapter 8
Examining the effects of mindfulness-based yoga instruction on positive embodiment and affective responses
Anne E. Cox, Sarah Ullrich-French, Catherine Cook-Cottone, Tracy L. Tylka, and Dianne Neumark-Sztainer
Eating Disorders, volume 28, issue 4 (2020) pp. 458–475

Chapter 9
A yoga-based therapy program designed to improve body image among an outpatient eating disordered population: program description and results from a mixed-methods pilot study
Lisa Diers, Sarah A. Rydell, Allison Watts, and Dianne Neumark-Sztainer
Eating Disorders, volume 28, issue 4 (2020) pp. 476–493

Chapter 10
Yoga Practice in a College Sample: Associated Changes in Eating Disorder, Body Image, and Related Factors Over Time
Rachel Kramer and Kelly Cuccolo
Eating Disorders, volume 28, issue 4 (2020) pp. 494–512

Chapter 11
Yoga's impact on risk and protective factors for disordered eating: a pilot prevention trial
CR Pacanowski, L Diers, RD Crosby, M Mackenzie, and D. Neumark-Sztainer
Eating Disorders, volume 28, issue 4 (2020) pp. 513–541

Chapter 12
Future directions for research on yoga and positive embodiment
Catherine Cook-Cottone, Anne Elizabeth Cox, Dianne Neumark-Sztainer, and Tracy L. Tylka
Eating Disorders, volume 28, issue 4 (2020) pp. 542–547

For any permission-related enquiries please visit:
http://www.tandfonline.com/page/help/permissions

Notes on Contributors

Ashlye Borden, Department of Counseling, School, and Educational Psychology, University at Buffalo, State University of New York, USA.

Margaret A. Brennan, Department of Educational Psychology, University of Alberta, Edmonton, Canada; Department of Educational Psychology, University of British Columbia, Vancouver, Canada.

Catherine Cook-Cottone, Counseling, School, and Educational Ps, University at Buffalo, State University of New York, USA.

Anne E. Cox, Department of Kinesiology and Educational Psychology, Washington State University, Pullman, USA.

RD Crosby, Sanford Center for Bio-Behavioral Research, Fargo, USA.

Kelly Cuccolo, Department of Psychology, University of North Dakota, Grand Forks, USA.

Lisa Diers, Private Practice, Lisa Diers Yoga and Nutrition Consulting, LLC, Minneapolis, USA.

Rachel Kramer, Department of Psychology, University of North Dakota, Grand Forks, USA; Behavioral Medicine and Clinical Psychology, Cincinnati Children's Hospital Medical Center, Cincinnati, USA.

M Mackenzie, Department of Behavioral Health and Nutrition, University of Delaware, Newark, USA.

Dianne Neumark-Sztainer, Division of Epidemiology and Community Health, School of Public Health, University of Minnesota, Minneapolis, USA.

CR Pacanowski, Department of Behavioral Health and Nutrition, University of Delaware, Newark, USA.

Iris Perey, Chair of Sport and Health Management, Technical University of Munich, Germany.

Niva Piran, Department of Applied Psychology and Human Development Ontario Institute for Studies in Education, University of Toronto, Canada.

Courtney B. Rogers, UNC Charlotte Department of Psychological Science, USA.

Sarah A. Rydell, Division of Epidemiology and Community Health, School of Public Health, University of Minnesota, Minneapolis, USA.

Donald Sharpe, Department of Psychology, University of Regina, Canada.

Erin Vinoski Thomas, Georgia State University School of Public Health, Center for Leadership in Disability, Atlanta, USA.

Tracy L. Tylka, Department of Psychology, The Ohio State University, Columbus, USA.

Sarah Ullrich-French, Department of Kinesiology & Educational Psychology, Washington State University, Pullman, USA.

Allison Watts, Division of Epidemiology and Community Health, School of Public Health, University of Minnesota, Minneapolis, USA.

Jennifer B. Webb, UNC Charlotte Department of Psychological Science, USA.

William J. Whelton, Department of Educational Psychology, University of Alberta, Edmonton, Canada.

Introduction

Dianne Neumark-Sztainer, Catherine Cook-Cottone, Tracy L. Tylka, and Anne E. Cox

ABSTRACT

Studying the practice of yoga and its relationship to body image, embodiment, and eating disorders brings together the professional and personal aspects of our lives as yoga practitioners, researchers, and women living in bodies within a society that can be tough on body appreciation. Developing this edition on "Yoga for positive embodiment in eating disorder prevention and treatment" has been a work of love for all of us. As yoga practitioners, we have personally experienced the benefits of yoga in our own bodies and felt that there may be benefits for others. As researchers, we are dedicated to the exploration and utilization of evidence-based practices to enhance well-being, promote a positive body image and sense of embodiment, and both prevent and treat eating disorders. Our experiences as yoga practitioners, in conjunction with our curiosity as researchers, led us to explore the extant evidence for yoga as a tool for leading to improvements in body image, disordered eating behaviors, and eating disorders, and to embark on our own research in this area to fill necessary gaps in our knowledge base. Our long-term dedication to the fields of body image and eating disorders, in conjunction with our emerging interest in yoga as a potential tool, led us to the compilation of this edition on yoga and positive embodiment.

Empirical research and theoretical models on yoga and body image, embodiment, and eating disorders are in the early stages. Yet this edition includes scientific papers that clearly demonstrate the passion for the topic at hand, deep thought regarding processes of influence and best strategies, and the beginnings of important research. Furthermore, the articles in this edition set the stage for future directions (Cox, Cook-Cottone, Tylka, & Neumark-Sztainer, 2020). We have included a construct review paper that provides an overview of the psychological theories of embodiment and the practice of yoga (Perey & Cook-Cottone, 2020) and a theoretical paper that applies of the Developmental Theory of Embodiment specifically to the practice of yoga (Piran & Neumark-Sztainer, 2020). To support further research, we include a paper detailing a conceptual model exploring the mechanisms that connect yoga to positive embodiment (Cox & Tylka, 2020) and a perspective piece on social justice and intervention studies (Webb, Rogers, & Thomas, 2020). Along with the latest intervention studies (Brennan & Whelton, 2020; Cox, Ullrich-French, Cook-Cottone, Tylka, & Neumark-Sztainer, 2020; Diers, Rydell, Watts, & Neumark-Sztainer, 2020; Kramer, & Cucculo, 2020; Pacanowski, Diers, Crosby, Mackenzie, & Neumark-Sztainer, 2020), this special issue includes the most comprehensive review and meta-analysis on eating disorder and yoga to date (Borden & Cook-Cottone, 2020). You may choose to review all of the abstracts and then do a close read of one or two articles. Or, you may choose to read the whole edition from front to back to gain a rich perspective on the state of the field with regard to yoga and its potential to help with body image, a sense of embodiment, and eating disorders.

Given the strong intersection between the professional and the personal on the topics of yoga, body image, embodiment, and eating disorders, we take the unusual step here of providing some background on our own journeys through yoga both as a personal practice and an area of research interest. Some of us are clinicians; some of us are yoga instructors; and some of us have had body image concerns and/or eating disorders. All of us are serious yoga practitioners and researchers within the areas of body image and eating disorders. In studying yoga in relation to these health outcomes, we find ourselves in a situation where we have reached a state of "near-perfect union" between our personal and professional interests. Our personal experiences with yoga have greatly informed and enriched our theoretical writings and our empirical research. Yet, we know the importance of conducting strong research and avoiding bias in the design of studies, the implementation of data collection and intervention protocols, and interpretation of study findings. We have made every effort to avoid any bias in papers that we have either written or reviewed. But we also recognize the potential for bias. Thus, we share brief summaries of our own body image, yoga, and yoga research journeys, given that others on similar paths may be interested in our stories, and to be transparent about our own personal involvement in the topic at hand.

Anne E. Cox PhD writes: My struggle with body image started at the end of the first year of college when I had put on a tiny bit of weight. I was a college basketball player but instead of focusing on feeling good and supporting my performance, all I could think about was being thinner and lighter. It dominated my thinking and planning throughout the day. During the 15 years after college, I slowly healed somehow, but still ideas of having eaten too much or not burning enough calories would run through my head. The external focus did continue to loosen its grip. I remember one poignant moment when I felt so pleased to be a size smaller (compared to before pregnancy) a couple months after having my child. It quickly dawned on me that I was smaller because I had lost so much muscle. The ridiculousness of feeling good about that sat like a weight in my bones—another nail in the coffin housing my body image concerns. There were many such nails, but yoga was the final one. I started practicing at a yoga studio 6.5 years ago when my daughter had just turned 5. I really can't remember why I was drawn to it, but each and every class was a revelation. As a researcher, I would sit and contemplate why I was feeling so damn good in my own skin. And the unique experience of being instructed to be in my body, breathe in my body, feel my body without judgment or comparison set this form of movement apart from anything I had ever experienced as an athlete or exerciser. I was hooked! It only took a few months before I really felt like my external, objectifying focus on my body became almost completely internal. So now I practice yoga almost every day and I never have negative thoughts or emotions about my body. It doesn't take up space in my thinking throughout the day. I am free to just be and live and experience. I am now teaching yoga and researching the effects of yoga on body image and physical activity motivation in the hopes of helping others on their journey.

Tracy Tylka PhD shares the following: I struggled with disrupted embodiment from a very early age. My sister, who is 14 years older, was always on a "strict diet" and complained incessantly about her body. When I was 4 years old, she served as a template for how to experience my body in this world (as disconnected and a source of discomfort). I internalized her disrupted embodiment, which was fueled within family interactions laden with weight stigma. Cognitive-behavioral therapy eventually helped me arrive at a place of "neutrality" toward my body, meaning that I didn't have any recognizable symptoms of negative body image or disordered eating, but I didn't feel positively towards it either. Instead, I tried to not think about my body much. Self-care was more mechanistic at this point, such as following a food plan with little attention of what my body needed beyond its most basic requirements. Rooted in my personal experiences and my interest in psychology, I began conducting research on body image and disordered eating in my undergraduate and graduate research in psychology. After I joined the Department of Psychology at The Ohio State University, I started wondering if there was a place beyond "body neutrality" and I started studying positive body image, which including developing a measure of it, the Body Appreciation Scale. My research had a side benefit of helping me shift my attitude towards my body from neutral to positive. Yet, reflecting back, I don't think that I experienced positive embodiment at this point (i.e., I appreciated my body, but was not particularly connected to it or comfortable with or within it). A few years after I was promoted to full professor, when I was separated from my husband, I started yoga at a nearby studio at the suggestion of a friend. Through yoga, I physically worked through my difficult emotions surrounding the separation and my body discomfort and disconnection—I was finally "in my body." I felt these emotions, which were once stuck inside, work their way up from my core to the surface and were released in my movement through the asanas. In addition to sweat, my mat would include my fallen tears. Yoga helped orient me toward my body in a way that I never felt before—as a source of strength, connection, and comfort. It also provided patience and forgiveness, as well as space for me to sort out my confusing thoughts and experiences. Unfortunately, I had to recently postpone vinyasa flow due to a broken metatarsal, severe toe arthritis, surgery, and recovery, but other yoga practices have kept me centered, focused, calm, and appreciative during this time of restricted body function. For me, yoga has been the therapy that has lifted me to positive embodiment, picking up where more traditional Western thera-peutic approaches and even studying body appreciation left off. I view yoga as a gift to my body, an intentional practice to build and maintain positive embodiment.

Catherine Cook-Cottone, PhD, E-RYT 500 shares: In 9th grade I was officially diagnosed with an eating disorder, culminating years of at-risk behavior, negative body image, and an embattled relationship with my body. Because of my not-good-enough body, I was a failed dancer, a soccer player who flinched rather than scored, and a swimmer who wasn't ever quite fast enough. My body, despite my ongoing efforts to oppress it, was also not thin enough, pretty enough, or generally enough in any way. By the time I was a tenure-track researcher, through counseling and my own personal work, I was relatively recovered, except that I still was not at home in my own body and sometimes, to be completely truthful, still hated it (and I know hate is a strong word).

Early in my career as a professor, one of my students who was also in yoga teacher training invited me to take one of her yoga classes. She said that my ideas, theories, and approaches were very aligned with yoga. I demonstrated my forward fold, to show her one of my body's many inadequacies and explained that yoga was not for me. Disagreeing, she said anyone could do yoga. I said that "Maybe. Maybe, I will come to your class." A year later, I registered for her beginners' yoga class. We started out in Corpse Pose. "Morbid," I thought. I now see this as perfect. Death and rebirth—start in corpse—perfect. We placed one hand on our bellies and one hand on our hearts. She showed us how to breathe. For those of you who were born yogis this might sound ridiculous, but these breaths were miraculous to me. I wanted to cry. After class, I was, well, a few things. I declared to all who would listen, "This is the best I have felt without a few glasses of red wine in years, perhaps ever." And I felt successful, "I can do yoga!"

So, here I am, 20 years later, embodying self-love. After two decades of yoga, my body and my mind have gotten to know each other. It was in that first yoga class that I began to see and know my body in a new way and not from my outward, judgmental gaze. I began in inhabit, sense, and move from my body. I did not know the term at the time, but I was moving toward what is now called positive embodiment. I have researched eating disorders and yoga for many years. More importantly, I do yoga. I practice nearly every day. I also teach yoga. I want as many people as possible to feel like I feel when I do yoga. When I look out at the class in final resting pose, I can only imagine that these deeply personal and embodied transformations will make the world a much happier place.

Dianne Neumark-Sztainer PhD MPH RD RYT-500 writes: My yoga journey began nearly 40 years ago on a kibbutz in Israel. I loved the practice of yoga, but it got shelved for many years, as life got busy. I returned to yoga about 15 years ago—this time in Minnesota. I took up yoga for physical reasons (i.e., lower back pain), but continued the practice for a combination of physical, energetic, mental, emotional, and spiritual reasons. Through practicing yoga I became more in touch with sensations in my body and found myself better able to respond to them throughout my day. Over a few years, my yoga practice grew from participating in weekly classes at a community center to trying different classes at a local yoga studio, seeking extended yoga workshops and retreats, and developing a regular home practice. My curiosity grew with regard to the potential value of this practice for the fields of body image and eating disorders. I decided that I wanted to learn more so I took a sabbatical leave from my academic career and embarked on a deep study of yoga, including participating in an advanced yoga teacher-training program. For a few years, I had the amazing experience of teaching yoga to individuals with body image concerns at an eating disorders treatment program. And, I began to develop a line of research in this area. The knowledge gained from my personal practice, the teacher-training programs, and the experience of working within an eating disorders treatment program has guided the research questions that we are exploring. I have been involved in a few intervention studies, but the bulk of my work is linked to my ongoing longitudinal population-based study, Project EAT, to which we added questions on yoga. Perhaps of less relevance to this edition, but of great relevance to my life, when I became Chair of a large academic department and had to deal with many challenging situations, my yoga practice served me well. The personal and the professional have certainly come together for me.

We hope you will enjoy reading the articles in this edition as much as we have enjoyed compiling the edition. More importantly, we hope it will serve as a jump-off point for your own personal and professional explorations of the topic of yoga and its potential to help improve body image, a sense of embodiment, and eating disorders. We welcome your thoughts!

Dianne

Catherine

Tracey

Anne

References

Borden, A., & Cook-Cottone, C. P. (2020). Yoga and eating disorder prevention and treatment: A comprehensive review and meta-analysis. Eating Disorders: The Journal of Treatment and Prevention, 28(4), 400–437.

Brennan, M. A., & Whelton, W. J. (2020). Benefits of yoga in the treatment of eating disorders; Results of a randomized controlled trial. Eating Disorders: The Journal of Treatment and Prevention, 28(4), 438–457.

Cox, A. E., Cook-Cottone, C. P., Tylka, T. L., & Neumark-Sztainer, D. (2020). Future Directions for Research on Yoga and Positive Embodiment. Eating Disorders: The Journal of Treatment and Prevention, 28(4), 542–547.

Cox, A. E., Ullrich-French, S., Cook-Cottone, C. P., Tylka, T. L., & Neumark-Sztainer, D. (2020). Examining the effects of mindfulness-based yoga instruction in positive embodiment and affective responses. Eating Disorders: The Journal of Treatment and Prevention, 28(4), 458–475.

Cox, A. E., & Tylka, T. L. (2020). A conceptual model describing the mechanism for how yoga practice may support positive embodiment. Eating Disorders: The Journal of Treatment and Prevention, 28(4), 376–399.

Kramer, R., & Cucculo, K. (2020). Yoga practice in a college sample: Associate changes in eating disorder, body image, and related factors over time. Eating Disorders: The Journal of Treatment and Prevention, 28(4), 494–512.

Pacanowski, C. R., Diers, L., Crosby, R. D., Mackenzie, M., & Neumark-Sztainer, D. (2020). Yoga's impact on risk and protective factors for disordered eating: A pilot prevention trial. Eating Disorders: The Journal of Treatment and Prevention, 28(4), 513–541.

Perey, I., & Cook-Cottone, C. P. (2020). Eating disorders, embodiment, and yoga: A conceptual overview. Eating Disorders: The Journal of Treatment and Prevention, 28(4), 315–329.

Piran, N., & Neumark-Sztainer, D. (2020). Yoga and the experience of embodiment: A discussion of possible links. Eating Disorders: The Journal of Treatment and Prevention, 28(4), 330–348.

Webb, J. B., Rogers, C. B., & Thomas, E. V. (2020). Realizing yoga's all-access pass: A social justice critique of Westernized yoga and inclusive embodiment. Eating Disorders: The Journal of Treatment and Prevention, 28(4), 349–375.

Theoretical and empirical considerations

Eating disorders, embodiment, and yoga: a conceptual overview

Iris Perey and Catherine Cook-Cottone

ABSTRACT

Yoga and its relation to embodiment and disordered eating has only recently received research attention. Nevertheless, early research indicates that yoga is an effective tool in the prevention and treatment of eating disorders. It is assumed that yoga ameliorates eating disorder symptoms and facilitates a shift from negative towards positive body image and well-being by cultivating positive embodiment (i.e., the ability to feel a sense of connection between mind and body). In order to provide the context of the constructs of disordered eating, embodiment, and yoga, this article presents a brief overview and conceptualization of these constructs. The three major eating disorders and current treatment methods are described. Further, the philosophical roots and theoretical models of embodiment are delineated and their communal core features are outlined. Lastly, the origin, basic principles, and modern interpretations of yoga are discussed.

Clinical Implications

- Provides practitioners working in eating disorder prevention and treatment a conceptual overview of eating disorders, embodiment, and yoga.
- Provides a conceptual context for understanding yoga as a tool for prevention of and as an adjunctive treatment for eating disorders.
- Theoretical models of embodiment present useful frameworks for explaining the positive effects of yoga in eating disorder prevention and treatment.

Introduction

Over the past few decades, yoga has become increasingly popular as an adjunctive support in the treatment of eating disorders (EDs), presenting an accessible, cost-effective, and stigma-free approach (Ariel-Donges et al.,

2018; Domingues & Carmo, 2019; Neumark-Sztainer, 2014). In addition, yoga has also been incorporated as a method to prevent the development of ED symptomatology and associated risk factors, including body dissatisfaction, body surveillance, self-objectification, and appearance evaluation (Ariel-Donges et al., 2018; Cook-Cottone et al., 2017; Cox et al., 2017; Scime & Cook-Cottone, 2008).

It is theorized that yoga supports recovery and disrupts the onset of EDs by facilitating positive embodiment (Cook-Cottone, 2020). Quantitative and qualitative research suggests that yoga practice promotes positive ways of experiencing the body, such as increased body awareness and responsiveness, body connectedness, body appreciation, and body satisfaction (Daubenmier, 2005; Halliwell et al., 2019; Neumark-Sztainer et al., 2018). Experiencing body connection and attunement may strengthen an individual's capacity to respond to body- and eating-related challenges in adaptive ways (Cook-Cottone, 2020). Indeed, positive embodiment has been found to serve as a protective factor against negative body image and disordered eating (Levine & Smolak, 2016). Further, a positive way of being in and with the body is considered an essential perquisite to ED recovery (Cook-Cottone, 2020; Menzel & Levine, 2011; Piran, 2002, 2017).

This special issue is dedicated to the review of the relevant research on yoga for promoting positive embodiment as a pathway to ED prevention and treatment. In order to support a shared understanding of the fundamental ideas behind yoga, embodiment, and EDs, we provide a brief overview of the three major EDs, an introduction to the philosophical roots and the theoretical work in the area of embodiment, as well as a short history and description of the practices of yoga.

Eating disorders

EDs are complex mental disorders marked by a disturbance in food- and body-related attitudes, cognitions, and behaviors that are evoked by a range of biological, psychological, and sociocultural factors (American Psychiatric Association, 2013). EDs are, in essence, a disordered manifestation of an individual's experience of being in and with the body (Cook-Cottone, 2020). This presents behaviorally as dysfunctional eating behaviors (i.e., bingeing and restriction), the misuse of pharmaceuticals (i.e., laxatives and diuretics), and excessive exercise (American Psychiatric Association, 2013). Clinical EDs are associated with physiological (e.g., impaired organ and bodily functions), psychological (e.g., emotional distress and anxiety) and social (e.g., social isolation and poor school and work performance) difficulties, as well as an increased mortality risk (Smink et al., 2013).

Three major types of EDs are usually considered, namely anorexia nervosa (AN), bulimia nervosa (BN), and binge eating disorder (BED). AN involves a distorted perception of the body, which causes individuals with AN to deny their objectively low body weight and to pursue an unattainable ideal of thinness. Driven by an intense fear of gaining weight, individuals suffering from anorexia restrict their food intake and frequently ignore hunger cues and other bodily signals (American Psychiatric Association, 2013). Diagnostically, the restricting and the binge-eating/purging subtypes are differentiated (American Psychiatric Association, 2013).

BN is marked by destructive thoughts about food and body, as well as a cycle of bingeing and compensatory purging behaviors to prevent weight gain (American Psychiatric Association, 2013). Pathological behaviors frequently go unnoticed even by friends and family members since individuals with BN may act in secrecy, presenting the self as effectively functioning (Hay & Claudino, 2015). Similar to individuals with AN, sufferers from BN exceedingly base their self-evaluation on their physical appearance and inhabit the body as object rather than sensing and experiencing it (American Psychiatric Association, 2013; Cook-Cottone, 2015a). In contrast, individuals with BN typically maintain a normal weight or are overweight (Bulik et al., 2012).

Symptomatology of BED is characterized by episodes of uncontrolled bingeing with distress but without the compensatory behaviors seen in BN (American Psychiatric Association, 2013). Bodily cues are ignored as food is consumed rapidly until feeling uncomfortably full or in the absence of hunger (Cook-Cottone, 2015a, 2015b). Binges frequently occur in response to stressful life events or emotional struggles (Brewerton, 2004). Although BED is associated with overweight and obesity (Grucza et al., 2007; Wilson et al., 2010), it is distinct in that quality of life levels are lower in individuals with BED and obesity is not considered a clinical psychopathology (Smink et al., 2013).

Treatment of eating disorders

The multi-faceted nature of EDs indicates the imperative of a multidisciplinary approach to treatment, targeting biological, psychological, behavioral, as well as social factors (Brewerton, 2004; Rosen, 2010). Disturbances in the experience of the body are typically addressed within the psychological and behavioral elements of treatment. Empirically supported psychological interventions for individuals with AN include cognitive behavioral therapy (CBT), interpersonal therapy (IPT), and family-based treatment (FBT) for adolescents (Linardon et al., 2016; Lock & Le Grange, 2015; Watson & Bulik, 2013). In individuals with BN, the use of CBT, IPT, as well as Dialectic Behavioral Therapy (DBT), a mindfulness-based therapy focusing on emotion regulation and distress tolerance, has shown to be effective (Erford et al., 2013; McIntosh et al., 2011; Poulsen et al., 2014;

Tanofsky-Kraff & Wilfley, 2010). Although research on BED intervention methods is still in its infancy, CBT, IPT, and DBT have been found to effectively reduce bingeing (Amianto, Ottone, Daga & Fassino, 2015; Iacovino et al., 2012; Wilson et al., 2010).

In a recent review on the treatment of EDs, Murray (2019) concludes that the majority of patients do not achieve full and lasting recovery. Empirically supported treatment methods for EDs mainly target improving eating behavior, self-regulation, and interpersonal relationships. The individual's embodied experience, which is central to the development and maintenance of all EDs, is disregarded (Cook-Cottone, 2015a; Cook-Cottone, 2016). In order to provide patients with a pathway towards true healing, instead of the mere alleviation of symptoms, it is imperative to incorporate strategies that support positive embodiment above and beyond the traditional treatment goal to manage dysfunctional cognitions about the body (Cook-Cottone, 2015b; Cook-Cottone, 2016; Domingues & Carmo, 2019; Piran & Teall, 2012).

Positive embodiment, the ability to feel a sense of connection between mind and body, may be critical to full recovery (Cook-Cottone & Douglass, 2017; Piran & Teall, 2012). Giving form to positive embodiment involves integrating awareness of one's internal needs and environmental demands, as well as intentional engagement in embodied practice (Cook-Cottone, 2015a). By these means, judgement, objectification and ignorance of the body may be replaced with actively *experiencing* it (Cook-Cottone, 2020). Eventually, positively inhabiting the body is accompanied by sustained mental and physical health. Current methods of treatment for individuals with EDs may thus be enriched by incorporating embodied approaches that help patients cultivate an authentic experience of their bodies (Cook-Cottone, 2015a, 2019, 2020; Piran & Neumark-Sztainer, 2020).

Philosophical roots and psychological theories of embodiment

Philosophically, embodiment presents a developing, evolving experience of self (Cook-Cottone, 2020). More than a way of being in the body, many assert that embodiment is what we know as the experience of self (e.g., Merleau-Ponty, 2013). Historically, philosophers and theologians assumed that human embodiment is the consequence of a fall from grace, an originally superior state of pure mental or ethereal existence (Cook-Cottone, 2020; Smith, 2017). Superior, the mind was considered closer to what was understood as God. The body was the seat of sin, the mortal drives, and human frailties (Cook-Cottone, 2020). From this perspective, embodiment is a state of being a subject or entity, coexisting with, captaining, or even imprisoned in a body (Smith, 2017). Accordingly, humans aspired to be free of the body, its burdens, limitations, and mortality (Cook-Cottone, 2020).

In the 20th century, philosophers started questioning the traditional notion of the body being inferior to the mind (Cook-Cottone, 2020; Smith, 2017). The lived body was brought to the center of human experience not as a difficulty to be overcome, but as *the self* (Merleau-Ponty, 2013). In 1946, another important contribution came from Viktor Frankl who detailed his experiences in the Auschwitz concentration camp during World War II in his book *Man's Search for Meaning* (Frankl, 1959). Frankl (1959) proposed that life questions each of us and our answers must be embodied in right action. It is through the body that the ideas of our heart and mind (e.g., passions, beliefs, and values) manifest in action. Frankl's concept of *tri-dimensional ontology* (1969) suggests that the self constitutes an anthropological unity, composed of somatic (i.e., body), psychic (i.e., mental), and noetic (i.e., spiritual) aspects (Cook-Cottone, 2020; Stankovskaya, 2014).

Attempts at defining embodiment as a measurable, psychological construct have yielded multifaceted theories that are anchored in and inspired by these early discussions of embodiment. Contemporary theoretical models integrate the internal and external experiences, as well as the relational, developmental, contextual, cultural, and existential aspects of the self (Cook-Cottone, 2020).

Piran's developmental theory of embodiment

Inspired by the feminist existentialist Simone de Beauvoir's writings on the loss of embodiment in adolescence, Niva Piran began studying embodiment 20 years ago (Piran, 2017). Her *Developmental Theory of Embodiment* (DTE; Piran, 2002, 2016, 2017; Piran & Teall, 2012) examines the relationship between social interactions and girls' and women's embodied experiences while engaging in the world around them. The theory is informed by a mixed-method research program conducted by Piran and colleagues (e.g., Piran, 2016, 2017; Piran & Teall, 2012). Their work includes 171 interviews with girls and women, 116 focus groups with school girls, and quantitative surveys with women, exploring the quality of embodied lives and the factors that shape them.

With regards to the quality of embodied lives, the narratives of participants revealed a multi-dimensional core construct, termed *Experience of Embodiment* (EE; Piran, 2016, 2017, 2019a). This construct ranges from positive embodiment, defined as "positive body connection and comfort, embodied agency and passion, and attuned self-care" (Piran, 2016, p. 47), to negative embodiment, described as "disrupted body connection and discomfort, restricted agency and passion, and self-neglect or harm" (Piran, 2016, p. 47). The quality of a girl or woman's EE is organized along five dimensions: (a) Body connection and comfort, (b) agency and functionality, (c) experience and expression of bodily desires, (d) attuned self-care, and (e) inhabiting the body as a subjective (vs. objective) site (Piran, 2019b). This conceptualization proposes that actively engaging in behaviors such as positive self-talk, exercising with agency, appreciating bodily functions, connecting to and expressing bodily desires, attending and responding to internal cues, and inhabiting the body with a sense of subjective immersion, allows a shift from negative towards positive embodiment (Piran, 2016, 2019a). EE and its dimensions can be measured by the 34-item Experience of Embodiment Scale (EES; Piran, 2019a).

Next, the EEs described by girls and women indicated protective and risk factors that shape embodied lives via three key pathways: Experiences in the physical domain, experiences in the mental domain, and experiences related directly to social power and relational connections (Piran & Teall, 2012). Protective factors include, for example, the engagement in physical activity for enjoyment (i.e., physical domain), the freedom to act self-determined (i.e., mental domain), and the freedom from prejudicial treatment (i.e., social power and relational connections domain; for a detailed description of protective and risk factors, see Piran, 2017).

By providing a theoretical framework for understanding disruptive and facilitative factors that define how the body is inhabited, this theory is influential in that it moves beyond the negative body image construct. Piran (2016), Piran (2019b) considers embodiment as inclusive of constructs such as agency, functionality, comfort, pleasure, and connection, thus presenting a positive approach with an actionable quality that offers implications for constructive change and the treatment of EDs.

Menzel and Levine's embodiment model of positive body image

Following the work of Piran (2002), Jessie Menzel and Michael Levine proposed the Embodiment Model of Positive Body Image (Menzel & Levine, 2007) proposed the *Embodiment Model of Positive Body Image*. In their work, embodiment is defined this way, "Embodiment refers to an integrated set of connections in which a person experiences her or his body as comfortable, trustworthy, and deserving of respect and care because the person experiences his or her body as a key aspect of—and expresses through her physicality—competence, interpersonal relatedness, power, self-expression, and well-being" (Menzel & Levine, 2007, p. 1). Thus, they suggest that embodiment does not equal the absence of disembodiment, but rather refers to a beneficial state of being that overlaps with the construct of positive body image.

In their theoretical model, Menzel and Levine (2007) identify experiences and activities that encourage embodiment as a key factor in the development of positive body image. *Embodying activities* are those that foster an integration of the mind and body, increase body awareness and responsiveness, and build a sense of physical empowerment and competence, potentially resulting in a state of flow (Mahlo & Tiggemann, 2016; Menzel & Levine, 2011). In addition to cultivating embodiment and positive body image directly, it is proposed that embodying conditions may work indirectly, by protecting against self-objectification (i.e., the internalization of an observer's perspective upon one's own body; Fredrickson & Roberts, 1997; Mahlo & Tiggemann, 2016; Menzel & Levine, 2011). Although the theory is grounded in a conceptual analysis of competitive athletics, activities such as hiking, climbing, martial arts, horseback riding, and yoga are presented as potential further embodying activities (Mahlo & Tiggemann, 2016; Menzel & Levine, 2011).

Recently, Menzel et al. (2019) took a quantitative approach in developing the Physical Activity Body Experiences Questionnaire (PABEQ) to explore the relation between embodying activities and embodiment. The scale measures the two constructs Mind-Body Connection (e.g., perceived connection with the body, mind, and self) and Body Acceptance (e.g., perceived experience of feeling good inside of the body) and has been shown to effectively predict body awareness, body responsiveness, positive body image, body satisfaction, self-objection, disordered eating, and positive body image (Menzel et al., 2019).

Cook-Cottone's embodied self-model

In order to make the concept of embodiment more easily comprehensive and accessible for clinicians and researchers, Catherine Cook-Cottone developed the *Embodied Self Model* (Cook-Cottone, 2006, 2015a, 2020). In this model, embodiment is defined as "a way of being (non-dualistic conceptualization self) in which being is understood as residing in and manifesting from the body as one experiences the internal (i.e., physiological, emotional, cognitive), external (i.e., interpersonal, social, and cultural), and existential dimensions of life" (Cook-Cottone, 2020, p. 22). Internal and external dimensions are interconnected by a process termed *attunement*, which is based on Daniel Siegel's definition of attunement as a reciprocal process of mutual influence and co-regulation (Siegel, 2007). According to Cook-Cottone (2020), the quality of an individual's embodiment (i.e., positive vs. negative) depends on whether the inner and outer aspects of the self are attuned or misattuned. Positive embodiment requires the ability to (a) nurture an awareness of and maintenance of attunement with the internal aspects of self and (b) engaging effectively within the context of relationships across each of the ecological domains (Cook-Cottone, 2015a). Fundamentally, attunement within an individual's inner and outer dimensions is created and maintained by the embodiment of ongoing behavioral patterns—the way in which an individual actively constructs the self and engages with the environment (Cook-

Cottone, 2006, 2015a, 2020). In other words, embodiment is developed through actionable practice.

A variety of influences from the internal and external systems may collectively cause the loss of attunement and an authentic sense of the self, creating the risk for EDs. The Embodied Self-Model (Cook-Cottone, 2006, 2015a, 2020) suggests that resilience and recovery are not the product of diminished maladaptive or disordered behaviors and cognitions, but instead can be achieved through participation in practices that promote positive embodiment. Three practices that facilitate a positive way of being are offered: (a) mindful awareness and presence, (b) mindful self-care, and (c) purpose and mission. Mindful awareness and presence means noticing what is present without judgement, and doing so with an attitude of kindness and curiosity (Cook-Cottone, 2020). Mindful self-care involves awareness of internal needs and external demands as well as the intentional engagement in self-care practices to address these needs and demands (e.g., intuitive eating, relaxation, exercise, and yoga; Cook-Cottone, 2015a, 2020). Purpose and mission can be defined as having a sense of meaning in life (Cook-Cottone, 2020).

The engagement in these practices enables individuals to experience embodiment. Cook-Cottone (2015a, 2020) stresses that, above and beyond the cessation of dysfunctions, these forms of active practice hold the potential for flourishing (i.e., a state in which individuals experience fulfillment in life, accomplish meaningful tasks, and connect with others at a deeper level; Seligman, 2011) and well-being. By taking a salutogenic perspective, she emphasizes that those struggling with EDs can seek for a healthy, positive relationship with the own body.

Launeanu and Kwee's existential analysis of embodiment

Rooted in Frankl's (1969) tri-dimensional model of the human being, Mihaela Launeanu and Janelle Kwee take a theoretical and clinical approach to delineate embodiment and the fundamental existential motivations (Launeanu and Kwee 2018). In their *existential analysis* view of the body, embodiment is understood as "a holistic, integrated experience of body, mind, and spirit" (Launeanu & Kwee, 2018, p. 51). The body itself represents a constitutive dimension of being that serves as the physical structure of human existence; sensual connection to life, ourselves, and others; the expression of personality; and the agent for action in the world (Launeanu & Kwee, 2018).

According to Launeanu and Kwee (2018), structure for existence is given by four fundamental motivation dimensions, which each correspond to existential questions: The motivations to *be* (i.e., Can I be? Do I have the necessary space, protection, and support?), to experience *value* (i.e., Do I like to live? Do I feel my emotions and experience the value of my life?), to *be oneself* (i.e., May I be myself? Am I free to be me?), and to *search for meaning* (i.e., What am I here for? What do I live for? What gives my life meaning?). Across each of these dimensions, those suffering from EDs have difficulties experiencing "I am a body" and overcompensate this through an excessive focus on "I have a body" (p. 41), creating distance from and treating the own body as object (Launeanu & Kwee, 2018).

In this model, disordered eating is not seen as a range of dysfunctional habits related to food and eating, but rather as a disturbance to identify how to exist as a living body in the world. This disturbance impacts the body on all levels of the embodied human existence: Physical, emotional, relational, personal, and spiritual (Launeanu & Kwee, 2018). Groundedness, sensuality, agency, freedom, movement, and creativity of the body are lost (Cook-Cottone, 2020). Accordingly, treatment requires the promotion of an authentic experience of the body at all of the levels of embodiment.

Embodiment: bringing it all together

The psychology of embodiment and its importance in the prevention and treatment of EDs is a recently emerging field (Cook-Cottone, 2020; Underwood, 2013). When comparing the current approaches, it is apparent that theorists and researchers generally agree upon that embodiment can be seen as the manifestation of a person's inner and outer worlds as they negotiate their lived experience. Further, across theories there is an acknowledgement that embodiment varies in quality and can be negative, self-destructive, violated, and abandoned, as well as positive, unifying, and liberating. Overall, the psychological theories of embodiment share several core features (see Table 1).

Table 1. Core features of embodiment theories.

1 There is no, or minimal, distinction between mind and body (i.e., non-dualism).
2 The body is experienced as a subjective site.
3 The body is the source of lived experience.
4 The body is the home of sensing and sensuality.
5 The body is essential in the feeling and experiencing of, and response to, emotions.
6 The personal experience of connection with the body, attunement to the body, and embodiment varies.
7 The body can be a source of pain, limitation, and discomfort as well as a source of sanctuary, pleasure, and resources for coping and decision making.
8 The body provides functionality, agency, and vocation to act in the world.
9 The body is situated in relational, familial, cultural, social, power, and political contexts.
10 There is purpose and meaning in embodiment.

Informed by (Cook-Cottone, 2006, 2015a; Launeanu & Kwee, 2018; Menzel & Levine, 2007; Piran, 2002, 2016, 2017; N. Piran & Teall, 2012).

Origin, basic principles, and modern interpretations of yoga

Yoga is eclectic, comprising physical, spiritual, and moral dimensions (Feuerstein, 2013). It is believed that yoga originated in India more than 4,000 years ago (Anderson & Sovik, 2000; Simpkins & Simpkins, 2011; Stephens, 2011; Weintraub, 2004). With elements being found in Hinduism, Jainism, and Buddhism, yoga is not limited to any particular philosophical or religious system (Simpkins & Simpkins, 2011; Stephens, 2011). In its traditional essence, yoga is a multitude of philosophical ideas concerned with the path leading to recognition of the true self (Costin & Kelly, 2016; Douglass, 2007). The term yoga derives from the Sanskrit verb *yuj* and means to join or unite (Anderson & Sovik, 2000; Iyengar, 1996). The experience of the self is believed to rest in two realms: An inner realm of thoughts, emotions, and sensations; and an outer realm with which we interact (Anderson & Sovik, 2000; Strauss, 2005). Being capable of living in both realms paves the way to move past suffering and towards physical and mental thriving (Gard et al., 2014).

Rather than merely providing a methodology to strengthen and stretch the body, yoga facilitates the development of the connection between mind and body as well as our inner and outer experiences of the self (Costin & Kelly, 2016; Halliwell et al., 2019). The Yoga Sutras define the fundamental elements of yoga theory and practice in *eight limbs* (Feuerstein, 2013). The first five limbs are considered the external limbs of yoga and include practices associated with the external aspects of the self. They provide guidance on handling the physical body as well as on social interactions and are intended to prepare mind and body for the three later practices (Anderson & Sovik, 2000; Feuerstein, 2013; Weintraub, 2004). The external limbs include ethical disciplines (i.e., *yamas* and *niyamas*), physical postures (i.e., *asanas*), breath work (i.e., *pranayama*), and inward attention (i.e., *pratyahara*). The last three limbs (i.e., *dharana, dhyana,* and *samadhi)* are considered the internal limbs and describe various stages of meditation that may ultimately lead to self-awareness (Anderson & Sovik, 2000; Feuerstein, 2013; Gard et al., 2014).

Yoga's history is long and rich, marked with continuous adaptations to diverse cultures, traditions, lifestyles, and applications (McCall, 2007; Simpkins & Simpkins, 2011). Today, yoga is taught in yoga studios, gyms, shopping malls, churches, schools, and prisons; and has become utilized in the prevention and treatment of mental disorders (Domingues & Carmo, 2019; Khalsa, 2013). Accordingly, adaptations were made to suit the practice to its different uses. A wide array of forms and styles of yoga (e.g., *Hatha, Ashtanga, Iyengar, Vinyasa, Power yoga*) is now offered. In modern interpretations, yoga is regarded as a practice to promote physical and mental well-being and is mainly associated with physical postures (i.e., *asanas*), breath work (i.e., *pranayama*), and meditation (i.e., *dyana*; Domingues & Carmo, 2019; Gard et al., 2014). The variety in interpretation and implementation of yoga in present times indicates that the use of yoga remains complex, multifaceted, and heterogeneous (Cook-Cottone, 2015b). At the same time, this diversity points to the value of enhancing mental and physical health and improving well-being in individuals with varied needs.

Eating disorders, embodiment, and yoga

The body of work shared in this special issue suggests that yoga may help facilitate positive embodiment, prevent EDs, and support recovery (Cook-Cottone, 2020). As an active practice, yoga offers the experience of being with and in the body, inclusive of all the sensations, emotions, and cognitions that are present. This experience provides means to inhabit the body as a subjective site, in which the self holds the capability of exerting functionality, agency, and volition in the world. Eventually, yoga allows practitioners to connect with and attune their bodies to personal experiences and others around them. For patients with EDs, yoga provides a tool to perceive the body as a source of sanctuary, pleasure, and competence; serving purpose and meaning (Mahlo & Tiggemann, 2016).

As you will read in the articles presented in this special issue, there is a social justice context to this practice. Further, there is a need for more research specifically exploring the experience of embodiment during yoga practice and the factors that can support or hinder embodiment (Cox & Tylka, 2020; N. Piran & Neumark-Sztainer, 2020). In addition, researchers must continue to seek a better understanding of and measures for the key mechanisms involved in how yoga as an embodied practice affects disordered eating (e.g., mindfulness, breath work, attention training, self-regulation, self-compassion, body appreciation, interoceptive awareness; Ariel-Donges et al., 2018; Cox & Tylka, 2020; Kramer & Cuccolo, 2020; N. Piran & Neumark-Sztainer, 2020). Even though the study of yoga and its relation to embodiment and disordered eating presents a young area of research, early findings indicate that yoga provides a promising path for the prevention and treatment of EDs.

References

American Psychiatric Association. (2013). *Diagnostic and statistical manual of mental disorders* (5th ed.).

Amianto, F., Ottone, L., Daga, G. A., & Fassino, S. (2015). Binge-eating disorder diagnosis and treatment: A recap in front of DSM-5. *BMC Psychiatry*, *15*(1), 70. https://doi.org/10.1186/s12888-015-0445-6

Anderson, S., & Sovik, R. (2000). *Yoga: Mastering the basics.* The Himalayan Institute.

Ariel-Donges, A. H., Gordon, E. L., Bauman, V., & Perri, M. G. (2018). Does yoga help college-aged women with body-image dissatisfaction feel better about their bodies? *Sex Roles*, *80*(1–2), 41–51. https://doi.org/10.1007/s11199-018-0917-5

Brewerton, T. D. (Ed.). (2004). *Clinical handbook of eating disorders: An integrated approach.* CRC Press.

Bulik, C. M., Marcus, M. D., Zerwas, S., Levine, M. D., & La Via, M. (2012). The changing "weightscape" of bulimia nervosa. *American Journal of Psychiatry, 169*(10), 1031–1036. https://doi.org/10.1176/appi.ajp.2012.12010147

Cook-Cottone, C. (2016). Embodied self-regulation and mindful self-care in the prevention of eating disorders. *Eating Disorders: The Journal of Treatment and Prevention, 24*(1), 98–105. https://doi.org/10.1080/10640266.2015.1118954

Cook-Cottone, C., & Douglass, L. L. (2017). Yoga communities and eating disorders: Creating safe space for positive embodiment. *International Journal of Yoga Therapy, 27(1),* 87–93. https://doi.org/10.17761/1531-2054-27.1.87

Cook-Cottone, C., Talebkhah, K., Guyker, W., & Keddie, E. (2017). A controlled trial of a yoga-based prevention program targeting eating disorder risk factors among middle school females. *Eating Disorders, 25*(5), 392–405. https://doi.org/10.1080/10640266.2017.1365562

Cook-Cottone, C. P. (2006). The attuned representation model for the primary prevention of eating disorders: An overview for school psychologists. *Psychology in the Schools, 43*(2), 223–230. https://doi.org/10.1002/pits.20139

Cook-Cottone, C. P. (2015a). Incorporating positive body image into the treatment of eating disorders: A model for attunement and mindful self-care. *Body Image, 14,* 158–167. https://doi.org/10.1016/j.bodyim.2015.03.004

Cook-Cottone, C. P. (2015b). *Mindfulness and yoga for self-regulation: A primer for mental health professionals.* Springer Publishing Company.

Cook-Cottone, C. P. (2019). Brain integration, embodied mindfulness, and movement-based approaches to facilitate positive body image and embodiment. In T. L. Tylka & N. Piran (Eds.), *Handbook of positive body image and embodiment* (pp. 337–346). Oxford University Press.

Cook-Cottone, C. P. (2020). *Embodiment and the treatment of eating disorders: the body as a resource in recovery.* New York, NY: W. W. Norton.

Costin, C., & Kelly, J. (Eds.). (2016). *Yoga and eating disorders: Ancient healing for modern illness.* Routledge.

Cox, A. E., & Tylka, T. L. (2020). A conceptual model describing mechanisms for how yoga practice may support positive embodiment. *Eating Disorders: The Journal of Treatment and Prevention, XX,* XX–XX. https://doi.org/10.1080/10640266.2020.1740911

Cox, A. E., Ullrich-French, S., Howe, H. S., & Cole, A. N. (2017). A pilot yoga physical education curriculum to promote positive body image. *Body Image, 23,* 1–8. https://doi.org/10.1016/j.bodyim.2017.07.007

Daubenmier, J. J. (2005). The relationship of yoga, body awareness, and body responsiveness to self-objectification and disordered eating. *Psychology of Women Quarterly, 29*(2), 207–219. https://doi.org/10.1111/j.1471-6402.2005.00183.x

Domingues, R. B., & Carmo, C. (2019). Disordered eating behaviours and correlates in yoga practitioners: A systematic review. *Eating and Weight Disorders-Studies on Anorexia, Bulimia and Obesity, 24*(6), 1015–1024. https://doi.org/10.1007/s40519-019-00692-x

Douglass, L. (2007). How did we get here? A history of yoga in America, 1800-1970. *International Journal of Yoga Therapy, 17*(1), 35–42. https://doi.org/10.17761/ijyt.17.1.180p845622653856

Erford, B. T., Richards, T., Peacock, E., Voith, K., McGair, H., Muller, B., ... Chang, C. Y. (2013). Counseling and guided self-help outcomes for clients with bulimia nervosa: A meta-analysis of clinical trials from 1980 to 2010. *Journal of Counseling & Development, 91,* 152–172. https://doi.org/http://dx.doi.10.1002/j.1556-6676.2013.00083.x

Feuerstein, G. (2013). *The yoga tradition: Its History, literature, philosophy, and practice.* Hohm Press.

Frankl, V. (1959). *Man's search for meaning.* Beacon Press.

Frankl, V. (1969). *The will to meaning: Foundations and applications of logotherapy.* The World Publishing Company.

Fredrickson, B. L., & Roberts, T. A. (1997). Objectification theory: Toward understanding women's lived experiences and mental health risks. *Psychology of Women Quarterly*, *21*(2), 173–206. https://doi.org/10.1111/j.1471-6402.1997.tb00108.x

Gard, T., Noggle, J. J., Park, C. L., Vago, D. R., & Wilson, A. (2014). Potential self-regulatory mechanisms of yoga for psychological health. *Frontiers in Human Neuroscience*, *91*(2), 152-172. https://doi.org/10.3389/fnhum.2014.00770

Grucza, R. A., Przybeck, T. R., & Cloninger, C. R. (2007). Prevalence and correlates of binge eating disorder in a community sample. *Comprehensive Psychiatry*, *48*(2), 124–131. https://doi.org/10.1016/j.comppsych.2006.08.002

Halliwell, E., Dawson, K., & Burkey, S. (2019). A randomized experimental evaluation of a yoga-based body image intervention. *Body Image*, *28*, 119–127. https://doi.org/10.1016/j.bodyim.2018.12.005

Hay, P. J., & Claudino, A. M. (2015). Bulimia nervosa: online interventions. *BMJ Clinical Evidence*, *2015*, 1009. https://www.ncbi.nlm.nih.gov/pmc/articles/PMC4356174/pdf/2015-1009.pdf

Iacovino, J. M., Gredysa, D. M., Altman, M., & Wilfley, D. E. (2012). Psychological treatments for binge eating disorder. *Current Psychiatry Reports*, *14*(4), 432–446. https://doi.org/10.1007/s11920-012-0277-8

Iyengar, B. K. S. (1996). *Light on yoga.* Schocken Books.

Khalsa, S. B. S. (2013). Yoga for psychiatry and mental health: An ancient practice with modern relevance. *Indian Journal of Psychiatry*, *55*(3), S334-S336. https://pubmed.ncbi.nlm.nih.gov/24049194https://pubmed.ncbi.nlm.nih.gov/24049194

Kramer, R., & Cuccolo, K. (2020). Yoga practice in a college sample: Associated changes in eating disorder, body image, and related factors over time. *Eating Disorders: The Journal of Treatment and Prevention*, *XX*, 1–19. https://doi.org/10.1080/10640266.2019.1688007

Launeanu, M., & Kwee, J. L. (2018). Embodiment: A non-dualistic and existential perspective on understanding and treating disordered eating. In H. L. McBride & J. L. Kwee (Eds.), *Embodiment and eating disorders: Theory, research, prevention, and treatment* (pp. 35–52). Routledge.

Levine, M. P., & Smolak, L. (2016). The role of protective factors in the prevention of negative body image and disordered eating. *Eating Disorders*, *24*(1), 39–46. https://doi.org/10.1080/10640266.2015.1113826

Linardon, J., Brennan, L., & De la Piedad Garcia, X. (2016). Rapid response to eating disorder treatment: A systematic review and meta-analysis. *International Journal of Eating Disorders*, *49*(10), 905–919. https://doi.org/10.1002/eat.22595

Lock, J., & Le Grange, D. (2015). *Treatment manual for anorexia nervosa: A family-based approach.* Guilford Publications.

Mahlo, L., & Tiggemann, M. (2016). Yoga and positive body image: A test of the Embodiment Model. *Body Image*, *18*, 135–142. https://doi.org/10.1016/j.bodyim.2016.06.008

McCall, T. (2007). *Yoga as medicine: The yogic prescription for health & healing.* Bantam Dell, Random House.

McIntosh, V. V., Carter, F. A., Bulik, C. M., Frampton, C. M., & Joyce, P. R. (2011). Five-year outcome of cognitive behavioral therapy and exposure with response prevention for bulimia nervosa. *Psychological Medicine*, *41*(5), 1061–1071. https://doi.org/http://dx.doi.10.1017/S0033291710001583

Menzel, J., & Levine, M. P. (2011). Embodying experiences and the promotion of positive body image: The example of competitive athletics. In R. Calogero, S. Tantleff-Dunn, & J. K. Thompson (Eds.), *Self-objectification in women: Causes, consequences, and counteractions* (pp. 163–186). American Psychological Association.

Menzel, J., & Levine, M. P. (2007). *Female athletes and embodiment: Development and validation of the athlete body experiences questionnaire.* Poster presented at the annual convention of the American Psychological Association, San Francisco, CA.

Menzel, J. E., Thompson, J. K., & Levine, M. P. (2019). Development and validation of the physical activity body experiences questionnaire. *Bulletin of the Menninger Clinic, 83*(1), 53–83. https://doi.org/10.1521/bumc.2019.83.1.53

Merleau-Ponty, M. (2013). *Phenomenology of perception.* Routledge.

Murray, S. B. (2019). Updates in the treatment of eating disorders in 2018: A year in review in eating disorders: The Journal of Treatment & Prevention. *Eating Disorders: The Journal of Treatment and Prevention, 27*(1), 6–17. https://doi.org/10.1080/10640266.2019.1567155

Neumark-Sztainer, D. (2014). Yoga and eating disorders: Is there a place for yoga in the prevention and treatment of eating disorders and disordered eating behaviours? *Advances in Eating Disorders: Theory, Research and Practice, 2*(2), 136–145. https://doi.org/10.1080/21662630.2013.862369

Neumark-Sztainer, D., Watts, A. W., & Rydell, S. (2018). Yoga and body image: How do young adults practicing yoga describe its impact on their body image? *Body Image, 27,* 1–13. https://doi.org/10.1016/j.bodyim.2018.09.001

Piran, N. (2002). Embodiment: A mosaic of inquiries in the area of body weight and shape preoccupation. In S. Abbey (Ed.), *Ways of knowing in and through the body: Diverse perspectives on embodiment* (pp. 211–214). Soleil Publishing.

Piran, N., & Teall, T. (2012). The developmental theory of embodiment. In G. McVey, M. Levine, N. Piran, & B. Ferguson (Eds.), *Preventing eating-related and weight-related disorders: Collaborative research, advocacy, and policy change* (pp. 169–198). Wilfrid Laurier University Press.

Piran, N. (2016). Embodied possibilities and disruptions: The emergence of the experience of embodiment construct from qualitative studies with girls and women. *Body Image, 18,* 43–60. https://doi.org/10.1016/j.bodyim.2016.04.007

Piran, N. (2017). *Journeys of embodiment at the intersection of body and culture: The developmental theory of embodiment.* Elsevier.

Piran, N. (2019a). The experience of embodiment construct: Reflecting the quality of embodied lives. In T. L. Tylka & N. Piran (Eds.), *Handbook of positive body image and embodiment* (pp. 11–21). Oxford University Press.

Piran, N. (2019b). The developmental theory of embodiment: Protective social factors that enhance positive embodiment. In T. Tylka & N. Piran (Eds.), *Handbook of positive body image and embodiment* (pp. 105–117). Oxford University Press.

Piran, N., & Neumark-Sztainer, D. (2020). Yoga and the experience of embodiment: A discussion of possible links. *Eating Disorders: The Journal of Treatment and Prevention,* 1–19. https://doi.org/10.1080/10640266.2019.1701350

Poulsen, S., Lunn, S., Daniel, S. I., Folke, S., Mathiesen, B. B., Katznelson, H., & Fairburn, C. G. (2014). A randomized controlled trial of psychoanalytic psychotherapy or cognitive-behavioral therapy for bulimia nervosa. *American Journal of Psychiatry, 171* (1), 109–116. https://doi.org/10.1176/appi.ajp.2013.12121511

Reynolds, J., & Roffe, J. (2018). Neither/Nor: Merleau-Ponty's ontology in 'the intertwining/ the chiasm'. In A. Mildenberg (Ed.), *Understanding Merleau-Ponty, understanding modernism* (pp. 100–116). Bloomsbury Academic.

Rosen, D. S. (2010). Identification and management of eating disorders in children and adolescents. *Pediatrics, 126*(6), 1240–1253. https://doi.org/10.1542/peds.2010-2821

Scime, M., & Cook-Cottone, C. (2008). Primary prevention of eating disorders: A constructivist integration of mind and body strategies. *International Journal of Eating Disorders, 41*(2), 134–142. https://doi.org/10.1002/eat.20480

Seligman, M. E. P. (2011). *Flourish: A visionary new understanding of happiness and well-being.* Simon & Schuster.

Siegel, D. J. (2007). *The mindful brain, reflection and attunement in the cultivation of well-being.* WW Norton & Company.

Simpkins, A. M., & Simpkins, C. A. (2011). *Meditation and yoga in psychotherapy: Techniques for clinical practice.* Wiley.

Smink, F. R., van Hoeken, D., & Hoek, H. W. (2013). Epidemiology, course, and outcome of eating disorders. *Current Opinion in Psychiatry, 26*(6), 543–548. https://doi.org/10.1097/YCO.0b013e328365a24f

Smith, J. E. H. (2017). *Embodiment: a history.* Oxford: Oxford University Press.

Stankovskaya, E. (2014). *Embodiment: Thoughts from an existential-analytic perspective.* Basic Research Program, National Research University Higher School of Economics.

Stephens, M. (2011). *Teaching yoga: Essential foundations and techniques.* North Atlantic books.

Strauss, S. (2005). *Positioning yoga: Balancing acts across cultures.* Berg/Oxford.

Tanofsky-Kraff, M., & Wilfley, D. E. 2010. Interpersonal psychotherapy for bulimia nervosa and binge-eating disorder. C. M. Grilo & J. E. Mitchell, Eds. *The treatment of eating disorders: A clinical handbook.* (pp. 271–293). Guilford Press.

Underwood, M. (2013). Body as choice or body as compulsion: An experiential perspective on body-self relations and the boundary between normal and pathological. *Health Sociology Review, 22*(4), 377–388. https://doi.org/10.5172/hesr.2013.22.4.377

Watson, H. J., & Bulik, C. M. (2013). Update on the treatment of anorexia nervosa: Review of clinical trials, practice guidelines and emerging interventions. *Psychological Medicine, 43*(12), 2477–2500. https://doi.org/http://dx.doi.10.1017/S0033291712002620

Weintraub, A. (2004). *Yoga for depression: A compassionate guide to relieve suffering through yoga.* Broadway Books.

Wilson, G. T., Wilfley, D. E., Agras, W. S., & Bryson, S. W. (2010). Psychological treatments of binge eating disorder. *Archives of General Psychiatry, 67*(1), 94–101. https://doi.org/10.1001/archgenpsychiatry.2009.170

Yoga and the experience of embodiment: a discussion of possible links

Niva Piran and Dianne Neumark-Sztainer

ABSTRACT

The impact of yoga on body image and embodiment has been a recent area of focus in the field of body image and eating disorders. This paper comprises a theoretical discussion of how the practice of yoga can lead to positive ways of inhabiting the body, specifically through the lens of the Developmental Theory of Embodiment. Yoga may enhance the overall experience of embodiment, by having a positive impact on each of its five dimensions: body connection and comfort, agency and functionality, attuned self-care, subjective immersion (resisting objectification), and experience and expression of desires. The article therefore describes examples of teacher-related practices during yoga that can enhance each of these dimensions. Further, yoga teachers can consider the varied protective physical and social factors delineated by the Developmental Theory of Embodiment to facilitate positive embodiment. Future research should explicitly integrate embodiment theory with yoga interventions, as well as measures that assess both possible mechanisms of change and positive ways of living in the body.

Clinical Implications

- Yoga has the potential to foster positive embodiment through the enhancement of positive body connection, body functionality, attuned self-care, and subjective immersion in the body.
- Highlighting flexibility in the practice of yoga, by adapting and selecting poses in line with practitioners' needs, provides them with opportunities to feel comfortable and positive in their bodies.
- Diversity in class composition in terms of body weights, shapes, abilities, and varied dimensions of social locations, supports experiences of body acceptance.
- The inward emphasis in the practice of yoga is important for all individuals living in a culture that places much importance on appearance and other external characteristics.

Introduction

Yoga is a practice that involves physical postures, focused breathing, mindfulness, and meditation. Yoga has the potential to influence all ways of life, including our daily thoughts and actions, how we understand ourselves at a deep level, and our interactions with the world around us. Although commonly considered a physical practice, yoga has the potential to extend well beyond physical engagement into all aspects of life. Indeed, yoga is an eight-limbed practice that involves asanas (physical postures), pranayama (breathing and energy work), pratyahara (internalization of the mind and senses), dharana (concentration), dhyana (meditation), samadhi (absorption or unity consciousness), yamas (ethical attitudes and observances) and niyamas (Frawley, 2018; Yoga's Ethical Guide to Living). The Sanskrit word 'yoga' has various meanings and is derived from the Sanskrit root "yuj," meaning "work," "coordination," and "integration" (Frawley). Yoga is defined as "union," which may be interpreted as a state of oneness with our innermost self. Yoga is often described as the practice of uniting the different parts of ourselves—our physical, energetic, mental, emotional, and spiritual selves.

The impact of yoga on body image and embodiment, described here as individuals' lived experiences in their bodies as they engage with the world (see Piran, 2017), has been a recent area of focus in the field of body image and eating disorders (e.g., Cook-Cottone, 2019; Neumark-Sztainer, 2019). A number of quantitative studies suggest that the practice of yoga is associated with positive ways of living in the body, with yoga practitioners having higher body satisfaction (Neumark-Sztainer, MacLehose, Watts, Pacanowski, & Eisenberg, 2018) and body responsiveness and awareness (Daubenmier, 2005). In a qualitative study, participants indicated that yoga had a mainly positive impact on their body image via perceived physical changes, gratitude for one's body, a sense of accomplishment within one's yoga practice, self-confidence, and witnessing different types of bodies practicing yoga (Neumark-Sztainer, Watts, & Rydell, 2018). This growing area of study needs to be further informed by research, including well-designed epidemiological, qualitative, and intervention studies that are informed by strong theoretical frameworks.

A comprehensive, research-based theoretical framework for understanding both the development and experience of embodiment is the Developmental Theory of Embodiment (DTE) (Piran, 2002, 2016, 2017; Piran & Teall, 2012). This paper comprises a theoretical discussion of how the practice of yoga can lead to positive ways of inhabiting the body, specifically through the lens of the DTE. We start with a description of theoretical constructs related to embodiment and the DTE and continue by linking dimensions of embodiment, and the factors that shape them, to the practice of yoga. Our goals for this paper are three-fold.

First, linking theoretical constructs of the DTE, especially dimensions of positive embodiment and protective factors, with yoga practices, can highlight processes through which yoga can contribute to positive embodiment; teachers and practitioners can then deliberately enhance these processes to amplify the positive effects of yoga. Second, a greater understanding of DTE and its relevance to the practice of yoga could be helpful in informing theoretically based research exploring the relationship between yoga and embodiment. Third, addressing both risk and protective factors to positive embodiment, the DTE has a range of implications to treatment and prevention (Piran, 2017). Examining the DTE in relation to yoga provides an opportunity to examine its utility in relation to a specific type of intervention.

Theoretical constructs related to embodiment and the developmental theory of embodiment

The construct of embodiment in critical theory

The current understanding of the construct of embodiment is grounded in the writings of the French phenomenologist Merleau-Ponty (1962). In contrast to Cartesian ontology that viewed the mind and body as distinct, the body as a material object and the mind as a thinking subject (Crossley, 1995), as well as the mind as superior to the body (Bordo, 1993), Merleau-Ponty (1962) proposed that the mind and body were equivalent, intertwined and inseparable (Csordas, 1994; Howe, 2003). Further, he viewed the body not only as sensational but also as sentinel in perceiving, interpreting, and experiencing the world meaningfully (Crossley, 1995). For Merleau-Ponty, therefore, the body is the site of subjectivity, and embodiment refers to the "perceptual experience of engagement of the body in the world." This interpretive "perceptual experience" is always in relation to a particular location of the body in the world; a dialectical relationship therefore exists between body and culture, and inner and outer, such that the body performs culturally informed practices, and, in turn, shapes culture (Crossley, 1995).

Foucault (1995) extended the theoretical discussion of embodiment, by examining the role of power in shaping embodiment. In particular, he suggested that modern societies exert power through restrictive social discourses which individual citizens internalize, such that they learn to live in docile, compliant bodies. Feminist scholars highlighted the role of gender inequity, in particular, in producing docile female bodies (Bartky, 1988; Bordo, 1989). De Beauvoir (1974) problematized the way in which a girl's adolescent's body is, "taken away from her" (p. 346) and Bordo (1989) described the experience of "insufficiency, of never being good enough" (p. 14). The disciplinary power embedded in social discourses relates not only to gender, but to all dimensions of social location, including social class, ethnicity/race and immigration, sexual orientation, gender identities, weight, health and physical ability, and other factors. For example, hooks (1997) problematized the continued disciplining and exploitation of African American women's bodies through sexist/racist objectification. Individuals' experiences of inhabiting their bodies are therefore shaped by intersecting dimensions of social locations (Buchanan, Settles, & Woods, 2019; Piran, 2017).

The embodiment research program

Anchored in the discussions of embodiment and power in philosophy and critical theory, Piran and colleagues (e.g., Piran, 2002, 2016, 2017; Piran & Teall, 2012) conducted a mixed-method research program that explored, first, the quality of embodied lives and, second, the factors that shaped them. Theoretical constructs and pathways that emerged through a constructivist grounded theory analysis (Charmaz, 2006) of 171 interviews with 69 girls and women (e.g., Piran, 2017), and that were therefore anchored in girls' and women's narratives, were also tested using a range of quantitative cross-sectional methodologies (e.g., structural equation modeling: Piran & Thompson, 2008; multiple regression: Piran & Cormier, 2005; and scale construction: Piran, 2019; Teall, 2015).

Experience of embodiment: assessing the quality of embodied lives

Regarding the quality of embodied lives, Piran (e.g., 2016, 2017) described the emergent multi-dimensional Experience of Embodiment (EE) construct, which ranges from positive embodiment: "positive body connection and comfort, embodied agency and passion, and attuned self-care" (Piran, 2016, p. 47) to negative embodiment: "disrupted body connection and discomfort, restricted agency and passion, and self-neglect or harm" (Piran, 2016, p. 47). EE depends on the quality of experiences on each of its five dimensions: (a) body connection and comfort; (b) agency and functionality; (c) attuned self-care; (d) inhabiting the body as a subjective site (vs. objectification); and (e) experience and expression of bodily desires (see also Table 1). EE and its dimensions can be measured using the Experience of Embodiment Scale (EES) (Piran, 2019). EE as a whole, and, in particular, its first dimension of Positive Connection and Comfort, relates conceptually to other constructs that measure positive ways of living in the body, such as: body appreciation (Tylka & Wood-Barcalow, 2015), body flexibility (Sandoz, Wilson, Merwin, & Kellum, 2013), and functionality appreciation (Alleva, Tylka, & Kroon Van Diest, 2017); however, the construct of positive embodiment is broader in scope (Piran, 2016, 2019; Tylka & Piran, 2019), and also suggests the continuity of experiences between negative and positive embodiment, allowing to trace shifts in EE across the life span (Piran, 2016). While most of the research on EE has been conducted to date among cisgender girls and women of diverse backgrounds, studies with the EES in Sweden (Holmqvist Gattario, Frisén, & Piran, 2018) and Norway (Sundgot-Borgen et al., 2019) suggest that the scale has good psychometric qualities among adolescent and adult men.

The DTE: delineating protective experiences

The DTE provides an integrated, research-based, critical social theory into both protective and risk processes that shape EE (and its five dimensions) as one engages with the world (Piran, 2002, 2016, 2017). In line with the DTE, these risk and protective processes shape EE via three core pathways: the physical domain, the mental domain of social discourses and expectations, and the social power and relational connections domain.

For the purpose of this article, we focus on a brief description of the protective factors in each of these domains (for a detailed labeling and description of these factors, see Piran, 2017):

(A) Physical Domain: (A1) immersed and joyful engagement in physical activities (non-objectifying/sexualizing; not aimed at achieving idealized bodies); (A2) safety; (A3) opportunities to practice attuned care of the body; and (A4) exposure to experiences that support and validate desire.
(B) Mental Domain of Social Discourses: A limited exposure to, and a critical stance towards, widely disseminated stereotypes about gender, race/ethnicity, and other dimensions of social locations. For girls and women, the DTE describes the protective role of resistance to: (B1) experiencing the body as a deficient object; and (B2) acting in a docile manner (submissive, demure, small, not too powerful/loud/assertive/in control, and being other – rather than self-oriented).
(C) In the social power and relational connections domain, the DTE highlights: (C1) freedom from prejudicial treatment; (C2) non-appearance-related sources of social power; (C3) the presence of empowering relationships (especially with individuals of similar social location); and (C4) membership in communities of equity.

According to the DTE, all these factors, concurrently, shape the experience of embodiment.

The practice of yoga and the experience of embodiment

Both the Experience of Embodiment construct and the list of protective factors delineated by the DTE can be useful towards fostering positive embodiment through the practice of yoga. First, the EE intra-individual construct suggests that yoga teachers and practitioners should be mindful

Table 1. Dimensions of the experience of embodiment, examples of practices that enhance them, and protective physical and social factors that are operating to enhance dimensions of embodiment through the exemplified practices.

Dimensions of the Experience of Embodiment	Examples of Facilitative Yoga Practices	Activated DTE Protective Factors (Domain)
Dimension 1:	The practice of mindful "noticing" (e.g., of breath, impact of postures)	– Attuned, immersed, joyful physical engagement (Physical)
Body Connection and Comfort	Choice and flexibility in practices (e.g., related to ability, comfort, safety)	– Safety (Physical) – Opportunities to practice attuned care of the body (Physical) – Empowering relationships (Social Power)
	Practicing in diverse communities (e.g., weight, ethnicity, ability)	– Membership in communities of equity (Social Power) – Non-appearance-related social power (Social power) – Freedom from prejudicial treatment – (Social Power)
Dimension 2: Agency and Functionality	Practicing with the experience of accomplishment (e.g., implementing a new pose, taking a pose just one inch deeper, or feeling joy in movement)	– Attuned, immersed, joyful physical engagement (Physical) – Countering learned social constructions (e.g., women's bodies as deficient objects) (Mental)
	Engagement in Empowering poses (e.g., Warrior I & II), supplemented with empowering self-talk (optional)	– Countering learned social constructions (e.g., women as submissive, docile) (Mental)
Dimension 3: Attuned Self-Care	Emphasizing self-study in the process of practice (e.g., svadhyaya), while prioritizing body-anchored insights over a thinking mind	– Opportunities to practice attuned care of the body (Physical) – Countering learned social constructions (e.g., women as other- vs. self-attuned) (Mental)
Dimension 4: Inhabiting the Body as a Subjective Site (resisting objectification)	Internal attunement during practice to the integrated working of different body parts and breathing, and to other body sensations and internal experiences (through teachers' verbal guidance, and class norms)	– Attuned, immersed, joyful physical engagement (Physical)
	De-emphasizing external appearance of poses	– Countering learned social constructions (e.g., women's bodies as deficient objects) (Mental) – Non-appearance-related social power (Social power)

(Continued)

Table 1. (Continued).

Dimensions of the Experience of Embodiment	Examples of Facilitative Yoga Practices	Activated DTE Protective Factors (Domain)
Dimension 5: Experience and Expression of Desire	Attunement to desires as an aspect of enhanced body- and inward- focus during practice (e.g., teacher can encourage responding to experienced needs to nourish the body& hydrate, during physical practices)	– Attuned, immersed, joyful physical engagement (Physical) – Opportunities to practice attuned care of the body (Physical) – Countering learned social constructions (e.g., women's bodies as deficient objects) (Mental)

of, and enhance, different dimensions of EE towards the goal of facilitating the overall positive embodiment. We therefore organize our discussion of yoga and embodiment by discussing each of these dimensions and exemplifying the potential impact of particular yoga practices on them. Second, the list of protective factors delineated by the DTE can help highlight what particular facilitative physical and social experiences may be activated during particular yoga practices. Therefore, after describing suggested yoga practices, we highlight particular protective factors that are associated with them. This information is summarized in Table 1.

Body connection and comfort

This first dimension addresses both the quality of connection with, and the feelings towards, the body. At the positive end, individuals experience a positive connection to their bodies and a range of positive feelings towards their bodies, such as pride, appreciation (of functioning, health, wisdom, etc.), care, or joy. At the negative end, individuals experience negative connection with, or disconnection from, their bodies. They also experience a host of negative feelings towards their bodies, such as shame, fear, anger, or hate.

Yoga, as a physical, energetic, mental, and spiritual practice, has the potential to help enhance positive connection and comfort with one's body, as well as a host of positive feelings towards the body, in line with the protective DTE factor, immersed and joyful engagement in physical activities. Mindful attunement to the body during practice, or "noticing", is a central aspect of the practice of yoga, enhancing the connection to the body. For example, the practice of yoga often starts and ends with sitting and noticing the breath, whereby a teacher invites participants to notice the breath prior to beginning the asana practice and at the end of the class, noting changes that may have taken place. A teacher can enhance such attunement by pausing in between physical poses and inviting students to examine the impact of the poses on a changed experience of the body. For example, in a yin practice in which yoga practitioners lie on the ground and work only with one leg at a time (e.g., using a strap to hold the leg vertical and then to each side for a few minutes in each pose), a teacher can ask students to pause and notice differences between the experience of their legs. The teacher may also cue for certain reactions (e.g., "you may notice that one leg feels longer than the other, or warmer, or that there is a sense of tingling, increased energy flow, or prana"). For yoga practitioners who practice on their own at home, it can be helpful to build in moments of pause in between postures, movement, and breathwork, to notice what one is feeling and enhance the connection with one's breath and body. Yoga teachers can also remind students about how yoga practice can be taken "off the mat" such that they will continue to notice and respond to shifts in the experience of the body elsewhere, for example, pausing and deciding how to react in a social situation when one's heart is beating more strongly and when feeling anxious.

Concurrently with strengthening one's connection with the body, yoga has the potential to enhance comfort and a host of other positive feeling towards one's body. The increased comfort lies in the wide range of poses and practices available for people of different physical abilities. This flexibility can provide opportunities to practice attuned care of the body, another protective factor in the physical domain of the DTE. The teacher can enhance such attuned and caring practice by acknowledging that some poses may not feel comfortable or safe for some students and offer ways to modify poses, encouraging students' mindful attunement to their experiences and inviting their autonomy in deciding whether to modify, or not do, a pose. For example, poses in which the legs are spread wide may not feel comfortable for students who have been sexually violated and students should be given options of modifying the pose or doing a completely different pose. Similarly, rather than telling students to close their eyes during particular practices it can be helpful for teachers to say, "If you feel comfortable, you may close your eyes, to come inward, or you may focus your gaze with your eyes open." Such available choices enhance the experience of physical safety, an additional protective factor in the physical domain of the DTE.

Within a culture that idealizes particular objectified body forms, challenging such norms and nurturing acceptance of diverse body characteristics works towards establishing the class as a community of equity, a protective factor for positive embodiment in the DTE's social power domain. Further, the acceptance of diversity of body forms and movement establishes students' experience of social power *with* others as free of appearance-based social power. Diversity in class composition and teacher in relation to a range of social locations (e.g., age, ethnicity, size) may reinforce equity and freedom from appearance-dependent acceptability. In interviews with young adults of different body sizes who practice yoga, they noted that witnessing different types of bodies practicing yoga helped them feel comfortable with their own bodies (Neumark-Sztainer, Neumark-Sztainer et al., 2018). Yoga studios need to take active steps to ensure that students of all shapes, sizes, and abilities, and those from diverse ethnic/racial backgrounds, will feel welcome. Yoga teachers can also emphasize that while poses may look different on the outside, their impact on the inside does not depend on the external appearance of the pose (e.g., how far one can stretch forward). Accepting and cherishing each student's body and journey with yoga establish, as well, important empowering relationships of teachers with their students, and students' acceptance of, and positive feelings towards, their bodies.

Agency and functionality

The second dimension of the EE addresses experiences of agency and functionality in the world, ranging from acting in the world with a sense of power through voice and physical competence to experiencing ineffectiveness and restraint.

Yoga can help enhance the experience of physical agency and functionality through engendering a sense of accomplishment associated with the immersed and joyful engagement in physical activities protective factor of the DTE's physical domain. A sense of accomplishment or greater agency may come from implementing a new pose, taking a pose just one inch deeper or simply feeling joy in movement. Specific physical poses can help the practitioner to feel more powerful, stronger, and more confident, and language by the teacher and self-talk can enhance the impact of the poses on one's sense of agency. For example, Warrior I and II are very powerful poses. Their impact can be enhanced by the teacher's use of language, encouraging students to feel their own power in these poses. In particular, the impact of these poses can be enhanced by linking the movement to breathe and to qualities that one wants to enhance and engaging in positive self-talk (i.e., mantras). For example, in Warrior I, on the exhale, the practitioner can bring one's hands, breath, and sense of confidence into the solar plexus area or the third chakra, inhale, and say out loud or silently, "I breathe in confidence."

Practicing poses such as Warrior I and II, denoting strength and assertiveness can help counter internalized disempowering social discourses among individuals exposed to social messages in relation to various dimensions of social location, such as gender, age, ethnocultural heritage, or physical ability. Specifically in relation to gender, the poses can help counter the docility discourse transmitted to girls and women. The powerful positive process of relearning to inhabit the body with agency through performing movements of strengths and resistance that have been arrested due to exposure to adverse social processes of restriction and trauma has been highlighted by the sensorimotor approach to therapy (Ogden, Minton, &

Pain, 2006). Yoga therefore can support in countering restrictive social expectations that disrupt the experience of embodiment.

Attuned self-care

Attuned self-care reflects the degree of attunement and responsiveness to the embodied self and its physical, emotional, relational, aspirational, and spiritual needs. Attuned self-care ranges from awareness and responsiveness to internal cues and needs to disconnection and non-responsiveness to such cues.

Yoga can enhance attuned self-care through providing multiple avenues of attunement to physical, social, spiritual, and other needs, as well as opportunities to practice such care. The physical practice of yoga, as described above in the Body Connection and Comfort, allows for attuned physical engagement and opportunities for individuals to take care of themselves during this physical engagement.

The practice of yoga further encourages one to come inward and explore oneself through self-study. The breathwork of yoga, for example, is a practice of attunement as one notices the speed, depth, and sound of the breath. Further, the ethical guidelines of yoga, as described in Pantajali's sutras (Carrera, 2006) are the yamas and niyamas. Yamas have been described as self-regulating behaviors regarding interactions with other people and the world at large. Niyamas are personal practices that relate to one's inner world ("Yoga's ethical guide", n.d.). One of the niyamas of relevance to the dimension of attunement is svadhyaya, translated as self-study or inner exploration. For example, restorative yoga that involves getting into a comfortable physical pose and staying in it, invites the practitioner to engage in an inner exploration. Questions posed during restorative yoga or during meditation, can include, "What is it I really need to know? What does my heart desire?" One is then encouraged to listen to the answers that emerge from within as one is in restorative body position. When teachers pose the questions, it can be helpful to let students know that just the act of asking is enough, since an answer will not always emerge. It can also be helpful for teachers to remind students that instead of trying to answer the question from one's thinking mind, it can be helpful to feel what emerges within one's body (e.g., a sense of fatigue may indicate a need for rest, slowing down, and/or a strong desire for an internal sense of equanimity).

The invitation to engage in self-exploration and care can provide a balancing force to living in a culture that focuses on external actions and symbols of achievement. Further, for individuals who have learned to prioritize the care of others over self-attunement and care, such an invitation in yoga to practice care of oneself can be particularly important. For example, women often learn, since girlhood, to be other-(rather than self-) attuned and provide most of the care of others (Cerrato & Cifre, 2018; Piran, 2017; Ussher & Perz, 2010). As these and other authors indicate, the pattern of overriding and renouncing own needs, associated with the women as docile discourse cluster in the mental domain, has adverse long-term implications to women's well-being. The practice of yoga then can counter these social expectations, and enhance the care of oneself and positive embodiment.

Inhabiting the body as a subjective site (vs. as an objectified site)

This dimension refers to inhabiting the body as a subjective site, ranging from immersion in subjectively perceived embodied experiences and meaningful pursuits to inhabiting the body as an object to be gazed at and engaging in ongoing activities aimed at compliance with appearance expectations, overriding comfort, safety, and pleasure.

The practice of yoga can be powerful in developing an inward lens in inhabiting one's body. Practicing asanas requires an internal attunement to the integrated working and positioning of different body parts (e.g., muscles, spinal column, internal organs) to patterns of breathing. Concurrently, practitioners attune to other experiences associated with asanas and pranayamas, such as freedom, safety, power, relaxation, and pleasure or joy from sensing movement. Such internal attunement can be enhanced by teachers through linguistic guidance and the establishment of related class norms. Teachers can encourage students to listen to their bodies, trust their sensations, and learn to discern between helpful and unhelpful sensations. For example, with regard to the prior example of Warrior II, the teacher can help students further extend their arms out to the sides by suggesting that they adjust the pose in a manner that helps them breath more fully ("move so you can deepen your breath") or feel a greater sense of opening in the heart region. Teachers can encourage students to notice emotions as they move into different poses such as feelings of joy, sadness, uplifting or relaxation. Language by teachers can help students notice these feelings or sensations, be curious about what they might mean in the greater context of one's life, and to try not to judge the feelings as being desirable or undesirable.

The inward emphasis in the practice of yoga is important for all individuals living in a culture that places much importance on appearance and other external characteristics. Women, in particular, are exposed since childhood to social discourses that encourage them to inhabit their bodies as objects to be gazed at and to view their bodies as deficient, requiring ongoing surveillance and repair (Fredrickson & Roberts, 1997; Piran, 2017). In yoga, three DTE protective factors combine, providing opportunities to resist objectification and be immersed in one's subjective embodied experiences. First, yoga is a physical practice with a strong inward and positive focus, in line with the DTE protective factor of immersed and joyful engagement in physical activities (non-objectifying, non-sexualizing, and non-appearance or weight-related). Second, the practice of yoga, through its inward focus, and the valuing of the impact of asanas on internal experiences of the body rather than on the external appearance of poses, directly counter the constraining appearance-related discourses: the body as a deficient object. Third, as norms of de-emphasizing external appearance in yoga class are established, social power and connections *with* others become unrelated to appearance, in line with the protective factor of non-appearance-related sources of social power.

Experience and expression of bodily desires

The fifth, and final, dimension addresses connection to appetite and sexual desire, ranging from experiencing bodily desires and responding to them in attuned, self-caring, and joyful ways, to experiencing disrupted connection to desire and its association with negative emotions.

Engagement in attuned, immersed, and joyful physical practices, opportunities to practice attuned self-care, experiencing physical safety, countering objectifying pressures, and other DTE delineated protective factors involved in yoga, can enhance not only connection with the body but also attunement to bodily experiences of desire. Regarding appetite, an increased attunement to one's body may help in the recognition of signs of hunger and satiety, in addition to eating in accordance with one's bodily needs. In an intervention study examining the impact of yoga on binge eating, McIver and colleagues analyzed participants' comments in their personal journals for emerging themes (McIver, McGartland, & O'Halloran, 2016). Participants wrote about making healthier food choices due to a greater connection with the body and a greater understanding of the connection between what is eaten and how one feels as a result. Some participants wrote about enjoying food more. A mixed-methods study on a population-based sample of young adults found that yoga practitioners made healthier food choices; interview data revealed that yoga supported healthier eating through motivation to eat healthfully, greater mindfulness, management of stress and emotional eating, healthy food cravings, and the influence of the yoga community (Watts, Rydell, Eisenberg, Laska, & Neumark-Sztainer, 2018). In the second author's experience in teaching yoga within an eating disorder treatment center, one woman commented that due to yoga she had experienced hunger for the first time in many years.

Regarding sexual desire, Brotto and colleagues (Brotto, Mehak, & Kit, 2009) have suggested that the greater ability to maintain a focused and non-judgmental mindful attunement to the body during the physical practice of yoga may serve as a pathway to enhanced connection to desire. Such focused body awareness may help address the impact of distractions on women's sexual functioning (Dove & Wiederman, 2000). Further, studies suggest that self-objectification relates to self-consciousness during sexual contact and to decreased sexual functioning (Claudat & Warren, 2014; Steer & Tiggemann, 2008), and body shame is associated with lower sexual arousability and ability to reach orgasm (Quinn-Nilas, Benson, Milhausen, Buchholz, & Goncalves, 2016; Sanchez & Kiefer, 2007). It is therefore important that women practitioners of yoga have been found to be less likely to objectify their bodies, which also could enhance their desire (Impett, Daubenmier, & Hirschman, 2006), although further research is warranted.

The role of the yoga teacher in enhancing connections to desires is less clear-cut than for the other dimensions. It may be best for the practice itself to do its work with little needing to be said. Nonetheless, in therapeutic interventions with a yoga therapist, it may be helpful to ask clients about any changes they are noticing as a result of their yoga practice. For example, in working with clients with eating disorders, it may be helpful to ask questions about increased recognition of hunger and satiety cues, or increased enjoyment of eating, as a result of practicing yoga and coming inward to recognize and respond to one's body's needs. Further research is needed on the connection between yoga and experiences and expressions of desire, such as eating in response to hunger and enjoying the process of eating.

Conclusions and future directions

This article focuses on the practice of yoga and its potential contribution to positive embodiment, as informed by the Developmental Theory of Embodiment. As discussed, yoga may enhance the overall experience of embodiment by having a positive impact on each of its five dimensions: body connection and comfort, agency and functionality, attuned self-care, subjective immersion (resisting objectification), and experience and expression of desires. For yoga teachers, including teachers who use yoga towards therapeutic goals, these five dimensions can comprise *specific goals* (beyond a general goal of positive embodiment or body image) that can guide approaches to teaching, instructions, and language used during class, and the establishment of class norms. For this reason, in this article, we have described examples of teacher-related practices that could enhance each of these dimensions, such as enhancing positive connection with the body while engaging positively in asanas through appreciating its functioning. In addition to practice recommendation, we suggest that research studies that aim to study the impact of yoga practices include a range of ways to assess positive ways of living in the body, such as: experience of embodiment (total score and its subscales; Piran, 2019; Piran & Teall, 2012; Teall, 2015), body appreciation (Tylka & Wood-Barcalow, 2015), mindful self-care scale (Cook-Cottone & Guyker, 2017), or the appreciation of body functionality (Alleva et al., 2017).

Further, in addition to outlining the five dimensions of the experience of embodiment, which is a multidimensional intra-individual construct that reflects the quality of embodied lives, the DTE also delineates protective (and risk) factors in the physical and social environment that facilitate positive embodiment. A systematic consideration of these factors can suggest ways to further enhance the experience of embodiment through yoga. In the text and in Table 1, we provided examples of the protective factors that may be particularly relevant to each of the yoga practices that we described. Teachers may find the list of physical and social protective factors delineated by the DTE, such as practicing care of the body, safety, non-appearance-related social power, or membership in communities of equity, useful to their teaching practices. Yoga studios can make their settings more conducive to the promotion of a positive experience of embodiment through active steps at recruiting and retaining yoga practitioners of diverse body shapes and sizes, genders, sexual orientations, abilities and disabilities, and ethnic/racial and socioeconomic backgrounds (Cook-Cottone & Douglass 2017; Neumark-Sztainer, Neumark-Sztainer et al., 2018; Picket & Cunningham, 2017). The way in which yoga is portrayed also needs to be examined since challenging social processes may affect the practice of yoga adversely, limiting its potential contribution to positive experience of embodiment, and, even further, disrupting positive embodiment. For example, an analysis of the physical appearance attributes and attire worn by female cover models of a Yoga journal during the past 40 years found that more recent covers promoted objectified body competence and a drive for leanness (Webb, Vinoski, Warren-Findlow, Burrell, & Putz, 2017). As the experience of embodiment reflects the dialectical relationships between inner and outer, body and culture, yoga teachers and practitioners need to be mindful of the context within which yoga is portrayed and practiced.

The discussion of ways in which yoga may contribute positively to embodiment in this article relies on the application of constructs of the research-based DTE to the field of yoga, as informed by the second author 's (DNS) experiences as a yoga student, practitioner, and teacher. However, the suggested practices needed to be tested empirically through planned interventions. In terms of research, the outlined protective factors and related practices may operate as mechanisms of change mediating outcome observed in intervention studies involving yoga practices. Inconsistencies in the outcome of yoga interventions may relate to variations in the presence of protective factors explored in this article. Intervention studies may aim at constructing yoga classes that specifically address particular protective factors that enhance positive embodiment. In order to facilitate the evaluation of these factors in yoga intervention studies, we devised a scale of these protective factors as they may apply to yoga (DTE-informed Yoga Practice Experiences: DTEYPE; Piran & Neumark-Sztainer, 2019; see Appendix A). These items were developed by the first author and they follow the detailed list of research-based protective factors that enhance positive embodiment delineated by the DTE (see a summarized list of these factors in the "The DTE: Delineating Protective Experiences" section of this manuscript, and in Table 1.2 in Piran, 2017, p. 16). These protective factors emerged in three qualitative studies (Piran, 2017), and three quantitative studies (Piran, 2019; Piran & Cormier, 2005; Piran & Thompson, 2008; Teall, 2015). Further, the DTEYPE items resemble selected items from previously developed psychometrically tested measures of the physical, mental, and social power domains of the DTE (see Teall, 2015). The second author suggested revisions to the wording of the items based on her experience as a researcher and yoga instructor. However, the DTEYPE scale itself has not been administered or studied psychometrically. It therefore requires a series of psychometric studies before it can be used as a research measure in outcome evaluation studies or other research.

The study of yoga in relation to embodiment and positive body image is a growing field of research. The DTE comprises one lens through which to examine this relationship, suggesting the potential contribution of a research-based embodiment theory on exploring yoga-related processes. In particular, the research-based DTE addresses dimensions of positive embodiment that may be enhanced through specific yoga practices. The DTE further delineates protective factors that contribute to positive embodiment, and can inform yoga instructors. Further research in this area is needed, in particular, the exploration of DTE constructs among groups that have not been studied as extensively in embodiment research (such as men) and evaluation studies that explicitly integrate embodiment theory with yoga practices.

Acknowledgments

The work on the Developmental Theory of Embodiment was supported by the Social Sciences and Humanities Research Council of Canada to Niva Piran (PI) under grant numbers: 410-1999-1370, 410-2003-0280, 410-2007-0630, and 410-2011-0205. Dianne Neumark-Sztainer's time to write this manuscript was partially supported by Grant number R35HL139853 from the National Heart, Lung, and Blood Institute (PI: Dianne Neumark-Sztainer). The content is solely the responsibility of the authors and does not necessarily represent the official views of the National Heart, Lung, and Blood Institute or the National Institutes of Health.

Funding

This work was supported by the National Heart, Lung, and Blood Institute [R35HL139853].

References

Alleva, J. M., Tylka, T. L., & Kroon Van Diest, A. (2017). The Functionality Appreciation Scale(FAS): Development and psychometric evaluation in U.S. community women and men. *Body Image, 23*, 28–44. doi:10.1016/j.bodyim.2017.07.008

Bartky, S. L. (1988). Foucault, femininity and the modernization of patriarchal power. In I. Diamond & L. Quinby (Eds.), *Feminism and Foucault: Reflections on resistance* (pp. 61–86). Boston, MA: Northeastern University.

Bordo, S. (1989). The body and the reproduction of femininity: A feminist appropriation of Foucault. In A. M. Jaggar & S. R. Bordo (Eds.), *Gender/body/knowledge* (pp. 13–33). New Brunswick, NJ: Rutgers University.

Bordo, S. (1993). *Unbearable weight: feminism, western culture, and the body.* Berkeley: University of California Press.

Brotto, L. A., Mehak, L., & Kit, C. (2009). Yoga and sexual functioning: A review. *Journal of Sex & Marital Therapy, 35*, 378–390. doi:10.1090/00926230903065955

Buchanan, N. T., Settles, I. H., & Woods, K. C. (2019). Black women's positive embodiment in the face of race × gender oppression. In T. L. Tylka & N. Piran (Eds.), *Handbook of positive body image and embodiment* (pp. 191–200). New York, NY: Oxford University Press.

Carrera, J. (2006). *Inside the Yoga Sutras: A comprehensive sourcebook for the study and practice of Patanjali's yoga sutras.* Yogaville, Virginia: Integral Yoga Publications.

Cerrato, J., & Cifre, E. (2018). Gender inequality in household chores and work-family conflict. *Frontiers in Psychology. 9*:1330. Retrieved from https://www.frontiersin.org/arti cles/10.3389/fpsyg.2018.01330

Charmaz, K. (2006). *Constructing grounded theory: A practical guide through qualitativ analysis.* Thousand Oaks, CA: Sage.

Claudat, K., & Warren, C. S. (2014). Self-objectification, body self-consciousness during sexual activities, and sexual satisfaction in college women. *Body Image, 11*, 509–515. doi:10.1016/j.bodyim.2014.07.006

Cook-Cottone, C, & Douglass, L.L. (2017). Yoga communities and eating disorders: creating safe space for positive embodiment. Retrieved from. doi: https://www.ncbi.nlm.nih.gov/ pubmed/28492346doi:10.1776/IJYT2017_Methods_Cook-Cottone_Epub

Cook-Cottone, C. P. (2019). Brain integration, embodied mindfulness, and movement-based approaches to facilitate positive body image and embodiment. In T. L. Tylka & N. Piran (Eds.), *Handbook of positive body image and embodiment* (pp. 337–346). New York, NY: Oxford University Press.

Cook-Cottone, C. P., & Guyker, W. M. (2017). The development and validation of the mindful self-care scale (MSCS): An assessment of practices that support positive embodiment. *Mindfulness, 9*, 161–175. doi:10.1007/s12671-017-0759-1

Crossley, N. (1995). Merleau-Ponty, the elusive body and carnal sociology. *Body and Society, 1*, 43–63. doi:10.1177/1357034X95001001004

Csordas, T. J. (1994). *Embodiment and experience, the existential ground of culture and self.* Cambridge, UK: Cambridge University.

Daubenmier, J. J. (2005). The relationship of yoga, body awareness, and body responsiveness to self-objectification and disordered eating. *Psychology of Women Quarterly, 29*, 207–219. doi:10.1111/j.1471-6402.2005.00183.x

De-Beauvoir, S. (1974). The second sex. (2nd edition). Trans. H. Parshley. New York: Vintage.

Dove, N. L., & Wiederman, M. W. (2000). Cognitive distraction and women's sexual functioning. *Journal of Sex and Marital Therapy, 26*, 67–78. doi:10.1080/009262300278650

Foucault, M. (1995). *Discipline and punish: The birth of a prison* (2nd ed.). New York, NY: Vintage.

Frawley, D. (2018). *Yoga: A guide to the teaching and practices.* San Rafael, CA: Mandala.

Fredrickson, B. L., & Roberts, T. (1997). Objectification Theory: Toward understanding women's lived experiences and mental health risks. *Psychology of Women Quarterly, 21*, 173–206. doi:10.1111/j.1471-6402.1997.tb00108.x

Holmqvist Gattario, K., Frisén, A., & Piran, N. (2018, June). Embodiment: Cultural and gender differences and associations with life satisfaction. Paper presented at the Appearance Matters 8 Conference, Bath.

hooks, B. (1997). Selling hot pussy: Representations of Black female sexuality in the cultural marketplace. In K. Conboy, N. Medina, & S. Stanbury (Eds.), *Writing on the body: Female embodiment and feminist theory* (pp. 113–128). New York, NY: Columbia University Press.

Howe, L. A. (2003). Athletics, embodiment, and the appropriation of the self. *The Journal of Speculative Philosophy, 17*, 92–107. doi:10.1353/jsp.2003.0032

Impett, E. A., Daubenmier, J. J., & Hirschman, A. L. (2006). Minding the body: Yoga, embodiment and well-being. *Sexuality Research & Social Policy, 3*, 39–48. doi:10.1525/srsp.2006.3.4.39

McIver, S., McGartland, M., & O'Halloran, P. (2009). Overeating is not about the food": Women describe their experience of a yoga treatment program for binge eating. *Qualitative Health Research, 19*(9), 1234–1244. doi:10.1177/1049732309343954

Merleau-Ponty, M. (1962). *Phenomenology of perception.* (C. Smith, Trans). New York, NY: Humanities.

Neumark-Sztainer, D. (2019). The practice of yoga: Can it help in addressing body image concerns and eating disorders? In T. L. Tylka & N. Piran (Eds.), *Handbook of positive body image and embodiment* (pp. 326–336). New York, NY: Oxford University Press.

Neumark-Sztainer, D., MacLehose, R. F., Watts, A. W., Pacanowski, C. R., & Eisenberg, M. E. (2018). Yoga and body image: Findings from a large population-based study of young adults. *Body Image, 24*, 69–75. doi:10.1016/j.bodyim.2017.12.003

Neumark-Sztainer, D., Watts, A. W., & Rydell, S. (2018). Yoga and body image: How do young adults practicing yoga describe tis impact on their body image? *Body Image, 27*, 1–13. doi:10.1016/j.bodyim.2018.09.001

Ogden, P., Minton, K., & Pain, C. (2006). *Trauma and the body: A sensorimotor approach t psychotherapy.* New York, NY: W.W. Norton.

Picket, A. C., & Cunningham, G. B. (2017). Creating inclusive physical activity spaces: The case of body- positive yoga. *Research Quarterly for Exercise and Sport, 88*, 329–338. doi:10.1080/02701367.2017.1335851

Piran, N. (2002). Embodiment: A mosaic of inquiries in the area of body weight and shape preoccupation. In S. Abbey (Ed.), *Ways of knowing in and through the body: Diverse perspectives on embodiment* (pp. 211–214). Welland, ON: Soleil Publishing.

Piran, N., & Teall, T. L. (2012). The developmental theory of embodiment. In G. McVey, M. P. Levine, N. Piran, & H. B. Ferguson (Eds.), *Preventing eating-related and weight-related disorders: Collaborative research, advocacy, and policy change* (pp. 171–199). Waterloo, ON: Wilfred Laurier Press.

Piran, N. (2016). Embodied possibilities and disruptions: The emergence of the experience of embodiment construct from qualitative studies with girls and women. *Body Image, 18*, 43–60. doi:10.1016/j.bodyim.2016.04.007

Piran, N. (2017). *Journeys of embodiment at the intersection of body and culture: The developmental theory of embodiment.* San Diego, CA: Elsevier. doi:10.1016/c2015-0-04666-4

Piran, N. (2019). The experience of embodiment construct: Reflecting the quality of embodied lives. In T. L. Tylka & N. Piran (Eds.), *Handbook of positive body image and embodiment* (pp. 11–21). New York, NY: Oxford University Press.

Piran, N., & Cormier, H. (2005). The social construction of women and dis- ordered eating patterns. *Journal of Counseling Psychology, 52*, 549–558. doi:10.1037/a0021905

Piran, N., & Neumark-Sztainer, D. (2019). *The developmental theory of embodiment-informed yoga practice experiences (DTEYPE) scale.* Unpublished manuscript.

Piran, N., & Thompson, S. (2008). A study of the adverse social experiences model of the development of eating disorders. *International Journal of Health Promotion and Education, 46*, 65–71. doi:10.1080/14635240.2008.10708131

Quinn-Nilas, C., Benson, L., Milhausen, R. R., Buchholz, A. C., & Goncalves, M. (2016). The relationship between body image and domains of sexual functioning among heterosexual, emerging adult women. *Sexual Medicine, 4*, e182–189. doi:10.1016/j.esxm.2016.02.004

Sanchez, D. T., & Kiefer, A. K. (2007). Body concerns in and out of the bedroom: Implications for sexual pleasure and problems. *Archives of Sex Behavior, 36*, 808–820. doi:10.1007/s10508-007-9205-0

Sandoz, E. K., Wilson, K. G., Merwin, R. M., & Kellum, K. K. (2013). Assessment of body image flexibility: The Body-Image Acceptance and Action Questionnaire. *Journal of Contextual Behavioral Science*, *2*, 39–48. doi:10.1016/j.jcbs.2013.03.002

Steer, A., & Tiggemann, M. (2008). The role of self-objectification in women's sexual functioning. *Journal of Social and Clinical Psychology*, *27*, 205–225. doi:10.1521/jscp.2008.27.3.205

Sundgot-Borgen, C., Friborg, O., Kolle, E., Engen, K. M. E., Sundgot-Borgen, J., Rosenvinge, … Bratland-Sanda, S. (2019). The healthy body image (HBI) intervention: Effects of a school-based cluster-randomized controlled trial with 12-months follow-up. *Body Image*, *29*, 122–131. doi:10.1016/j.bodyim.2019.03.007

Teall, T. L. (2015). *A quantitative study of the developmental theory of embodiment: Implications to health and well being*. (Ph.D. thesis, University of Toronto, Toronto, Canada). Retrieved from http://research.proquest.com.myaccess.library.toronto.ca/docvie/

Tylka, T. L., & Piran, N. (2019). Focusing on the positive: An introduction to the volume. In T. L. Tylka & N. Piran (Eds.), *Handbook of positive body image and embodiment* (pp. 1–8). New York, NY: Oxford University Press.

Tylka, T. L., & Wood-Barcalow, N. L. (2015). The body appreciation scale: Item refinement and psychometric evaluation. *Body Image*, *12*, 53–67. doi:10.1016/j.bodyim.2014.09.006

Ussher, J., & Perz, J. (2010). Gender differences in self-silencing and psychological distress in informal cancer carers. *Psychology of Women Quarterly*, *34*, 228–242. doi:10.1111/j.1471-6402.2010.01564.x

Watts, A. W., Rydell, S. A., Eisenberg, M. E., Laska, M. N., & Neumark-Sztainer, D. (2018). Yoga's potential for promoting healthy eating and physical activity behaviors among young adults: A mixed-methods study. *International Journal of Behavioral Nutrition and Physical Activity*, *15*. doi:10.1186/s12966-018-0674-4

Webb, J. B., Vinoski, E. R., Warren-Findlow, J., Burrell, M. I., & Putz, D. Y. (2017). Downward dog becomes fit body, inc.: A content analysis of 40 years of female cover images of Yoga Journal. *Body Image*, *22*, xx–xx. doi:10.1016/j.bodyim.2017.07.001

Yoga's ethical guide to living: The Yamas and Niyamas (n.d.). The Kripalu Center. Retrieved from https://kripalu.org/resources/yoga-s-ethical-guide-living-yamas-and-niyamas

Appendix

DTE Yoga Practice Experiences (DTEYPE) (Piran & Neumark-Stzainer, 2019)[a]

During my yoga practice:

1. I felt immersed in (really into) the practice of the different postures and enjoyed it.
2. I could feel my body moving, stretching, or relaxing in ways that made me feel good about what the body can do.
3. I felt comfortable taking up physical space while practicing.
4. I felt safe in my body.
5. I felt the freedom and power to alter the practice in ways that fit for me.
6. I was encouraged, and felt able to, take care of my body (e.g., adjust the asanas to what I was comfortable with, rest when I needed).
7. I felt supported in being attuned to my bodily desires (e.g., hydrate or feed the body in response to thirst or hunger to enhance its ability to engage in the physical practice of yoga, and for general well being).
8. I felt freedom from looking at my body as an object that needs to appear a certain way.
9. I felt free from criticizing the appearance of my body.
10. I felt good about taking time and doing something good for myself (and not only taking care of others).
11. I felt comfortable feeling powerful and strong (e.g., during the warrior poses).
12. I felt free from prejudices about me or my background (because of my gender, ethnicity/race, weight, ability, sexual orientation, gender identity, social class, or other factors).
13. I felt an acceptance of diversity among group members
14. I felt I was treated equally to others
15. I felt empowered by others (teacher, other students)
16. I felt that physical appearance (or the way asanas looked) was not a source of social power (or social standing) in the class.

[a]Please contact the first author for permission to use the DTEYPE

Realizing Yoga's all-access pass: a social justice critique of westernized yoga and inclusive embodiment

Jennifer B. Webb, Courtney B. Rogers, and Erin Vinoski Thomas (iD)

ABSTRACT

In the 21st century, the ancient mind–body practice of yoga has surged in popularity among western enthusiasts for its numerous health benefits. Particularly, a growing evidence base supports yoga for cultivating positive embodiment and reducing risk for disordered eating. Nevertheless, amidst its rise are concerns about yoga's departure from its spiritual foundations and increasing assimilation into the appearance- and commercial-driven exercise and fitness culture. Consequently, an exclusionary identity has been perpetuated in shaping norms surrounding who can and does practice yoga, which contradicts earlier egalitarian visions of a yoga for all. Therefore, we adopt a social justice lens in offering a focused analysis of the intersection of yoga, embodiment, and inclusion for select marginalized social identities typically underrepresented among yoga practitioners and in yoga scholarship. Data are synthesized from both qualitative and quantitative sources and integrate an understanding of how confined media representations of "the yoga body" and other practical constraints may undermine the perceived access to the practice for members of diverse groups. We conclude with inviting future considerations towards fostering more interdisciplinary community-based research partnerships among the variety of stakeholders invested in advancing the accessibility and inclusion of yoga and positive embodiment for all bodies.

Clinical implications

- Yoga professionals are encouraged to assess how their business practices could be enhanced to invite greater access to practitioners from culturally-diverse backgrounds.
- Yoga researchers are invited to increase collaborative partnerships with yoga professionals within the community to improve access in yoga research participation.
- Yoga professionals may benefit from increased awareness and training in identifying body image and eating disorder symptoms among their students.

"Yoga does not discriminate: it embraces you where you are and people need to know that."—Dana A. Smith (Smith, 2018, p. 199)

Introduction

The ancient holistic practice of yoga has been catapulted to the forefront of contemporary science (Domingues & Carmo, 2019; Park, Braun, & Siegel, 2015) informed by current theory (e.g., Cook-Cottone, 2015; Menzel & Levine, 2011; Piran, 2017) as a major vehicle for cultivating positive embodiment in the prevention and treatment of disordered eating. Aligned with its original spiritual foundations, yoga encourages the integration of mind and body via meditation and physical asanas (i.e., postures) which in turn facilitate the experiences of embodied self-regulation and attunement (Cook-Cottone, 2015). These qualities of strengthening the individual's capacity to respond adaptively to the dynamic association continuously unfolding between the demands of one's internal (e.g., thoughts, feelings, physiology) and external (e.g., family, community, broader culture) experiential self-systems (Cook-Cottone, 2015).

When engaged in yoga from this stance, this discipline reinforces the value of body functionality and competence over prioritizing physical appearance (Cook-Cottone, 2015). Of note, an accumulating evidence base inclusive of experimental and naturalistic designs confirms yoga's positive links to aspects of positive body image and physical embodiment and inverse associations with negative body image and self-objectification (Domingues & Carmo, 2019).

Yoga's moral and ethical philosophy additionally invites practitioners to adopt complementary lifestyle behaviors that for instance support adaptive, socially conscious eating practices (Domingues & Carmo, 2019; Freeman, Vladagina, Razmjou, & Brems, 2017). Indeed, recent systematic reviews of the literature noted that yoga practitioners reported lower intake of fast food and sugary beverages in conjunction with more frequent consumption of fruits and vegetables and adherence to a vegetarian or a vegan diet relative to non-practitioners (Cramer, Sibbritt, Park, Adams, & Lauche, 2017; Domingues & Carmo, 2019; Park et al., 2015). Individuals who practice yoga further evidenced greater engagement in mindful eating and a robust positive link between body awareness and intuitive eating (Domingues & Carmo, 2019). Meanwhile, the collective experience of participating as a member of a supportive practice community has the potential to capitalize on existing resources for stimulating positive embodiment with greater intentionality of reducing risk for disordered eating (Cook-Cottone & Douglass, 2017; Neumark-Sztainer, 2019).

Nevertheless, heightened concerns over yoga's assimilation into the highly appearance-focused exercise and fitness culture have emerged alongside its rapid growth in the West (Freeman et al., 2017; Lacasse, Santarossa, & Woodruff, 2019; Markula, 2014). Unfortunately, such a dramatic shift away from its spiritual roots towards greater commercialization and secularization may ironically expose individuals to factors which could confer augmented risk for disembodying experiences such as body image disturbance and dysfunctional eating patterns (Kauer, 2016; Neumark-Sztainer, 2019). For instance, yoga practice may increase the likelihood of engaging in body/appearance comparison, body hypervigilance, excessive exercising, and symptoms of orthorexia (i.e., an obsession with healthy or clean eating; Domingues & Carmo, 2019; Musial, 2016). Moreover, recent content analyses of mainstream media depictions of the "yoga body" reveal narrowly defined representations exemplified by the portrayal of *objectified body competence* (i.e., image attributes reflecting the duality of body functionality and sexual objectification: Bhalla & Moscowitz, 2019; Blaine, 2016; Boccio, 2012; Lacasse et al., 2019; Webb et al., 2017a).

Importantly, the widespread perpetuation of such media images and the corresponding limited representation of individuals reflecting an array of marginalized social identities in current yoga scholarship and among yoga practitioners and professionals may serve as perceived barriers (Park et al., 2015; Strings, Headen, & Spencer, 2019). Consequently, entire segments of the population may be unintentionally disenfranchised from experiencing its health benefits more generally and in particular averting risk for negative embodiment (e.g., disordered eating). This current western trend in advancing an exclusionary identity of the modern yoga practitioner parallels the historical exclusion of women from the practice in India prior to Latvian native Indra Devi's groundbreaking efforts to transcend the gender barrier in the late 1930s (see Bhalla & Moscowitz, 2019 for a discussion). Yet it also marked a radical departure from Swami Vivekananda's original vision to make yoga publicly available to the masses as a means of promoting anti-capitalist reform when he introduced the practice to the West during India's British colonial period (Page, 2016).

Therefore, inspired by these forerunners in the inclusive yoga movement, the primary goal of this article is to adopt the social justice lens previously advocated by leading experts (e.g., Berila, Klein, & Jackson Roberts, 2016; Cook-Cottone & Douglass, 2017; Klein, 2018; Klein & Guest-Jelley, 2014; Lipton, 2017; Neumark-Sztainer, Watts, & Rydell, 2018) in, p. 1) considering how stigmatization of marginalized identities contribute to the experiences of disordered eating and negative embodiment, 2) providing a brief window into the experience of yoga among select social identities typically underrepresented in contemporary western yoga research and yoga communities from both quantitative and qualitative sources (i.e., individuals from lower socioeconomic status, racial/ethnic minorities, males, transgender and gender non-conforming individuals, individuals of higher weight, sexual minorities, individuals with physical disabilities, and older adults), 3) highlighting existing gaps in the literature along with identified barriers and facilitators to the practice for members of marginalized groups, and 4) concluding with a roadmap offering potential future directions aimed at bolstering ongoing efforts in stimulating community-driven scientific initiatives to improve the inclusion and accessibility of yoga for its benefits to health, well-being, and embodiment for all.

Lower socioeconomic status

Popular perceptions endure in problematizing disordered eating as exclusive to those of higher socioeconomic means (Olsen, 2017). Nevertheless, a growing body of scholarship contends that the risk for eating and associated body image disturbance does not discriminate based on class or socioeconomic status (SES). Indeed, epidemiological data drawn from large-scale population-based samples have shown that rates of clinically significant forms of disordered eating were not distinguished by SES in adolescent girls (Rogers, Resnick, Mitchell, & Blum, 1997) and that eating disorder symptomatology was distributed equitably across various indicators of SES (e.g., income level, education, indigenous status, urbanicity) in adults (Mulders-Jones, Mitchison, Girosi, & Hay, 2017). Meanwhile, recent emerging evidence has observed that higher levels of food insecurity (prevalent among individuals living poverty) are associated with more frequent binge eating, dietary restraint, and compensatory behaviors (Becker, Middlemass, Taylor, Johnson, & Gomez, 2017) along with a higher likelihood of clinically elevated binge eating disorder (Rasmusson, Lydecker, Coffino, White, & Grilo, 2018) among low-income adults. Notably, as food insecurity worsened so did the severity of internalized weight self-stigma highlighting the critical intersectionality of the experience of weight and SES (Becker et al., 2017). Concerns regarding access to yoga and its benefits from a socioeconomic standpoint in the West were evident among its early leaders.

Hindu monk Swami Vivekananda was instrumental in planting the seeds for the transmission of yogic principles and practices to western culture (Page, 2016). Originally, he envisioned increasing access to the spiritual discipline for all as a vehicle to promote social liberation mirroring the earlier sociopolitical role of the wandering yoga spiritual leader in the resistance to subvert British colonization of India (Page, 2016). However, these social justice-driven ideals were undermined as the intended ascetic discipline became increasingly seen as an entrepreneurial opportunity for educated women of Eurocentric heritage rendering the formerly communal openness of the practice as exclusive and enclosed (Page, 2016). Similarly, among the first students of Indra Devi were female Hollywood celebrities which contributed to the entrenched notion that yoga was accessible only to the elite and financially well-off (Bhalla & Moscowitz, 2019).

Critics of the growing commercialization of yoga in western circles decried the bifurcation of the practice from its spiritual origins in favor or more consumerist-driven priorities selling commodified embodiment (Bhalla & Moscowitz, 2019; Blaine, 2016; Boccio, 2012; Freeman et al., 2017; Kauer, 2016; Markula, 2014). For instance, a recent national survey estimated that U.S. yoga practitioners spent over $16 billion on the practice in 2016 (Ipsos Public Affairs, 2016). Among the ramifications of this changing zeitgeist included the juxtaposition of contradictory representations of the spiritualism and secularization of the discipline revealing myriad goods (e.g., high-end apparel, gear, nutritional supplements, etc.), services (e.g., yoga studio management, etc.) and experiences (e.g., costly retreats, travel, etc.) advertised within the pages (Vinoski Thomas et al., 2017) and featured on the covers (Webb et al., 2017a) of mainstream yoga lifestyle print media.

Collectively, such a commercial focus and advocacy by famous celebrity practitioners may convey the idea that yoga is more of a luxury activity reserved for the rich. This emphasis reinforces the erroneous assumption that expensive products and clothing are required, thereby serving as barriers for individuals of modest economic means for believing there is space for them to be able to enter into and benefit from the practice (Page, 2016; Remski, 2012; Rosenfeld, 2016). Additionally, the cost and typical fee structure of attending classes in or becoming a member of a yoga studio are prohibitive for a large segment of society (Page, 2016; Rosenfeld, 2016). In line with this commentary, existing research confirms that yoga practitioners tend to be higher educated than non-practitioners and have a higher median household income relative to the US national median household income (Park et al., 2015).

Despite the limited representation of individuals of lower SES among current yoga practitioners, researchers have recently directed resources to prioritize their inclusion in contemporary yoga scholarship. Findings from yoga intervention research with lower-income multi-ethnic participants have demonstrated improvements in sleep-related attributes, stress, mood and anxiety symptoms, physical activity, and dietary behavior (Bertisch et al., 2019; Falsafi & Leopard, 2015; Pierce et al., 2017). Qualitative data further supported the acceptability and feasibility of these yoga-based protocols alongside providing useful insights into additional personal and structural barriers to consider when attempting to engage more economically disadvantaged groups with the practice (e.g., increasing affordability, convenience, and reach, for example, through online and smartphone-based technology, encouraging family-based practices, peer-led instruction, and other strategies that facilitate the integration of yoga into everyday life; Bertisch et al., 2019; Tenfelde, Hatchett, & Saban, 2018).

Concurrently, experts have called for a return to the activist roots of yoga and have suggested a number of practical strategies to encourage making yoga accessible regardless of financial means (e.g., offering a sliding scale and

charitable, donation-based classes, transforming the incentivization of indivi-
dualistic models of yoga studio financial infrastructure to cooperative community-based ones, making a kitchen an essential space within the yoga studio, etc.;
Kauer, 2016; Remski, 2012). Otherwise, Remski (2012) cautions: " … yoga will
continue to market itself as a consumer-class consolation, offering fashionable
inner peace to a preciously small fraction of humanity." (p. 121). In aspiring to
advance greater economic inclusion among practitioners within the broader
yoga community non-profit organizations like the Give Back Yoga Foundation,
the Hands to Heart Center, Yoga 4 Change, and Street Yoga are making access
more affordable and bringing yoga directly to the people in a range of diverse
settings both locally and globally (e.g., public housing, detention centers, home-
less shelters, etc.; Rosenfeld, 2016; Schware, 2016). Importantly, it will be fruitful
for subsequent investigations to more directly evaluate the potential utility of
yoga for enhancing embodiment (e.g., improving mindful and intuitive eating,
reducing binge eating, etc.) amidst the complex realities of living with hunger,
food insecurity, and the stigma of poverty.

Racial and ethnic minorities

Although significant attention has been paid to the experience of White
individuals, body image concerns and disordered eating occur across racial
and ethnic groups. In addition to societal appearance pressures, a well-
established risk factor, minority and acculturative stress may also play a role
in increasing vulnerability among diverse racial and ethnic groups (Claudat,
White, & Warren, 2016; Rodgers, Berry, & Franko, 2018). Disordered eating
may serve, in part, as an attempt to ameliorate identity-related distress.
Notably, a greater sense of ethnic identity is inversely related to body image
disturbance and body dissatisfaction and positively linked to body appreciation. This relationship appears to be partially mediated by lower perceived
pressure to attain societal appearance ideals (Cotter, Kelly, Mitchell, & Mazzeo,
2015; Rodgers et al., 2018).

   Although somewhat limited, extant research examining yoga practice
among ethnic and racial minorities demonstrates the benefits of this activity
for psychosocial and physical wellbeing (see Burnett-Zeigler, Schuette,
Victorson, & Wisner, 2016 for a review of the use of mind-body approaches
in these groups). Yoga may serve as an alternative outlet for coping with
general minority and acculturative stress. Regarding body image, engagement
in yoga may also encourage authenticity and embodiment, counteracting
negative effects of identity-related stressors (Bondy, 2014; Haddix, 2016).

   As part of the westernization of yoga, it has been characterized as
a predominately non-Hispanic White practice (Clarke, Black, Stussman,
Barnes, & Nahin, 2015; Smith & Atencio, 2017; Strings et al., 2019). Indeed,
racial and ethnic minorities were represented on only 26% of the covers of 3

leading yoga lifestyle magazines between 2010–2015 (Webb et al., 2017a) and nationally derived data corroborate the link between yoga practice and White race in western samples (Park et al., 2015). These phenomena hold implications for People of Color in western society in how they view, access, and experience a yoga practice (Bondy, 2014). For example, in one investigation of a 12-week yoga intervention intended to improve quality of life among breast cancer patients, 56% of Hispanic women, 26% of African American women, and 17% of White women chose not to attend any of the offered classes (Moadel et al., 2007). Although this lack of participation was likely due to a variety of factors (such as health of participants), it is possible that perceptions about the inclusivity and fit of yoga also discouraged these individuals from engaging with the practice.

In addition to perceptions about inclusivity, other barriers to engaging in the practice likely also exist. A qualitative study by Spadola et al. (2018) examined barriers to yoga practice in racial and ethnic minorities. Identified barriers included perceptions of yoga as a low-effort physical activity (i.e., with limited benefits for physical health) and perceived lack of ability to safely and competently engage in the practice. Perceived lack of time was also an issue, especially as compared to engagement in activities that were viewed as more spontaneous (e.g., walking). Although at-home practice may provide a feasible alternative to in-person instruction, there may also be perceived barriers to this such as lack of space, a mat, and instructional materials.

Spadola et al. (2018) also noted facilitators of yoga practice in racial and ethnic minority groups. Many of these facilitative factors were environmental in nature. For instance, participants noted that having access to classes that were perceived as accessible to beginners was important. Moreover, perceiving that a yoga instructor was knowledgeable, interpersonally capable, and relatable also encouraged engagement in yoga practice. Relatability may be linked to the availability of instructors from diverse racial and ethnic backgrounds, further supporting the importance of identity representation across various levels of yoga practice (e.g., by instructors, in the media; Middleton et al., 2017). Inclusion of marginalized persons in the organized practice also necessitates deliberate effort. Yoga instructor Marcelle Haddix (2016, p. 26) notes, "My challenge has been to encourage people of color from my local community to attend my yoga classes despite socially and historically constructed ideas that this is an activity that they do not participate in or that these are spaces where they do not belong. To do this, I was intentional in centering the interests and needs of black women with a deliberate stance that what is good for black women is good for all."

A series of personal essays have emerged describing the numerous benefits of yoga for body image and embodiment among racial and ethnic minority women (e.g., Bondy, 2014; Smith, 2014, 2016, 2018; Stanley, 2018). Yet it is surprising that published research has yet to specifically focus on providing complementary evaluations of yoga's impact on embodiment in these target groups. Additionally, scholarship remains to investigate the potential embodiment-related benefits of yoga practice for those who identify as multiracial. This may be an especially important area to address given the possible negative consequences of navigating multiple identities (Yoo, Jackson, Guevarra, Miller, & Harrington, 2016). Further research is also needed to understand attitudes toward yoga practice by racial and ethnic minority communities (Middleton et al., 2017; Spadola et al., 2018). Existing efforts by the peer-reviewed journal *Race and Yoga* and communities such as Black Girl in Om (http://blackgirlinom.com), Black Yoga Teacher's Alliance (http://blackyogateachersalliance.org), and South Asian American Perspectives on Yoga in America (http://saapya.wordpress.com) may also be beneficial to consider. Ideally, this work can inform guidelines for creating more accessible and inclusive yoga spaces for all individuals.

Males

Although men (especially those that identify as heterosexual) report lower rates of disordered eating as compared to women, body dissatisfaction remains a salient issue among this group. Men may perceive societal pressures to obtain a muscular appearance ideal which has been associated with strength and masculinity (Frederick et al., 2007). Participation in yoga may counteract body image disturbances and support a positive body image for men (Baskauskas, 2014); however, they may be reluctant to engage in this practice. In the United States, contrary to other parts of the world, yoga is perceived as a female-dominated activity (Clarke et al., 2015; Smith & Atencio, 2017). This phenomenon persists likely in part due to Indra Devi's, Swami Vivekananda's and other leaders' groundbreaking efforts to improve access to the discipline to (White) women who are currently disproportionately represented among western yoga practitioners (Bhalla & Moscowitz, 2019; Ipsos Public Affairs, 2016; Page, 2016; Park et al., 2015). Although these historical developments were seen as progressive at the time, the modern feminization of yoga in the West (also reflected in the declining and scarce representation of men on the covers of yoga lifestyle print media: Strings et al., 2019; Thompson, 2012; Webb et al., 2017b) has inadvertently deterred men from pursuing the practice and experiencing its health benefits. Indeed, those that identify as male may feel as if yoga is not inclusive to them or that it does not align with their perceptions of masculinity (Kest, 2014; McGraw, 2014). For example, when discussing his initial perceptions of the practice, McGraw (2014, p. 241) wrote, " ... I was convinced that yoga was not for me. After all, I was a male high school senior, and in my mind yoga was a flowery workout that was reserved for women."

Preliminary research indicates that male yoga practitioners report higher body satisfaction than men who engage in aerobics/weight-training (e.g., Flaherty, 2014). Nevertheless, more investigation is needed to understand whether these benefits extend to other aspects of embodiment, potential underlying mechanisms, and barriers to engagement in the practice. Organizations that specifically focus on the experience of men in westernized yoga may also be important in changing male perceptions about yoga practice. For example, efforts by companies such as Yoga for Men (http://yogaformen.com/blogs/yoga-for-men) normalize the participation in yoga by men and offer tailored suggestions for practice to this population.

Transgender and gender non-conforming

Beyond those that identify as cisgender, other individuals along the gender continuum may also benefit from the practice of yoga. In addition to these individuals being at increased risk for general psychological distress (Lee, 2000), body image concerns and disordered eating are also noteworthy to consider. In a large-scale study of college students ($N = 289,024$), those who identified as transgender endorsed the highest rates of disordered eating behaviors (Diemer, Grant, Munn-Chernoff, Patterson, & Duncan, 2015). This increased risk may be due to internalized shame regarding their appearance, especially if there is a discrepancy between their actual and desired appearance. Furthermore, disordered eating behaviors may serve as an attempt by transgender and gender non-conforming individuals to approximate their desired appearance (Diemer et al., 2015).

Although mainstream media representations and data documenting the numbers of transgender or gender non-conforming individuals who currently practice yoga are lacking, participation in yoga may provide a means for these individuals to connect with their body in an authentic, accepting manner (Ballard, 2018). For example, social justice advocate Jacoby Ballard shared, "My practice has allowed me to be all of myself, and to let all of myself be seen, without regret, guilt, or shame." (Ballard, 2018, p. 143). Despite the obvious potential benefits of yoga for the body image of these individuals, there is minimal research on the use of yoga in this population. Unfortunately, this exclusion of transgender and gender non-conforming persons from yoga research also reflects the reality that organized yoga is not always perceived as accommodating or inclusive to them.

As noted by Ballard and Kripalani (2016, p. 300), "If we are truly practicing yoga, whose root means union, united, or unity, then how can we exclude people in this way?" Further research on yoga participation by this population is needed to elucidate the potential benefits and accessibility of practice. Despite the current lack of empirical evidence, anecdotal writings by those within the community can be used to inform yoga instructors and studio owners on how to make the practice more inclusive (e.g., Ballard & Kripalani, 2016; Danis, 2018; Krieger, 2013). For example, the first steps in creating an inclusive space might involve instructing teachers to use gender-neutral language, supplying gender-neutral restrooms, and asking each student for their preferred name and pronouns. When possible, community members and organizations should be viewed as stakeholders in this process and consulted for guidance (Marglin, 2017); in addition, larger-scale organizations such as Trans Folx Fighting Eating Disorders (T-FEED; http://www.transfolxfighteds.org) also offer relevant resources and support. Relatedly, existing organizations such as Decolonizing Yoga (http://decolonizingyoga.com) offer a space to highlight the voices of individuals in marginalized communities and serve as informative resources.

Higher weight

In western culture thinness and lean muscularity are idealized and equated not only with physical attractiveness but are also often used as unsophisticated proxies for health status (Tylka et al., 2014). Therefore, individuals of higher weight [e.g., who possess a body mass index (BMI) of 25 or greater] whose bodies do not conform to these ideals are overtly dehumanized (Kersenberger & Robinson, 2019) and face unrelenting pressure from myriad sources (e.g., media, family, health-care providers, etc.) to engage in weight loss efforts in pursuit of these unrealistic appearance standards (Lee, Gonzalez, Small, Thompson, & Kavushansky, 2019; Tylka et al., 2014). Frequently, these dieting attempts fueled by stigma avoidance set in motion a vicious cycle of restrained eating, short-term unsustainable weight loss, feelings of deprivation, dysregulated eating patterns (e.g., binge eating), and disruptions in neuroendocrine physiology ultimately resulting in weight regain (Aamodt, 2016). What is more, such weight-cycling stemming from chronic "yo-yo dieting" undermines health via cardiometabolic dysregulation and is further associated with increased mortality risk (Rhee, 2017; Tylka et al., 2014). Importantly, research has confirmed that the weight-related oppression experienced by higher-weight individuals and its internalization are directly tied to higher levels of disordered eating and body image disturbance (e.g., Lee et al., 2019).

In efforts to counteract the dominant weight-centric philosophy indelible to modern biomedical and public health disciplines' framing of disease prevention, an alternative approach known as the weight-neutral stance on health promotion has emerged and gained momentum in both popular culture and academic circles (Tylka et al., 2014). One evidence-based manifestation of this contemporary framework is known as Health at Every Size®, which prioritizes the pursuit of living well regardless of one's size over weight loss as core to its mission (Association for Size Diversity and Health; ASDAH, 2013). Notably, this shifting zeitgeist has served as the impetus behind the burgeoning size-inclusive/body-positive yoga movement (Pickett & Cunningham, 2017; Webb et al., 2017a).

Analysis of media representations of who practices yoga as featured on the covers and within the pages of both specialized yoga lifestyle magazines (Vinoski

Thomas et al., 2017; Webb et al., 2017a) and more general mainstream outlets (Bhalla & Moscowitz, 2019) typically reflected the overt exclusion of larger bodies. For instance, only a single issue of *Yoga Journal* featured a cover model with a BMI over 25 during the 40-year span of 1975–2015 (Webb, Vinoski, Warren-Findlow, Burrell, & Putz, 2017b). Similarly, research conducted with both nationally-/regionally representative and convenience samples noted lower BMIs among yoga practitioners relative to non-practitioners (Park et al., 2015). Perceptions that yoga was not a good fit one's body type was reported by 12% of non-practitioners in a recent large-scale national survey as a potential barrier to the practice (Ipsos Public Affairs, 2016). The juxtaposition of conflicting media messages of yoga as both a tool promoting self-acceptance and disciplining fatness further contributes to the marginalization of larger bodies in this context (Strings et al., 2019).

Meanwhile, qualitative accounts further enrich our understanding of the obstacles faced by individuals of higher weight as they persisted in their journeys with the practice towards greater self-acceptance. These challenges included frequent misperceptions of their ability and the perpetual social critique of their bodies (e.g., Bondy, 2014; Dark, 2016; Guest-Jelley, 2014; Veer, 2018). Findings from one interview-based yoga study additionally revealed a stronger vulnerability to engage in self-critical body and physical ability comparisons among their higher-weight undergraduate participants relative to those of lower-weight status (Neumark-Sztainer et al., 2018). Similarly, after holding onto the belief that her body's appearance needed to change in order to gain from yoga, Curvy Yoga founder Anna Guest-Jelley arrived at this transformative realization in her practice: "Wait a minute ... what if the problem isn't my body? What if the problem is just that my teachers don't know how to teach me or other people with bigger bodies?" (Guest-Jelley, 2014, p. 57). Meanwhile, the scarce yoga research that specifically targeted the inclusion of higher-weight individuals has indicated several psychological and behavioral benefits. These preliminary outcomes have included reduced body shame and binge eating alongside gains in a sense of accomplishment regarding physical competence and physical well-being, positive body image, physical activity engagement, the behavioral commitment to exercise amidst experiencing normative discomfort, and the nutritional quality of food choices (McIver, McGartland, & O'Halloran, 2009a; McIver, O'Halloran, & McGartland, 2009b; Neumark-Sztainer et al., 2018; Webb, Padro, Rogers, Vinoski, Etzel, & Putz, 2018a).

In this context, those trailblazers at the forefront of the grassroots size-inclusive yoga movement have strategically infiltrated alternative spaces such as books (e.g., *Mega Yoga;* Garcia, 2006; *Yes! Yoga Has Curves: Volumes 1 and 2;* Smith, 2014, 2016; *Curvy Yoga*: Guest-Jelley, 2017; *Every Body Yoga*: Stanley, 2017; *Fat Yoga*: Harry, 2017), popular social media platforms (e.g., Instagram: Stanley, 2018; Webb et al., 2018b; Webb, Vinoski, Bonar, Davies, & Etzel, 2017c) along with web-based (e.g., Curvy Yoga: www.curvyyoga.com; Body Positive Yoga: www.bodypositiveyoga.com) and smartphone-based applications (e.g., Jessamyn Stanley's The Underbelly: www.theunderbelly.com) to extend their reach and accessibility to a wider audience. This phenomenon has also gained increased visibility and solidarity through the development of community-based organizations such as the Yoga and Body Image Coalition (ybicoalition.com). To overcome a more practical constraint that limited individuals of larger bodies from engaging with the practice, initiatives have been spearheaded to improve the availability of yoga clothing and athleticwear at larger sizes (e.g., Superfit Hero, Gaiam, Old Navy, Manifesta, and Athleta). Nevertheless, the time is ripe for partnering with body-positive yoga professionals making inroads in inspiring individuals of diverse body sizes and shapes to come to the practice (Pickett & Cunningham, 2017). Further, it is critical to expand the limited corpus of yoga scholarship focused on strengthening the experiences of positive embodiment and adaptive eating behavior among higher-weight individuals (McIver et al., 2009a, 2009b; Neumark-Sztainer et al., 2018; Webb et al., 2018a).

Sexual minorities

The prevalence of disordered eating and body image concerns is noteworthy among those of sexual minority status (Diemer et al., 2015). Cultural appearance pressures are significant risk factors to consider for both men and women in sexual minority groups (Huxley, Clarke, & Halliwell, 2014; Smith, Telford, & Tree, 2017). For instance, for gay men, achieving an idealized (but unrealistic) version of "male beauty" may serve as a means to overcome disempowerment due to minority status and increase social capital (Hospers & Jansen, 2005; Siconolfi, Halkitis, Allomong, & Burton, 2009). In a study by Siconolfi et al. (2009), engagement in disordered eating behavior by gay men was significantly predicted by factors such as desire for acceptance by others and concerns about social judgment. Minority stress (e.g., via discrimination) and internalized homophobia by those in sexual minority groups may also contribute to even greater risk for body image disturbance and overall psychological distress as compared to their heterosexual counterparts (Calzo, Blashill, Brown, & Argenal, 2017; Szymanski & Chung, 2003).

Yoga practice may assist individuals of different sexual orientations in coping with environments that are hostile due to their identity (Ballard & Kripalani, 2016). For example, it may serve a grounding function by allowing for vulnerability as well as authenticity in being, which can serve as a welcome contradiction to feeling as if one's identity is inherently offensive. This was the case for Bilger (2014, p. 256), who stated, "Warrior pose ... is about allowing yourself to be vulnerable, fiercely offering your heart to the world, and braving the possibility—the near certainty, even—of rejection, judgment, hostility." Nevertheless, limited available quantitative evidence indicates that more heterosexual than lesbian women participate in yoga (Park et al., 2015) and mainstream media depictions of yoga practitioners who identify as sexual minorities are scarce.

Although the theoretical links among sexual minority status, related stress, and improved body image via yoga are becoming more clear, further research is needed in this area. Existing research has often categorized those that identify with a given sexual orientation as belonging to a homogenous group; moreover, moving forward, research may benefit from utilizing a more intersectional lens. For instance, little is known about the experience of those that identify as both transgender and a sexual minority (Calzo et al., 2017). A greater understanding of perceived inclusivity and accessibility of yoga for these groups is also needed in order to inform future intervention work (see www.decolonizingyoga.com for additional resources and critiques).

Disability

Over one-quarter of US adults have some type of disability (Okoro, Hollis, Cyrus, & Griffin-Blake, 2018). People with disabilities experience significant health disparities; for example, individuals with disabilities are more likely to have cardiovascular disease and mental health symptoms than those without disabilities (Krahn, Klein Walker, & Correa-De-Araujo, 2015). People with disabilities may also experience poorer body image compared with individuals without disabilities (Pfaffenberger et al., 2011). Body image concerns among individuals with disabilities can be linked to both appearance and body functionality and can be related or unrelated to the primary disability (Bailey, Gammage, van Ingen, & Ditor, 2015; Taub, Fanflik, & McLorg, 2003; Vinoski Thomas et al., 2019b). A review of case studies describing eating disorders among individuals with a range of disabilities suggested those with disabilities may experience specific body image concerns that lead to the emergence of eating disorders, and that people with disabilities may engage in disordered eating to cope with or compensate for their disabilities, emphasizing the role *ableism* plays in fostering challenges to embodiment (Cicmil & Eli, 2014).

As such, yoga may be a beneficial practice for people with disabilities who seek to connect with their bodies in a positive manner and cope with the stress of living in a marginalized body. Benefits of yoga for people of all ages with a range of disabilities are documented, empirically and anecdotally. Studies exploring outcomes related to yoga participation among people with multiple sclerosis and spinal cord injury, for example, suggest that participants experienced postintervention improvements in quality of life, self-compassion, depressive symptoms, and various measures of physical and psychological functioning (Cohen et al., 2017; Curtis et al., 2017). Qualitatively, individuals with disabilities have documented how yoga has improved their connection to and awareness and acceptance of their bodies (McGraw, 2014; Wojtowicz, 2018). Emily Wojtowicz, a yoga teacher and practitioner, described how yoga facilitated this process of body and disability acceptance: "I wanted to learn to embrace my disability and the way my body looked and worked … And yoga helps me toward that acceptance, toward that integrated wholehearted perspective of my different physical body" (Wojtowicz, 2018, p. 221).

Despite the documented benefits of yoga practice among people with disabilities, gaps in representation, accessibility, and inclusivity for people with disabilities in yoga spaces still remain (Bondy, 2019; Heyman, 2019). First, the lack of disability representation in yoga media may convey to those with disabilities that they are unwelcome in yoga spaces and deter them from attempting to access the practice. A study analyzing disability representation within the text and images in a prominent yoga magazine found many references to mobility limitations within the text, but no evidence of visual representation of disability (Vinoski Thomas, Warren-Findlow, & Webb, 2019). It may be useful for future research to explore how people with disabilities perceive and react to their representation within yoga media and spaces. It may also be fruitful to explore how and through what outlets yogis with disabilities access information such as how to safely modify asanas or where to access accessible studios and trained teachers.

For people with disabilities who wish to practice, finding accessible and inclusive yoga spaces may be challenging. Most studies exploring outcomes of yoga participation for people with disabilities expose participants to a series of yoga classes designed *specifically for* individuals with disabilities as part of an intervention. Few studies have explored the outcomes of people with disabilities participating in *inclusive* or "mixed-ability" yoga classes (Bevis, Waterworth, & Mudge, 2018). The emergence of several organizations (e.g., AccessibleYoga.org, All Ability Yoga, Accessible Yoga Teacher Training) and self-help books (e.g., Bondy, 2019; Heyman, 2019) are working to increase positive disability representation and provide information and training about accessibility in yoga spaces.

Lastly, clinicians, researchers, and yoga professionals who work on yoga and disability must be cautious that they do not recommend yoga for people with disabilities solely as a means to "cure" or reduce disability, which is in itself ableist. Distinctions between therapeutic yoga and accessible or adaptive yoga should be clarified (Moonaz, 2016). Further, studies exploring the benefits of yoga for people with disabilities should assess psychological benefits (e.g., body appreciation, body compassion, reduced stress, coping with ableism, etc.) in addition to physical and functional changes.

Advancing age

The prevailing stereotype of the typical individual who is impacted by disturbances of eating and body image conjures up images of an adolescent or young adult female (Muhlheim, 2019). Contrary to this popular notion, a growing body of scholarship in western populations has revealed that individuals both men and women as they age are not immune to these experiences of negative embodiment (see Roy & Payette, 2012 for a systematic review). Indeed, approximately 13% of women at midlife and beyond are suffering from an eating disorder (Pietrangelo, 2018) and an increasing number of this demographic are presenting for eating disorder treatment (Hofmeier et al., 2017). Nevertheless, although both the importance of physical appearance and body dissatisfaction tends to persist among aging populations, research suggests this trend also corresponds with an increase in the prioritization of maintaining body functionality (Roy & Payette, 2012). Pursuing this goal is seemingly well-aligned with engaging in the practice of yoga with advancing age.

Unlike other social identities discussed here, it would appear that individuals (particularly women) at midlife (i.e., between 40 and 64 years old) are well-represented among US yoga practitioners comprising 43% of a nationally-derived sample (Park et al., 2015). However, the actual representation was minimal for individuals 65 and older (4%; Park et al., 2015). Despite this pattern, research indicates that middle-aged yoga practitioners are more likely to disclose social anxiety and fear of embarrassment as deterrents to the practice than their older adult peers (Wertman, Wister, & Mitchell, 2016). In line with this observation, Babette a 78-year-old yoga practitioner observed that although she is likely the oldest in her yoga studio and among the participants attending a recent yoga workshop, she has come to accept this disparity (Lipton, 2017). Rather than being preoccupied with comparing herself against the younger bodies present, she focuses on how the practice reinforces self-acceptance amidst reminders of what her own body used to look like in decades past: " … but I am more self-conscious about how I look as an older person when I'm in front of my own mirror at home and I see that my skin isn't the way it was twenty or thirty years ago. But when I'm doing yoga, I don't even think about that." (Lipton, 2017, p. 20).

Similarly, media representations of yoga practitioners are in step with these demographic trends. Whereas traditional images of leaders in the yoga community would prominently feature the frequently venerated male yogi swami or sage, contemporary images typically portray the yoga practitioner as female perceived to be on average in her 20s or 30s (Webb et al., 2017a). Such exclusionary practices by mainstream yoga media outlets have also been lamented by pioneering yoga teacher Cyndi Lee who entered the practice in the 1970s along with other major influencers: "We don't want to be told we should aspire to be like someone who is younger than we are … .I was consulted on who would be a good yoga model for my sequences, because evidently, at the age of 44+, I was too old to be photographed demonstrating yoga poses." (Lee, 2018, p. 247). As a form of empowered resistance, Lee and others like Lotta Sebzda and organizations such as DoYogaWithMe (https://www.doyogawithme.com/con tent/yoga-seniors) have taken to social media and other web-based platforms to provide alternative images (e.g., #selfie@sixty; Lee, 2018) and modified practices that celebrate the aging body and promote the practice of yoga for all bodies regardless of age or physical limitations (Majsiak, 2019). Meanwhile, authors have alerted those in the yoga community to the potential dangers of mixed messages conveyed in the articles of mainstream yoga media which juxtapose notions of "feeling younger" with "looking younger" as benefits of the practice (Strings et al., 2019).

The motivation to bolster the mobility and functionality of the normative aging body or one that is afflicted by a chronic illness are viewed as key determinants of why appreciable numbers of middle-aged individuals prac-tice yoga (Park et al., 2015). Yet given the notable underrepresentation of more senior yoga practitioners, recent scholarship has specifically targeted the inclusion of older adults within research demonstrating the benefits of the practice for improving both psychological (e.g., well-being, vitality, mood, sleep disturbances, self-efficacy; Bonura & Tenenbaum, 2014; Siddarth, Siddarth, & Lavretsky, 2014) and physiological (e.g., balance, endurance, flexibility, strength: Miller, Der Ananian, Hensley, & Ungar, 2017) health. Nonetheless, the exclusive focus on strengthening aspects of physical competence renders the potential gains in other dimensions of body image (e.g., acceptance of aging-related physical appearance changes) and positive embodiment (e.g., eating behavior) as a result of yoga practice highly underdeveloped in the aging population.

For instance, future research would benefit from investigating whether yoga practice with its emphasis on promoting greater body functionality is a protective factor against self-objectification, negative body image, and disordered eating among men and women at midlife and beyond. Doing so would more directly challenge assumptions that older yoga practitioners are unaffected by body image disturbances and disordered eating and would increase access to these critical conversations among yoga practitioners of advancing age. Pursuing this line of inquiry would further provide the unique opportunity to assess the degree to which effects are moderated by midlife versus more senior age status. This analysis would be particularly timely in light of recent evidence indicating that middle-aged adults are reportedly twice as likely as their older adult counterparts to identify weight loss as a motivation for engaging in the practice (Wertman et al., 2016).

Looking ahead: future directions in expanding inclusive embodiment in yoga in the west

As yoga has gained popularity in western culture for its wide-ranging health benefits, it has garnered particular appeal in strengthening positive embodiment and reducing risk for disordered eating (Domingues & Carmo, 2019; Neumark-Sztainer, 2019). Nevertheless, as this article underscored there are large segments of society possessing marginalized social identities who are underrepresented both among current yoga practitioners and among participants in contemporary yoga scholarship. Consequently, these individuals are inadvertently excluded from reaping the likely benefits to embodiment and well-being attributed to the practice. This phenomenon is especially concerning given that members of stigmatized groups are also vulnerable to body image disturbance and dysregulated eating behavior perhaps to a larger extent than previously assumed.

In closing, we offer three broad areas for consideration to further advance efforts to expand inclusive embodiment within yoga practice and scholarship:

Awareness, advocacy, and education

Across the multiple stakeholders who have a vested interest in promoting yoga and positive embodiment for all bodies, it will be critical to capitalize on the numerous outlets available to increase awareness of the benefits of the practice to as broad an audience as possible. Ways of enhancing the reach of the message include the expanding social media and online presence, books, and anthologies (e.g., *Yoga and Body Image*: Klein & Guest-Jelley, 2014; *Yoga Rising*: Klein, 2018; *Yoga Bodies*: Lipton, 2017) and other formats (e.g., smartphone applications) that increase exposure to greater diversification in our visual diet featuring more realistic portrayals of who practices and teaches yoga. Notably, *Yoga Journal* considered the leader in westernized mainstream yoga lifestyle media who came under fire for its role in perpetuating constrained representations of the "yoga body" recently renewed its commitment to use its status and platform to promote greater inclusion and accessibility and to earnestly approach dialoguing about complex and sensitive topics within the yoga community (e.g., controversial claims surrounding the Eurocentric cultural appropriation of the practice; Eichenseher, 2018, 2019a, 2019b).

Yoga professionals are encouraged to conduct a comprehensive self-assessment of their possible attitudes, biases, and practices that may undermine cultivating spaces of greater inclusion, accessibility, and positive embodiment for themselves and practitioners from marginalized groups (Cook-Cottone & Douglass, 2017). Yoga instructors are invited to seek additional training (e.g., www.yogaforalltraining.com; https://diannebondyyoga.com/diversity-training-for-yoga-teachers/) on how to attract and retain members of diverse groups within the studio environment (Cook-Cottone & Douglass, 2017). Similarly, organizations like Eat, Breathe, Thrive are part of an emerging movement to aid in strengthening yoga professionals' competency in integrating yoga, body image, and eating behavior within their instructional priorities and skill set (www.eatbreathethrive.org). Offering free or donation-based classes in community settings (e.g., libraries, public outdoor spaces, churches, low cost/free medical clinics, prisons, schools in low-income communities, minority-serving college campuses, senior centers and assisted living communities, etc.) are additional mechanisms for increasing awareness and educating the public about yoga. Providing reduced cost or scholarships for attending yoga teacher trainings and earning certifications along with instituting mentoring circles may help stimulate the recruitment and growth of yoga professionals from diverse backgrounds. Likewise, scientists and clinicians specializing in the interface between yoga and embodiment may opt to creatively disseminate and increase the visibility of relevant research findings also through a variety of in-person community venues (e.g., free lectures/presentations) as well as online environments (e.g., podcast interviews, blogs, publicly available academic research repositories like ResearchGate).

Meanwhile, the focus of this paper was on featuring the experiences and evidence-base targeting select marginalized social identities. Therefore, our efforts were not exhaustive nor did we offer insights on reconciling the challenges individuals reflecting intersecting identities face in the contexts of positive embodiment, disordered eating, and yoga practice. Thus, it is critical for future endeavors to more intentionally prioritize increasing awareness of the impact of intersectionality and to consider other identity or developmental factors that could negatively affect the experience of embodiment (e.g., body image and eating behavior) and for whom yoga may be a viable, complementary treatment approach (e.g., military veterans, women during pregnancy and the postpartum, individuals living with autoimmune conditions like rheumatoid arthritis, inflammatory bowel disease, etc. that are not only debilitating but also may carry social stigma).

Theoretical application and development

Several key theoretical frameworks have been offered to help define and explain what constitutes the multifaceted experience of embodiment. These include the Developmental Theory of Embodiment (DTE; Piran, 2017), the Attunement Model of Wellness and Embodied Self-Regulation (AMWESR; Cook-Cottone, 2015), the Embodiment Model of Positive Body Image (EMPBI; Menzel & Levine, 2011), and the Acceptance Model of Intuitive Eating (AMIE; Avalos & Tylka, 2006). Whereas the DTE and AMWESR specifically incorporate an understanding of how being embedded within the broader social context dynamically shapes the individual's experiences of embodiment, the EMPBI and AMIE tend to derive aspects of the construct as being primarily driven by more proximal inter- and intrapersonal core processes.

In keeping with the emphasis of this article, these existing theories could benefit from both greater application in the context of yoga and inclusive embodiment along with expansion to include target variables that describe perceptions of inclusion and acceptance within the context of practicing yoga. For instance, the DTE could be implemented as a useful framework among yoga practitioners of diverse social locations to reveal how their experiences of the embodiment are either manifested or undermined across the domains of mental freedom, social power, and physical freedom within the yoga community and beyond (Piran, 2017). Additionally, the AMIE highlights how the perceptions of how one's body is accepted by others are important in predicting other dimensions of positive body image and intuitive eating (Avalos & Tylka, 2006). It is advisable to consider how perceived body acceptance by others or conversely experiences of body shaming, for example, in the yoga studio could be operative within this original model as well as incorporated in other models of embodiment like the EMPBI (Menzel & Levine, 2011) studied in diverse samples. Indeed, informed by the EMPBI (Menzel & Levine, 2011) perhaps greater perceptions that others in a yoga practice setting accept one's body and hold a broad conceptualization of beauty (Tylka & Iannantuono, 2016) could be protective factors against self-objectification and support greater body appreciation among diverse yoga practitioners. Finally, it would be of interest to adapt the AMWESR (Cook-Cottone, 2015) to the specific context of negotiating the experience of marginalized social identities while practicing yoga to determine how attunement and mindful self-care may be disrupted at the hands of perceptions of body exclusion.

A social action research agenda

In all, the interdisciplinary focus of the intersection between the yoga practice community and embodiment research appears to be an optimal fit for implementing a community-based participatory research (CBPR) framework. Enacting this model would guide and facilitate the formation of greater partnerships that focus on conducting need assessments for all stakeholders involved (e.g., yoga professionals, members of disadvantaged groups, etc.) that empowers the inclusion of all voices. In doing so, these efforts would complement and extend traditional efficacy designs in this context through using mixed method protocols to bolster the feasibility, acceptability, and effectiveness of yoga-based embodiment interventions in sustainable, real-world community-based settings for members of marginalized groups. Such collaborations would require not only the social justice motivations of yoga professionals and embodiment scholars but also the incentivization and financial support of funding agencies at the local, state, regional, and national levels. Ultimately this line of social action research could influence health policy which in turn could result in a broader impact for the burgeoning inclusive embodiment movement in yoga.

Conclusions

Although notable progress has transpired much remains to be done to ensure that the empirically supported benefits of yoga for embodiment and health are available to traditionally underrepresented groups and that these individuals are more frequently included in the future, the evolving evidence base of yoga and embodiment scholarship. It is intended for this material to inspire reconnecting with earlier leaders' visions of a yoga for all, breaking down divisive barriers, and harnessing its potential to be a powerful vehicle for personal and social transformation for the masses. Nonetheless, in order for this shifting zeitgeist of augmenting diversity and inclusion in yoga embodiment to take root and flourish, it will necessitate prioritizing public health initiatives that are operating simultaneously at multiple levels/systems of the social ecology (i.e., individual, family, community, organizational/institutional, etc.). This cultural transformation will also require establishing greater interdisciplinary partnerships and engaging more socially empowered models of research to advance this social justice-based public health agenda at the crossroads of yoga, inclusion, and positive embodiment.

ORCID

Erin Vinoski Thomas ⓘ http://orcid.org/0000-0002-7154-8562

References

Aamodt, S. (2016). *Why diets make us fat: The unintended consequences of our obsession with weight loss.* New York, NY: Current.

Association for Size Diversity and Health (2013). *HAES® principles.* Retrieved from https://www.sizediversityandhealth.org/content.asp?id=76

Avalos, L. C., & Tylka, T. L. (2006). Exploring a model of intuitive eating with college women. *Journal of Counseling Psychology, 53,* 486–497. doi:10.1037/0022-0167.53.4.486

Bailey, K. A., Gammage, K. L., van Ingen, C., & Ditor, D. S. (2015). "It's all about acceptance": A qualitative study exploring a model of positive body image for people with spinal cord injury. *Body Image, 15,* 24–34. doi:10.1016/j.bodyim.2015.04.010

Ballard, J., & Kripalani, K. (2016). Queering yoga: An ethic of social justice. In B. Berila, M. Klein, & C. J. Roberts (Eds.), *Yoga, the body, and embodied social change: An intersectional feminist analysis* (pp. 293–319). Lanham, MD: Lexington Books.

Ballard, J. (2018). Learning to love the whole. In M. Klein (Ed.), *Yoga rising: 30 empowering stories from yoga renegades for every body* (pp. 137–144). Woodbury, MN: Llewellyn Publications.

Baskauskas, V. (2014). Work in progress. In M. Klein & A. Guest-Jelly (Eds.), *Yoga and body Image: 25 personal stories about beauty, bravery & loving your body* (pp. 63–71). Woodbury, MN: Llewellyn Publications.

Becker, C. B., Middlemass, K., Taylor, B., Johnson, C., & Gomez, F. (2017). Food insecurity and eating disorder pathology. *International Journal of Eating Disorders, 50,* 1031–1040. doi:10.1002/eat.22735

Berila, B., Klein, M., & Jackson Roberts, C. (2016). *Yoga, the body, and embodied social change: An intersectional feminist analysis.* Lanham, MD: Lexington Books.

Bertisch, S., Zhou, E. S., Qiu, X., Spadola, C., Rottapel, R., Guo, N., & Redline, S. (2019). Adapted behavioral sleep and yoga interventions for adults in low-income and racial/ethnic minority communities. *Sleep, 42*, A158. doi:10.1093/sleep/zsz067.389

Bevis, A., Waterworth, K., & Mudge, S. (2018). Participants' experiences of a mixed-ability yoga series. *New Zealand Journal of Physiotherapy, 46*, 29–35. doi:10.15619/NZJP/46.1.03

Bhalla, N., & Moscowitz, D. (2019). Yoga and female objectification: Commodity and exclusionary identity in U.S. women's magazines. *Journal of Communication Inquiry*, 1–19. doi:10.1177/0196859919830357

Bilger, A. (2014). Virabhadrasana in the academy: Coming out with an open heart. In M. Klein & A. Guest-Jelly (Eds.), *Yoga and body image: 25 personal stories about beauty, bravery & loving your body* (pp. 249–257). Woodbury, MN: Llewellyn Publications.

Blaine, D. Y. (2016). Mainstream representations of yoga: Capitalism, consumerism, and control of the female body. In B. Berila, M. Klein, & C. J. Roberts (Eds.), *Yoga, the body, and embodied social change: An intersectional feminist analysis* (pp. 129–140). Lanham, MD: Lexington Books.

Boccio, F. J. (2012). Questioning the "body beautiful": Yoga, commercialism, and discernment. In C. Horton & R. Harvey (Eds.), *21st century yoga: Culture, politics & practice* (pp. 45–56). Chicago, IL: Kleio Books.

Bondy, D. (2014). Confessions of a fat, black yoga teacher. In M. Klein & A. Guest-Jelly (Eds.), Yoga and body image: 25 personal stories about beauty, bravery & loving your body (pp. 73–81). Woodbury, MN: Llewellyn Publications.

Bondy, D. (2019). *Yoga for everyone: 50 poses for every type of body.* Indianapolis: Penguin Random House, LLC.

Bonura, K. B., & Tenenbaum, G. (2014). Effects of yoga on psychological health in older adults. *Journal of Physical Activity and Health, 11*, 1334–1341. doi:10.1123/jpah.2012-0365

Burnett-Zeigler, I., Schuette, S., Victorson, D., & Wisner, K. L. (2016). Mind-body approaches to treating mental health symptoms among disadvantaged populations: A comprehensive review. *The Journal of Alternative and Complementary Medicine, 22*, 115–124. doi:10.1089/acm.2015.0038

Calzo, J. P., Blashill, A. J., Brown, T. A., & Argenal, R. L. (2017). Eating disorders and disordered weight and shape control behaviors in sexual minority populations. *Current Psychiatry Reports, 19*, 49. doi:10.1007/s11920-017-0801-y

Cicmil, N., & Eli, K. (2014). Body image among eating disorder patients with disabilities: A review of published case studies. *Body Image, 11*, 266–274. doi:10.1016/j.bodyim.2014.04.001

Clarke, T. C., Black, L. I., Stussman, B. J., Barnes, P. M., & Nahin, R. L. (2015). Trends in the use of complementary health approaches among adults: United States, 2002–2012. *National Health Statistics Reports, 79*, 1–16.

Claudat, K., White, E. K., & Warren, C. S. (2016). Acculturative stress, self-esteem, and eating pathology in Latina and Asian American female college students. *Journal of Clinical Psychology, 72*, 88–100. doi:10.1002/jclp.22234

Cohen, E. T., Kietrys, D., Fogerite, S. G., Silva, M., Logan, K., Barone, D. A., & Parrott, J. S. (2017). Feasibility and impact of an 8-week integrative yoga program in people with moderate multiple sclerosis-related disability: A pilot study. *International Journal of MS Care, 19*, 30-9. doi:10.7224/1537-2073.2015-046

Cook-Cottone, C. (2015). *Mindfulness and yoga for self-regulation: A primer for mental health professionals.* New York, NY: Springer Publishing Company, LLC.

Cook-Cottone, C., & Douglass, L. L. (2017). Yoga communities and eating disorders: Creating safe spaces for positive embodiment. *International Journal of Yoga Therapy, 27*, 87–93. doi:10.17761/1531-2054-27.1.87

Cotter, E. W., Kelly, N. R., Mitchell, K. S., & Mazzeo, S. E. (2015). An investigation of body appreciation, ethnic identity, and eating disorder symptoms in Black women. *Journal of Black Psychology, 41*, 3–25. doi:10.1177/0095798413502671

Cramer, H., Sibbritt, D., Park, C. L., Adams, J., & Lauche, R. (2017). Is the practice of yoga or meditation associated with a healthy lifestyle?: Results of a national cross-sectional survey of 28,695 Australian women. *Journal of Psychosomatic Research, 101*, 104–109. doi:10.1016/j.jpsychores.2017.07.013

Curtis, K., Hitzig, S. L., Bechsgaard, G., Stoliker, C., Alton, C., Saunders, N., … Katz, J. (2017). Evaluation of a specialized yoga program for persons with a spinal cord injury: A pilot randomized controlled trial. *Journal of Pain Research, 10*, 999-1017. doi:10.2147/JPR.S130530

Danis, L. (2018). *How LGBTQ yoga can heal a community.* Retrieved from https://theestablishment.co/how-lgbtq-yoga-can-heal-a-community/

Dark, K. (2016). Fat pedagogy in the yoga class. In B. Berila, M. Klein, & C. J. Roberts (Eds.), *Yoga, the body, and embodied social change: An intersectional feminist analysis* (pp. 193–204). Lanham, MD: Lexington Books.

Diemer, E. W., Grant, J. D., Munn-Chernoff, M. A., Patterson, D. A., & Duncan, A. E. (2015). Gender identity, sexual orientation, and eating-related pathology in a national sample of college students. *Journal of Adolescent Health, 57*, 144–149. doi:10.1016/j.jadohealth.2015.03.003

Domingues, R. B., & Carmo, C. (2019). Disordered eating behaviours and correlates in yoga practitioners: A systematic review. *Eating and Weight Disorders-Studies on Anorexia, Bulimia and Obesity, 24*, 1015–1024. Advance online publication. doi:10.1007/s40519-019-00692-x

Eichenseher, T. (2018, November 12). Editor's letter: Selfless service. *Yoga Journal.*

Eichenseher, T. (2019a, February 8). Editor's letter: Begin again. *Yoga Journal.*

Eichenseher, T. (2019b, May–June 8). Editor's letter: Places you'll go. *Yoga Journal.*

Falsafi, N, & Leopard, L. (2015). Pilot study: use of mindfulness, self-compassion, and yoga practices with low-income and/or uninsured patients with depression and/or anxiety. *Journal Of Holistic Nursing, 33* (4), 289-297. doi: 10.1177/0898010115569351

Flaherty, M. (2014). Influence of yoga on body image satisfaction in men. *Perceptual and Motor Skills, 119*, 203–214. doi:10.2466/27.50.PMS.119c17z1

Frederick, D. A., Buchanan, G. M., Sadeghi-Azar, L., Peplau, L. A., Haselton, M. G., Berezovskaya, A., & Lipinski, R. E. (2007). Desiring the muscular ideal: Men's body satisfaction in the United States, Ukraine, and Ghana. *Psychology of Men & Masculinity, 8*, 103–117. doi:10.1037/1524-9220.8.2.103

Freeman, H., Vladagina, N., Razmjou, E., & Brems, C. (2017). Yoga in print media: Missing the heart of the practice. *International Journal of Yoga, 10*, 160–166. doi:10.4103/ijoy.IJOY_1_17

Garcia, M. (2006). *Mega yoga: The first yoga program for curvy women.* New York, NY: DK Publishing.

Guest-Jelley, A. (2014). Maybe the problem isn't my body. In M. Klein & A. Guest-Jelly (Eds.), *Yoga and body image: 25 personal stories about beauty, bravery & loving your body* (pp. 51–59). Woodbury, MN: Llewellyn Publications.

Guest-Jelley, A. (2017). *Curvy yoga: Love yourself & your body a little more each day.* New York, NY: Sterling Publishing Co., Inc.

Haddix, M. M. (2016). In a field the color purple: Inviting yoga spaces for black women's bodies. In B. Berila, M. Klein, & C. J. Roberts (Eds.), *Yoga, the body, and embodied social change: An intersectional feminist analysis* (pp. 17–28). Lanham, MD: Lexington Books.

Harry, S. (2017). *Fat yoga: Yoga for all bodies.* Chatswood, Australia: New Holland Publishers.

Heyman, J. (2019). *Accessible yoga: Poses and practices for every body.* Boulder, CO: Shambala Publications.

Hofmeier, S. M., Runfola, C. D., Sala, M., Gagne, D. A., Brownley, K. A., & Bulik, C. A. (2017). Body image, aging, and identity in women over 50: The gender and body image (GABI) study. *Journal of Women & Aging, 29*, 3–14. doi:10.1080/08952841.2015.1065140

Hospers, H. J., & Jansen, A. (2005). Why homosexuality is a risk factor for eating disorders in males. *Journal of Social and Clinical Psychology, 24*(8), 1188–1201. doi:10.1521/jscp.2005.24.8.1188

Huxley, C. J., Clarke, V., & Halliwell, E. (2014). A qualitative exploration of whether lesbian and bisexual women are 'protected' from sociocultural pressure to be thin. *Journal of Health Psychology, 19*, 273–284. doi:10.1177/135910531246849

Ipsos Public Affairs. (2016). *The 2016 yoga in America study.* Retrieved from https://www.yogaalliance.org/Portals/0/2016 Yoga in America Study RESULTS.pdf

Kauer, K. (2016). Yoga culture and neoliberal embodiment of health. In B. Berila, M. Klein, & C. J. Roberts (Eds.), *Yoga, the body, and embodied social change: An intersectional feminist analysis* (pp. 91–108). Lanham, MD: Lexington Books.

Kersenberger, I., & Robinson, E. (2019). Blatant dehumanization of people with obesity. *Obesity,* 1–8. doi:10.1002/oby.22460

Kest, B. (2014). Like father, like son. In M. Klein & A. Guest-Jelly (Eds.), *Yoga and body Image: 25 personal stories about beauty, bravery & loving your body* (pp. 231–239). Woodbury, MN: Llewellyn Publications.

Klein, M., & Guest-Jelley, A. (2014). *Yoga and body image: 25 personal stories about beauty, bravery & loving your body.* Woodbury, MN: Llewellyn Publications.

Klein, M. C. (2018). *Yoga rising: 30 empowering stories from yoga renegades for every body.* Woodbury, MN: Llewellyn Publications.

Krahn, G. L., Klein Walker, D., & Correa-De-Araujo, R. (2015). Persons with disabilities as an unrecognized health disparity population. *American Journal of Public Health, 105*, S198–S206. doi:10.2105/ajph.2014.302182

Krieger, N. (2013). *How radical is this practice?* Retrieved from http://www.decolonizingyoga.com/how-radical-is-this-practice/

Lacasse, J., Santarossa, S., & Woodruff, S. (2019). Yoga on Instagram: Understanding the nature of yoga in the online conversation and community. *International Journal of Yoga, 12*, 153–157. doi:10.4103/ijoy.IJOY_50_18

Lee, C. (2018). #Selfie@Sixty. In M. C. Klein (Ed.), *Yoga rising: 30 empowering stories from yoga renegades for every body* (pp. 241–254). Woodbury, MN: Llewellyn Publications.

Lee, M. S., Gonzalez, B. D., Small, B. J., Thompson, J. K., & Kavushansky, A. (2019). Internalized weight bias and psychological well-being: An exploratory investigation of a preliminary model. *PLoS ONE, 14*, e0216324. doi:10.1371/journal.pone.0216324

Lee, R. (2000). Health care problems of lesbian, gay, bisexual, and transgender patients. *Western Journal of Medicine, 17*, 403–408. doi:10.1136/ewjm.172.6.403

Lipton, L. (2017). *Yoga bodies: Real people, real stories & the power of transformation.* San Francisco, CA: Chronicle Books LLC.

Majsiak, B. (2019). *10 motivating yogis to follow on Instagram.* Retrieved from https://www.everydayhealth.com/fitness/motivating-yogis-follow-on-instagram/

Marglin, E. (2017). *Jacoby Ballard creates safe spaces for trans community.* Retrieved from https://www.yogajournal.com/lifestyle/good-karma-jacoby-ballard-creating-safe-spaces-transgender-community

Markula, P. (2014). Reading yoga: Changing discourses of postural yoga on the *Yoga Journal* covers. *Communication & Sport, 2*, 143.171. doi:10.1177/2167479513490673

McGraw, R. (2014). Doing more by doing less. In M. C. Klein & A. Guest-Jelley (Eds.), *Yoga and body image: 25 personal stories about beauty, bravery & loving your body* (pp. 241–248). Woodbury, MN: Llewellyn Publications.

McIver, S., McGartland, M., & O'Halloran, P. (2009a). "Overeating is not about the food": Women describe their experience of a yoga treatment program for binge eating. *Qualitative Health Research, 19*, 1234–1245. doi:10.1177/1049732309343954

McIver, S., O'Halloran, P., & McGartland, M. (2009b). Yoga as a treatment for binge eating disorder: A preliminary study. *Complementary Therapies in Medicine, 17*, 196–202. doi:10.1016/j.ctim.2009.05.002

Menzel, J. E., & Levine, M. P. (2011). Embodying experiences and the promotion of positive body image: The example of competitive athletics. In R. M. Calogero, S. Tantleff-Dunn, & J. K. Thompson (Eds.), *Self-objectification in women: Causes, consequences, and counteractions* (pp. 163–186). Washington, DC: American Psychological Association.

Middleton, K. R., Marana Lopez, M., Haaz Moonaz, S., Tataw-Ayuketah, G., Ward, M. M., & Wallen, G. R. (2017). A qualitative approach exploring the acceptability of yoga for minorities living with arthritis. 'Where are the people who look like me?'. *Complementary Therapies in Medicine, 31*, 82–89. doi:10.1016/j.ctim.2017.02.006

Miller, A. I., Der Ananian, C., Hensley, C., & Ungar, H. (2017). Evaluation of rewind yoga on physical function outcomes in older adults: A preliminary study. *Activities, Adaptation, & Aging, 41*, 291–300. doi:10.1080/01924788.2017.1326765

Moadel, A.B, Shah, C, Wylie-Rosett, J, Harris, M.S, Patel, S.R, Hall, C.B, & Sparano, J.A. (2007). Randomized controlled trial of yoga among a multiethnic sample of breast cancer patients: effects on quality of life. *Journal Of Clinical Oncology, 25* (28), 4387. 28 doi:10.1200/JCO.2006.06.6027

Moonaz, S. (2016). Yoga and dis/ability. In B. Berila, M. C. Klein, & C. J. Roberts (Eds.), *Yoga, the body, and embodied social change: An intersectional feminist analysis* (pp. 243–255). Lanham, MD: Lexington Books.

Muhlheim, L. (2019). *Midlife eating disorders: People of all ages are affected.* Retrieved from https://www.verywellmind.com/midlife-eating-disorders-4177137

Mulders-Jones, B., Mitchison, D., Girosi, F., & Hay, P. (2017). Socioeconomic correlates of eating disorder symptoms in an Australian population-based sample. *PLos ONE, 12*, e0170603. doi:10.1371/journal.pone.0170603

Musial, J. (2016). "Work off that holiday meal ladies!": Body vigilance and orthorexia in yoga spaces. In B. Berila, M. Klein, & C. J. Roberts (Eds.), *Yoga, the body, and embodied social change: An intersectional feminist analysis* (pp. 141–154). Lanham, MD: Lexington Books.

Neumark-Sztainer, D. (2019). The practice of yoga: Can it help in addressing body image concerns and eating disorders? In T. L. Tylka & N. Piran (Eds.), *Handbook of positive body image and embodiment: Constructs, protective factors, and interventions* (pp. 325–335). New York, NY: Oxford University Press.

Neumark-Sztainer, D., Watts, A. W., & Rydell, S. (2018). Yoga and body image: How do young adults practicing yoga describe its impact on their body image? *Body Image, 27*, 156–168. doi:10.1016/j.bodyim.2018.09.001

Okoro, C. A., Hollis, N. D., Cyrus, A. C., & Griffin-Blake, S. (2018). Prevalence of disabilities and health care access by disability status and type among adults – United States, 2016. *Morbidity and Mortality Weekly Report, 67*, 882–887. doi:10.15585/mmwr.mm6732a2

Olsen, H. B. (2017). *Yes, poor people have eating disorders, too.* Retrieved from https://everydayfeminism.com/2017/02/poor-people-eating-disorders/

Page, E. H. (2016). The gender, race, and class barriers: Enclosing yoga as a White public space. In B. Berila, M. Klein, & C. J. Roberts (Eds.), *Yoga, the body, and embodied social change: An intersectional feminist analysis* (pp. 41–65). Lanham, MD: Lexington Books.

Park, C. L., Braun, T., & Siegel, T. (2015). Who practices yoga? A systematic review of demographic, health-related, and psychosocial factors associated with yoga practice. *Journal of Behavioral Medicine, 38*, 460–471. doi:10.1007/s10865-015-9618-5

Pfaffenberger, N., Gutweniger, S., Kopp, M., Seeber, B., Sturz, K., Berger, T., & Gunther, V. (2011). Impaired body image in patients with multiple sclerosis. *Acta Neurologica Scandinavia, 124*, 165–170. doi:10.1111/j.1600-0404.2010.01460.x

Pickett, A. C., & Cunningham, G. B. (2017). Creating inclusive physical activity spaces: The case of body-positive yoga. *Research Quarterly for Exercise and Sport, 88*, 329–338. doi:10.1080/02701367.2017.1335851

Pierce, B., Bowden, B., McCullagh, M., Diehl, A., Chissell, Z., Rodriguez, R., … D'Adamo, C. R. (2017). A summer health program for African American high school students in Baltimore, Maryland: Community partnership for integrative health. *EXPLORE, 13*, 186–197. doi:10.1016/j.explore.2017.02.002

Pietrangelo, A. (2018). *Eating disorders plaguing older women*. Retrieved from https://www.healthline.com/health-news/eating-disorders-plaguing-older-women#6

Piran, N. (2017). *Journeys of embodiment at the intersection of body and culture: The developmental theory of embodiment*. Oxford, UK: Academic Press.

Rasmusson, G., Lydecker, J. A., Coffino, J. A., White, M. A., & Grilo, C. M. (2018). Household food insecurity is associated with binge-eating disorder and obesity. *International Journal of Eating Disorders, 52*, 28–35. doi:10.1002/eat.22990

Remski, M. (2012). Modern yoga will not form a real culture until every studio can also double as a soup kitchen and other observations from the threshold between yoga and activism. In C. Horton & R. Harvey (Eds.), *21st century yoga: Culture, politics & practice* (pp. 109–131). Chicago, IL: Kleio Books.

Rhee, E. (2017). Weight cycling and its cardiometabolic impact. *Journal of Obesity & Metabolic Syndrome, 26*, 237–242. doi:10.7570/jomes.2017.26.4.237

Rodgers, R. F., Berry, R., & Franko, D. L. (2018). Eating disorders in ethnic minorities: An update. *Current Psychiatry Reports, 20*, 90. doi:10.1007/s11920-018-0938-3

Rogers, L., Resnick, M. D., Mitchell, J. E., & Blum, R. W. (1997). The relationship between socio-economic status and eating-disordered behaviors in a community sample of adolescent girls. *International Journal of Eating Disorders, 22*, 15–23. doi:10.1002/(ISSN)1098-108X

Rosenfeld, J. (2016). *Yoga, but affordable: Some nonprofits insist that the practice can benefit everyone, not just those who have the money for classes and a mat*. Retrieved from https://www.theatlantic.com/business/archive/2016/01/yoga-expensive-affordable/423549/

Roy, M., & Payette, H. (2012). The body image construct among western seniors: A systematic review of the literature. *Archives of Gerontology and Geriatrics, 55*, 505–521. doi:10.1016/j.archger.2012.04.007

Schware, R. (2016). *Yoga for those living with poverty & trauma*. Retrieved from https://www.huffpost.com/entry/yoga-for-those-living-with-poverty-trauma_b_57f3e29ce4b03d61445c741b

Siconolfi, D., Halkitis, P. N., Allomong, T. W., & Burton, C. L. (2009). Body dissatisfaction and eating disorders in a sample of gay and bisexual men. *International Journal of Men's Health, 8*, 254–264. doi:10.3149/jmh.0803.254

Siddarth, D., Siddarth, P., & Lavretsky, H. (2014). An observational study of the health benefits of yoga or tai chi compared to aerobic exercise in community-dwelling middle-aged and older adults. *American Journal of Geriatric Psychiatry, 22*, 272–273. doi:10.1016/j.agp.2013.01.065

Smith, D. A. (2014). *Yes! Yoga has curves volume 1*. Upper Marlboro, MD: Spiritual Essence Yoga.

Smith, D. A. (2016). *Yes! Yoga has curves volume 2*. Upper Marlboro, MD: Spiritual Essence Yoga.

Smith, D. A. (2018). Never the perfect body. In M. C. Klein (Ed.), *Yoga rising: 30 empowering stories from yoga renegades for every body* (pp. 193–200). Woodbury, MN: Llewellyn Publications.

Smith, M. L., Telford, E., & Tree, J. J. (2017). Body image and sexual orientation: The experiences of lesbian and bisexual women. *Journal of Health Psychology*, 1–3. doi:10.1177/1359105317769448

Smith, S, & Atencio, M. (2017). "yoga is yoga. yoga is everywhere. you either practice or you don't": a qualitative examination of yoga social dynamics. *Journal Of Sport in Society: Cultures, Commerce, Media, Politics, 20* (9), 1167-1184. doi:10.1080/17430437.2016.1269082

Spadola, C. E., Rottapel, R., Khandpur, N., Kontos, E., Bertisch, S. M., Johnson, D. A., & Redline, S. (2018). Enhancing yoga participation: A qualitative investigation of barriers and facilitators to yoga among predominantly racial/ethnic minority, low-income adults. *Complementary Therapies in Clinical Practice, 29*, 97–104. doi:10.1016/j.ctcp.2017.09.001

Stanley, J. (2017). *Every body yoga: Let go of fear, get on the mat, love your body.* New York, NY: Workman Publishing Co., Inc.

Stanley, J. (2018). Instagram, yoga, and learning to love my big, black body. In M. C. Klein (Ed.), *Yoga rising: 30 empowering stories from yoga renegades for every body* (pp. 145–152). Woodbury, MN: Llewellyn Publications.

Strings, S., Headen, I., & Spencer, B. (2019). Yoga as a technology of femininity: Disciplining white women, disappearing people of color in *yoga journal. Fat Studies, 8*, 334–348. Advance online publication. doi:10.1080/21604851.2019.1583527

Szymanski, D. M., & Chung, Y. B. (2003). Internalized homophobia in lesbians. *Journal of Lesbian Studies, 7*, 115–125. doi:10.1300/J155v07n01_08

Taub, D. E., Fanflik, P. L., & McLorg, P. A. (2003). Body image among women with physical disabilities: Internalization of norms and reactions to nonconformity. *Sociological Focus, 36* (2), 159–176. doi:10.1080/00380237.2003.10570722

Tenfelde, S. M., Hatchett, L., & Saban, K. L. (2018). "Maybe black girls do yoga": A focus group study with predominantly low-income African American women. *Complementary Therapies in Medicine, 40*, 230–235. doi:10.1016/j.ctim.2017.11.017

Thompson, N. (2012). Bifurcated spiritualities: Examining mind/body splits in the North American yoga and Zen communities. In C. Horton & R. Harvey (Eds.), *21st century yoga: Culture, politics & practice* (pp. 57–72). Chicago, IL: Kleio Books.

Tylka, T. L., Annunziato, R. A., Burgard, D., Daníelsdóttir, S., Shuman, E., Davis, C., & Calogero, R. M. (2014). The weight-inclusive versus weight-normative approach to health: Evaluating the evidence for prioritizing well-being over weight loss. *Journal of Obesity, 82*, 8–15. doi:10.1155/2014/983495

Tylka, T. L., & Iannantuono, A. C. (2016). Perceiving beauty in all women: Psychometric evaluation of the Broad Conceptualization of Beauty Scale. *Body Image, 17*, 67–81. doi:10.1016/j.bodyim.2016.02.005

Veer, T. (2018). Finding the right fit: A journey to self-acceptance. In M. C. Klein (Ed.), *Yoga rising: 30 empowering stories from yoga renegades for every body* (pp. 67–76). Woodbury, MN: Llewellyn Publications.

Vinoski, E, Webb, J.B, Warren-Findlow, J, Brewer, K.A, & Kiffmeyer, K.A. (2017). Got yoga?: a longitudinal analysis of thematic content and models' appearance-related attributes in advertisements spanning four decades of yoga journal. *Body Image, 21*, 1-5. doi: 10.1016/j.bodyim.2017.01.006

Vinoski Thomas, E., Warren-Findlow, J., & Webb, J. B. (2019). Yoga is for every (able) body: A content analysis of disability themes in mainstream yoga media. *International Journal of Yoga, 12*, 68–72. doi:10.4103/ijoy.ijoy_25_18

Webb, J. B., Padro, M. P., Rogers, C. B., Thomas, E. V., Etzel, L., & Putz, D. Y. (2018a). *A preliminary evaluation of the yoga at every size program: A brief, minimally-guided yoga-based online intervention in college women of higher weight.* Oral Presentation, Appearance Matters 8 Conference, Bath, UK.

Webb, J. B., Thomas, E. V., Rogers, C. B., Clark, V. N., Burris, E. N., & Putz, D. Y. (2018b). Fitspo at every size?: A comparative content analysis of #curvyfit versus #curvyyoga Instagram images. *Fat Studies Journal Special Issue: Fat and Physical Activity.* Advance online publication. doi:10.1080/21604851.2019.1548860

Webb, J. B., Vinoski, E. R., Bonar, A. S., Davies, A. E., & Etzel, L. (2017c). Fat is fashionable and fit: A comparative content analysis of Fatspiration and Health at Every Size® Instagram images. *Body Image, 22,* 53–64. doi:10.1016/j.bodyim.2017.05.003

Webb, J. B., Vinoski, E. R., Warren-Findlow, J., Burrell, M. I., & Putz, D. Y. (2017b). Downward dog becomes fit body, inc.: A content analysis of 40 years of female cover images of *yoga journal. Body Image, 22,* 129–135. doi:10.1016/j.bodyim.2017.07.001

Webb, J. B., Vinoski, E. R., Warren-Findlow, J., Padro, M. P., Burris, E. N., & Suddreth, E. M. (2017a). Is the "Yoga Bod" the new skinny? A comparative content analysis of mainstream yoga lifestyle magazine covers. *Body Image, 20,* 87–98. doi:10.1016/j.bodyim.2016.11.005

Wertman, A., Wister, A. V., & Mitchell, B. A. (2016). On and off the mat: Yoga experiences of middle-aged and older adults. *Canadian Journal on Aging, 35,* 190–205. doi:10.1017/S0714980816000155

Wojtowicz, E. (2018). Focusing on ability in dis-ability of yoga. In M. C. Klein (Ed.), *Yoga rising: 30 empowering stories from yoga renegades for every body* (pp. 219–228). Woodbury, MN: Llewellyn Publications.

Yoo, H. C., Jackson, K., Guevarra, R. P., Miller, M. J., & Harrington, B. (2016). Construction and initial validation of the Multiracial Experiences Measure (MEM). *Journal of Counseling Psychology, 63,* 198–209. doi:10.1037/cou0000117

A conceptual model describing mechanisms for how yoga practice may support positive embodiment

Anne E. Cox and Tracy L. Tylka

ABSTRACT

Yoga practice has been associated with various indices of positive embodiment in correlational and intervention studies. Yet, systematic, theoretically-grounded models detailing specific mechanisms by which yoga supports positive embodiment are lacking. In this article, we present a conceptual model that describes mechanisms (i.e., mediators and moderators) that can be used to guide research to help answer how, for whom, and under what conditions yoga practice may promote positive embodiment. Based on existing theoretical frameworks and empirical findings, this model suggests that (a) yoga practice may cultivate embodying experiences during yoga (e.g., state mindfulness), (b) these embodying experiences may build stable embodying experiences that generalize beyond the yoga context (e.g., trait mindfulness), and (c) these stable embodying experiences may then promote embodying practices (e.g., mindful self-care). This mediational chain is likely moderated by the yoga context (e.g., instructional focus, presence of mirrors, diversity of bodies represented) and yoga practitioners' social identities (e.g., body size, physical limitations), social and personal histories (e.g., experiences with weight stigma and trauma), and personality traits and motives (e.g., body comparison, appearance-focused motives to practice yoga). Using the structure of this conceptual model, we offer researchers ideas for testable models and study designs that can support them.

Clinical implications

- Understanding the mechanisms by which yoga supports positive embodiment is key to designing interventions.
- Embodying experiences during yoga may support more general trait-like embodiment variables.
- The impact of yoga on positive embodiment is likely moderated by a number of individual and situational characteristics.

Introduction

Over the past decade, researchers have become increasingly interested in how yoga participation may support positive embodiment. This attention has developed both from a desire to understand the pathways by which yoga may be used as a tool to prevent or treat disordered eating (Neumark-Sztainer, 2014) as well as an interest in cultivating positive embodiment for its own inherent benefits (Cook-Cottone, 2015a, 2015b). Embodiment is a multi-faceted construct that includes a person's body image and their experience of engaging their body in the world—or the extent to which a person perceives that they can interact in the world with strength, functionality, and agency (Piran, 2016, 2017, 2019). Importantly, the environment shapes embodiment via the degree to which it accepts and welcomes a person and provides a safe place for their body. Thus, certain yoga contexts that offer a climate of body positivity, intentional inclusion and acceptance, strength, and community may help promote positive embodiment (Cook-Cottone & Douglass, 2017).

In her Developmental Theory of Piran (2002, 2016, 2017, 2019)) includes five dimensions and three processes that range from positive to disrupted embodiment. Because yoga has the potential to support positive embodiment (Cook-Cottone & Douglass, 2017; Impett et al., 2006; Mahlo & Tiggemann, 2016), we frame our discussion of yoga mechanisms in relation to the protective ends of these dimensions and processes. The first dimension, body connection and comfort, involves being connected to and comfortable with the body as it engages in the world. The second dimension, agency and functionality, is the ability to act assertively, expressively, and influentially in the world. The third dimension, experience and expression of desire, involves being in tune with the body's needs and desires and being able to express them within daily life and relationships. The fourth dimension, attuned self-care, entails responding to the body's needs in a nurturing way, such as moving the body in a joyful way for physical activity. The fifth dimension, inhabiting the body subjectively rather than objectively, is engaging with the world from a first-person perspective rather a third-person (i.e., observer's) perspective of the body—the focus is on how the body feels rather than looks. The protective processes include physical freedom, mental freedom, and social power. Physical freedom, or immersion in joyful physical activity, may best represent the path by which yoga can support positive embodiment. Yet, yoga can also serve mental freedom by creating a space for mindfulness and body-related agency, and social power via a safe community which to practice.

There is a rather robust literature linking yoga practice with variables that represent these dimensions and processes of positive embodiment. However, systematic, theoretically-grounded tests of specific mechanisms by which yoga supports positive embodiment are lacking. *Mechanisms* can be used to

Yoga Context
- Instructor Characteristics
  - Instructional focus
  - Physical features (body, dress)
- Physical/Social Environment
  - Mirrors Present
  - Diversity of participants
  - Type of yoga practiced
  - Clothing types promoted

Social Identities
- Body size
- Physical limitations
- Race
- Age
- Socioeconomic status
- Geographic limitations (far from studio)
- Gender

Social and Personal History
- Stigma due to body size/weight
- Exposure to environments that foster body acceptance and self-efficacy
- Trauma
- Dieting/disordered eating history
- Exercise history
- Experiences with exercise (mindful vs. gateway to weight loss)

Personality Traits and Motives
- Body comparison
- Gratitude (prior to yoga)
- Internalization of Sociocultural Body Ideals
- Body dissatisfaction (prior to yoga)
- Negative and positive affect
- Self-compassion (prior to yoga)
- Motives to practice yoga

Embodying Experiences During
- Reduced state self-objectification and body surveillance
- State mindfulness
- State self-compassion
- State body acceptance and appreciation
- State body image flexibility
- State perceived competence
- State joyful immersion and flow
- State connection to desire/pleasure

Stable Characteristics Built from Embodying Experiences
- Reduced trait self-objectification and body surveillance
- Trait mindfulness
- Trait self-compassion
- Trait body acceptance and appreciation
- Trait body image flexibility
- Trait perceived competence
- Joyful immersion and flow in everyday life
- Connection to desire/pleasure in everyday life

Embodying Practices
- Mindful self-care
- Intuitive eating
- Attuned exercise

Yoga Practice

Positive Embodiment

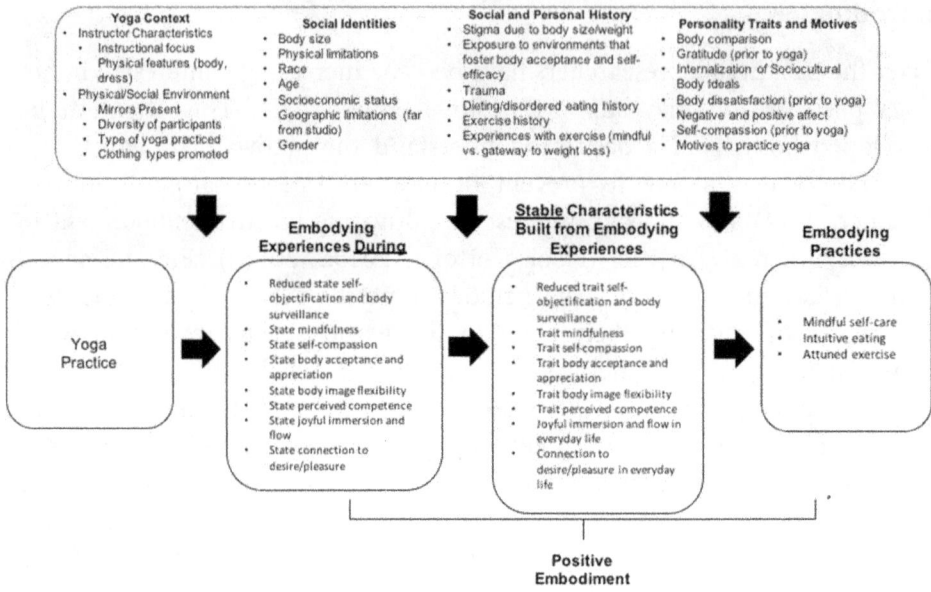

Figure 1. Conceptual model illustrating theoretically-grounded mediators and moderators as mechanisms of the link between yoga practice and positive embodiment. Bulleted variables are examples; they are not an exhaustive list.

understand and explain how changes come about—that is, how yoga may produce a change in positive embodiment. Therefore, in this paper, we present a conceptual model that can be used by researchers to study how, for whom, and under what conditions yoga practice may promote positive embodiment (see Figure 1).

In this model, we present potential mediators and moderators as mechanisms that help explain the relationship between yoga practice and positive embodiment. Embodying experiences during yoga are thought to build stable embodying experiences that generalize beyond the yoga context. These embodying experiences, in both state and trait form, may serve as *mediators* of the relationship between yoga practice and embodied practices (see Figure 1). For example, yoga practice may facilitate mindfulness both during and after practice, which then facilitates the embodied practices of eating mindfully and intuitively. Yet, perhaps yoga does not facilitate embodying experiences in everyone in every yoga context. Thus, we also have to consider *moderators*, or variables that can strengthen or weaken the links among yoga practice, its mediators, and embodying practices. Many mediators and moderators in Figure 1 have been identified as potential mechanisms of change within existing theory and research. Our conceptual model brings these mediators and moderators together in a framework that researchers can use to construct testable predictions for how yoga practice may promote positive embodiment. It is our hope that this

conceptual model provides a clear pathway forward for systematically investigating these mechanisms of change within specific theoretical frameworks.

Conceptual model of pathways from yoga to positive embodiment

Next, we review the variables and the pathways within our conceptual model
presented in Figure 1. These variables do not represent an exhaustive list;
instead, they have been identified within extant theory and research as
potentially important mechanisms in the relationship between yoga and
embodied practices. Future developments in theory and research will reveal
other possible variables, and we therefore encourage readers to use the
structure of our conceptual model to consider additional mechanisms (mediators and moderators) of the relationship between yoga practice and embodied practices.

Yoga practice

We define yoga practice as just that—practicing yoga. The word 'yoga' is
derived from the Sanskrit 'yuj,' which means to 'yoke' or 'join' the mind,
body, and spirit (Hewitt, 1977) and to join the internal with the external
(Neumark-Sztainer, 2019). In yoga, emphasis is placed on moving, stretching,
and balancing through a series of asanas (poses), pranayama (breathwork),
meditation (dhyana), and mindfulness (dharana). Asanas can be physically
challenging, with the potential for helping the practitioner feel empowered
and strong, and they can be gentle, with the potential for helping the
practitioner feel relaxed. These asanas, whether challenging or gentle, can
facilitate the journey 'inward' (i.e., greater connection to oneself) and provide
"an avenue for working with the physical body in a gentle, compassionate,
and positive manner" (Neumark-Sztainer, 2019, p. 328). Pranayama can
provide a foundation for the calming of the mind by observing the breath
as it is, changing the breath in tandem with a count, or breathing in what is
useful (e.g., gratitude for the body, confidence, strength, and calmness) and
breathing out what is not useful (e.g., negativity towards the self, stress).
Dhyana and dharana help practitioners meet their present-moment experience with openness, acceptance, and nonjudgment (Desikachar, 1995). In all
of these ways, yoga aids in quieting the fluctuations of the mind (Patañjali &
Feuerstein, 1989) and facilitates self-discovery through deep listening during
practice (Neumark-Sztainer, 2019). Through regular yoga practice, this deep
listening can be transferred "off the mat," to daily life, potentially providing
a heighted sense of body connection and body trust.

Embodied experiences and stable embodied characteristics

Yoga practice may enhance embodying experiences or states that, over time, build stable attitudes and approaches representative of positive embodiment. In our conceptual model, we separate embodied experiences into "embodied experiences during yoga" and "stable characteristics built from embodied experiences," with the proposition that state-based embodied experiences, when occurring regularly, will enhance trait levels of embodied characteristics (Garland et al., 2010). Research upholds this proposition. As an example, individuals who underwent an 8-week meditation intervention which activated regular state levels of mindfulness experienced, on average, higher trait mindfulness post-intervention (Kiken et al., 2015). The authors concluded that increasing state mindfulness over repeated meditation sessions may contribute to a more mindful disposition. In another study, women who listened to guided self-compassion meditation podcasts once a day for 3 weeks increased their trait levels of self-compassion over the course of the intervention, which was maintained at a 3-month follow-up (Albertson et al., 2015). Below, we review theory and research for both state and trait embodiment constructs together, but with an understanding that state embodied experiences will likely, over time, increase trait levels of embodied characteristics.

Reduced self-objectification and body surveillance

One of the most fundamental ways that yoga practice may support positive embodiment is by providing a context that directs individuals to inhabit their body as a subject rather than as an object. This subjective way of inhabiting the body means that one focuses more on internal bodily experiences rather than their external appearance (Piran, 2002, 2016, 2017). Impett et al. (2006) suggest that yoga may direct nonjudgmental attention to what the body does and how it feels, thereby reducing an emphasis on the external appearance of one's body. Yoga practitioners are also often encouraged to synchronize their breath with the physical movements of the practice, thereby increasing an internal awareness of bodily sensations—this internal focus is in opposition to the external focus on appearance that characterizes self-objectification.

Self-objectification refers to inhabiting the body as an object—that is, valuing one's body more for its aesthetic qualities rather than internal experiences such as sensation and function (Roberts et al., 2018). According to objectification theory, self-objectification is a consequence of the cultural emphasis placed on appearance, which prompts habitual body surveillance (i.e., closely monitoring one's appearance), which can then contribute to other disembodying experiences such as body shame, appearance anxiety, disordered eating, and depression (Fredrickson & Roberts,

1997). Research upholds the links from self-objectification and body surveillance to higher body shame, appearance anxiety, disordered eating, and negative affect (for a review, see Roberts et al., 2018) and lower body appreciation (Andrew et al., 2016; Avalos & Tylka, 2006; Cox et al., 2017), and focusing on internal body experiences is related to higher body appreciation (Oswald et al., 2017). Therefore, embodying physical activities such as yoga that encourage participants to be aware of and respond to the way their bodies feel rather than appear and to immerse themselves in the act of moving may support positive embodiment by reducing how often participants are mentally scanning or observing the appearance of their bodies (Daubenmier, 2005; Impett et al., 2006).

Evidence supports the association between yoga participation and lower self-objectification or body surveillance. For example, Mahlo and Tiggemann (2016) demonstrated significantly lower body surveillance in female yoga participants compared to a sample of university students. Furthermore, body surveillance partially explained the relationship between yoga participation and body appreciation. In longitudinal studies of yoga participants, significant decreases in body surveillance have been observed over eight, 12, and 16 weeks of yoga participation (Cox, Ullrich-French, Cole et al., 2016; Cox et al., 2017, 2019). These findings provide strong support for the inverse relationship between yoga participation and body surveillance; however, more rigorous experimental research designs that include a comparison group are needed to provide more robust evidence for the role yoga plays in reducing body surveillance as well as identifying characteristics of the yoga context that make this more likely to occur.

Mindfulness

The reduction in body surveillance over the course of sustained yoga participation may be due to the emphasis on paying attention to the physical sensations in the body while moving through the asanas or poses. Teachers often (but not always) encourage students to turn inward to tune into these physical sensations in order to make decisions that best serve the self in that moment. Daubenmier (2005) demonstrated some initial evidence for higher body awareness and responsiveness in yoga practitioners compared to non-practitioners. However, researchers have not delved deeply into how this may occur in yoga classes. Recent research on mindfulness may be one avenue through which we can begin understanding how specific experiences of yoga support lower body surveillance, more general improvement in self-care, and other embodying experiences and practices.

The body reflects a particular target of mindfulness. Whereas mindfulness more generally refers to open, nonjudgmental, and intentional focus on (or attention to) the present moment (Bishop et al., 2004; Tanay & Bernstein, 2013), mindfulness of the body applies this focus to bodily sensations and experiences (Cox, Ullrich-French, French et al., 2016; Tanay & Bernstein, 2013). Empirical evidence suggests that when one is more mindful of their bodily or physical experiences during yoga (i.e., state mindfulness), they experience greater declines in trait body surveillance and increases in physical self-worth over an 8-week period (Cox, Ullrich-French, French et al., 2016). State mindfulness of the body during yoga participation has been associated with lower state body surveillance in adolescents and adults (Cox, Ullrich-French, French et al., 2016; Cox et al., 2017). Finally, growth in trait mindfulness has been linked to growth in body appreciation over 16 weeks of yoga participation in a university sample (Cox & McMahon, 2019). However, the relationship between mindfulness during yoga practice and other embodying practices, such as self-care, has not been investigated and is a potential avenue for future research. Finally, the measure of state mindfulness that has been used focuses on awareness of and attention to physical sensations but not necessarily the quality of that attention (e.g., open, accepting, nonreactive, nonjudgmental). Developing measures that capture these other characteristics of mindfulness may more fully elucidate how it supports positive embodiment during the practice of yoga.

Self-compassion

Self-compassion is a multi-faceted construct that includes mindfulness, but also represents a more comprehensive response to pain, discomfort, or suffering that one experiences (Neff, 2003). The definition of self-compassion is grounded in how compassion more generally has been conceptualized and represents a fundamental attribute to be cultivated through yoga (Crews et al., 2016). There are three core components to self-compassion: (a) mindfulness (defined here as being able to hold painful or uncomfortable experiences such as thoughts and emotion with balance and clarity rather than ruminating or ignoring uncomfortable experiences altogether), (b) self-kindness (expressing care, comfort, and acceptance to the self rather than being self-critical), and (c) common humanity (having a greater sense that making mistakes, failure, and suffering are shared experiences among all human beings rather than feeling alone and isolated in pain and discomfort).

Self-compassion has been investigated as a potential mechanism explaining the relationships between yoga participation and stress (Gard et al., 2012; Riley & Park, 2015), body appreciation, and lower body surveillance (Cox et al., 2019). This work has demonstrated increases in self-compassion associated with yoga participation (Braun et al., 2012; Cox et al., 2019; Gard et al., 2012). In addition, empirical evidence links self-compassion to body image variables that are reflective of positive embodiment (see Braun et al., 2016), such as higher body appreciation, higher functionality appreciation, and lower body surveillance (Alleva et al., 2017; Cox et al., 2017;

Wasylkiw et al., 2012). Interventions have shown that extending more kindness to the self and less self-judgment helps women accept and appreciate their bodies (Albertson et al., 2015). Experiencing common humanity may also help women realize that almost no one fits cultural appearance ideals, and thus broaden their definition of beauty to be inclusive—that is, having more appreciation for varied expressions of internal and external beauty (Tylka & Iannantuono, 2016). Growth in self-compassion over the course of semester-long yoga classes in a university setting was found to associate with increases in body appreciation and declines in body surveillance (Cox et al., 2019). Collectively, these studies suggest that the extent to which self-compassion is promoted or facilitated within the context of yoga may be one pathway by which yoga supports positive embodiment.

Body appreciation

Body appreciation includes holding favorable opinions of the body regardless of actual physical appearance, accepting the body despite perceived imperfections, respecting the body by attending to its needs and engaging in healthy behaviors, and protecting the body by rejecting unrealistic societal appearance ideals (Avalos et al., 2005; Tylka & Wood-Barcalow, 2015). Thus, body appreciation encapsulates many characteristics illustrative of gratitude, acceptance, self-care, protection, love, and respect, which are offered unconditionally to the body. That is, the body does not need to look a certain way, function well, and have superior health to be accepted, loved, respected, treated well, and appreciated (Alleva et al., 2017; Wood-Barcalow et al., 2010). Body appreciation is distinct from body satisfaction: a person may not be satisfied with all, or even many, aspects of how their body looks, how their body functions, and their body's health, but still appreciate what their body provides for them and participate in practices to take care of it (Tylka & Wood-Barcalow, 2015).

Research has linked yoga practice to body appreciation. Mahlo and Tiggemann (2016) found that Iyengar and Bikram female practitioners reported higher levels of body appreciation than women who did not practice yoga. Moreover, they found that yoga participation was uniquely associated with body appreciation, even when body surveillance was considered as a mediator of this relationship. In a study about the perceived positive and negative effects of practicing yoga, Park et al. (2016) revealed that approximately 85% of 542 students who practiced yoga indicated that yoga had a positive impact on their level of body appreciation.

More recent studies have considered the changes in body appreciation that occur as a result of yoga practice. Cox and McMahon (2019) explored yoga practitioners' individual trajectories of change in trait body appreciation over a 16-week yoga course. They found average linear increases in body appreciation over the course, although not everyone experienced change at the same rate. It should be noted, though, that Cox et al. (2017) did not find an increase in body appreciation among high school students taking a yoga class over 12 weeks (in lieu of their traditional physical education course). Halliwell et al. (2019) conducted a 4-week yoga-based body image intervention which incorporated themes specially tailored to focus on positive body image. For example, themes included connection to the body, gratitude and appreciation of body function, body acceptance, and valuing the body by engendering respect and self-care. Participants in the yoga intervention reported increased body appreciation and body connectedness at post-test and at a 4-week follow-up.

Body image flexibility

Based in the psychological flexibility and acceptance and commitment therapy literature (Hayes et al., 2012), body image flexibility represents the ability to embrace rather than avoid, escape, or otherwise alter the content or form of distressing body-related thoughts and feelings in the present moment, while engaging in action toward chosen values even in times of great discomfort (Rogers et al., 2018; Sandoz et al., 2019). For instance, if a yoga practitioner high in body image flexibility notices that they have the largest body in a studio class, they are able to accept their discomfort without letting their thoughts and body-related distress overwhelm them as they continue their practice. Similar to psychological flexibility, body image flexibility is enhanced via six interdependent skills: present moment awareness (noticing the body's experiences), experiential acceptance (being open to the body's experiences even when uncomfortable), cognitive defusion (observing thoughts related to the body's experiences without them dominating attention or behavior), self-as-context (experiencing the self as more than the present body's experiences), valuing (choosing a purpose to guide action even when the body's experiences are painful), and committed action (engaging in behavior consistent with values, even when it results in increased contact with painful body experiences) (Sandoz et al., 2019).

The connection between yoga and body image flexibility has yet to be studied. We propose that yoga practice has the potential to provide a context for building these six skills. It may provide a context for yoga practitioners to begin to notice their body's experiences during yoga (e.g., they may notice their breathing become deeper and more regular, stretching sensations in their muscles). Some physical experiences may be unpleasant (e.g., emotional discomfort is often felt in certain asanas, noticing that an asana cannot be achieved or held). In yoga, the instructor may bring attention to this discomfort, create the space to invite it to surface, and meet it with compassion, which can help practitioners observe their thoughts without these thoughts dominating their practice. The act of practicing yoga, even when these unpleasant emotions arise, could represent committed action. Researchers may want to investigate these connections. Furthermore, given that self-compassion and mindfulness are emphasized in the six skills, researchers should determine whether they mediate the association between yoga practice and body image flexibility.

Perceptions of competence

Yoga may also facilitate perceptions of competence, such as self-efficacy and agency, that are characteristic of positive embodiment (Piran, 2016). Perceptions of competence can be conceptualized in more than one way. Achievement goal perspective theory (Nicholls, 1989; Seifriz et al., 1992) outlines two primary orientations or perspectives that individuals use to evaluate their own competence. The first is an ego goal orientation in which individuals compare their own abilities to others or a normative standard to evaluate their own competence. The second is a task goal orientation in which individuals use themselves as their own reference point and focus on skill mastery or improvement as indicators of competence. The degree to which yoga supports a sense of competence may depend in part on which perspective is emphasized by the yoga instructor (i.e., an ego-involving or task-involving climate). In physical activity settings, a task-involving climate is associated with greater enjoyment, effort, and self-confidence (e.g., Hogue et al., 2013).

In a yoga setting, instructors can create a task-involving climate that will support feelings of competence by emphasizing each participant's own unique path in yoga, finding modifications that work for each participant's body, and encouraging participants to listen to internal physical cues that may inform how much effort to put forth. It is common for yoga instructors to encourage participants to turn inward and make decisions that serve the body while still reaching for their edge to find personal challenge (see Neumark-Sztainer & Piran, this issue) and yoga participation has been associated with improvements in physical self-worth (Cox, Ullrich-French, Cole et al., 2016). These gains are exemplified by an interview response from a 29-year old yoga practitioner recovering from an eating disorder who noted how yoga led to, "a sense of competency and efficacy in my body and power and accomplishment" (Dittmann & Freedman, 2009, p. 283). However, creating a task-involving climate is certainly not universal in yoga settings and some participants have stated that practicing yoga actually prompted more social comparison and negative self-talk about their body (Neumark-Sztainer, Watts et al., 2018). Yoga instructors may inadvertently draw students' attention to social comparison or present a particular version of a pose as the one everyone should be striving for, thus creating more of an ego-involving climate. In this way, the approach of the instructor may moderate the impact of yoga practice on embodiment experiences and outcomes. Intentionally creating a task-involving climate in which one's personal path and improvement is emphasized and there is no greater value associated with certain versions of poses, may best support students' feelings of competence and agency in the yoga setting.

Even though many girls are immersed in physical activities in which they feel competent in their bodies, their physical agency and self-efficacy tend to get disrupted around puberty (Piran, 2016, 2017, 2019). The confluence of the maturing female body, pressure to conform one's external appearance to societal ideals, and increased sexualization and objectification of the female form contribute to declines in feelings of competence and increases in self-objectification (Piran, 2016). Yoga participation in adulthood may help women reclaim that sense of agency and develop a sense of competence for what their body can do and how they can progress in the physical postures. Although evidence is emerging on the relationship between yoga participation and a sense of physical competence, its ties to having a voice or agency more generally is lacking and represents and area for future research.

Joyful immersion and flow

The feelings of competence that can be cultivated in the context of yoga are also integral to the experience of being joyfully immersed in the experience of physical activity. The experience of being fully immersed in the act of moving one's body is reflected both in flow state and intrinsic motivation. The experience of flow is characterized by total absorption in a task or activity, high levels of concentration and functioning, and a sense of effortless control (Csikszentmihalyi et al., 2014). There is generally a complete loss of self-consciousness as the individual's awareness merges with the action and the participant is often not aware of the passage of time. For flow to occur, one's sense of competence must align with the degree of perceived challenge that one is encountering, goals must be clear, and feedback needs to be immediate and unambiguous. The degree to which participants experience a balance between their yoga abilities and the degree of challenge presented to them in class, the more likely they will be to experience flow. Yoga instructors can help students achieve flow through the creation of a task-involving climate that will support the development of competence as well as offering options that allow students to select an optimal level of challenge, and appropriate feedback that helps them meet the challenge. The practice of mindfulness throughout class may also improve their ability to concentrate and be in the present moment.

When individuals experience joyful immersion in physical activities, their behavior is likely being regulated from a place of intrinsic motivation. Intrinsic motivation represents the most adaptive and autonomous or volitional form of motivation as conceptualized within self-determination theory (Ryan & Deci, 2017). Individuals are intrinsically motivated when they participate in physical activity for the inherent rewards of the activity such as pleasure, enjoyment, satisfaction, or sense of accomplishment. This most internalized and integrated form of motivation is the strongest motivational predictor of sustained physical activity behavior (Teixeira et al., 2012) and supports feelings of enjoyment or pleasure (Hagger & Protogerou, 2018). Preliminary evidence suggests that more internal reasons (e.g., health) for exercise increase during eight weeks of yoga participation (Cox, Ullrich-French, French et al., 2016), and gains in body appreciation correspond with increases in intrinsic motivation over the course of 16 weeks of yoga participation (Cox et al., 2019). A recent study has found that gains in perceived competence and autonomy during yoga participation coincided with increases in more autonomous physical activity motivation (Cox et al., under review), thereby supporting strategies used by yoga instructors to facilitate the development of competence, feelings of autonomy, and intrinsic motivation.

Connection to desire and pleasure

Yoga practice also provides the opportunity to be aware of and connect with the body's sensations by potentially providing experiences of gratitude and positive affect as well as lowering negative affect. Gratitude is a habitual orientation toward noticing and being appreciative of the positive aspects of life (Wood et al., 2010), and could be beneficial to embodiment via amplifying a healthy and affirming connection to the body (Homan & Tylka, 2018; Tiggemann & Hage, 2019). Positive affect (e.g., feelings such as joy, interest, contentment, inspiration, and excitement) inspire approach behavior; that is, they prompt individuals to engage with their environments and partake in valued activities (Fredrickson, 2001). On the other hand, negative affect (e.g., feelings of distress, anxiety, fear, nervousness, worry, and sadness) tends to restrict engagement and concentration in non-threatening activities.

Gratitude predicts many aspects of well-being, such as life satisfaction, optimism, empathy, and hope (Emmons & McCullough, 2003; McCullough et al., 2002). The amplification model of gratitude suggests that gratitude enhances well-being by identifying the good things in life and magnifying them, bringing them into clear and sharp focus (Watkins, 2014). People are then motivated to think and behave in ways that will enhance these good things. Gratitude is linked to higher body appreciation, in part because it lowers social comparison and appearance and approval-contingent self-worth (Homan & Tylka, 2018). While gratitude is conceptualized as a trait (Wood et al., 2010), it can also be enhanced via practice (e.g., keeping daily gratitude lists (Emmons & McCullough, 2003). Given that yoga instructors may emphasize gratitude during practice (e.g., messages of being grateful for what is going well in life, messages of gratitude expressed toward the body), regular yoga practice containing these messages may support students' trait levels of gratitude. Indeed, yoga practice has been found to be related to trait levels of gratitude (Ivtzan & Papantoniou, 2014). Future research exploring state and trait gratitude shifts as a function of yoga interventions is needed.

Studies have provided evidence for the role of both short- and long-term yoga interventions in enhancing positive affect (Bershadsky et al., 2014; Halliwell et al., 2019; Impett et al., 2006; Kiecolt-Glaser et al., 2010) and reducing negative affect (Bershadsky et al., 2014; Felver et al., 2015; Impett et al., 2006; West et al., 2004). Yoga has also had beneficial effects on affect among cancer survivors. Positive affect (i.e., energy) increased and negative affect (i.e., tiredness, tension) decreased for a group of breast cancer survivors over a 7-week yoga intervention, and these effects were maintained or enhanced at the 6-month follow up (Mackenzie et al., 2013). In a sample of Stage II and III breast cancer survivors, those who attended at least three yoga sessions a week for six weeks experienced increased positive affect and decreased negative affect compared to those who were in a supportive therapy condition (Vadiraja et al., 2009).

Embodying practices

The abovementioned embodying states and stable characteristics encouraged by yoga practice may, in turn, facilitate embodied practices. Embodied practices consist of behaviors that involve listening to the body and trusting its signals. Three embodied practices have received research attention relative to yoga: mindful self-care, intuitive eating, and attuned exercise.

Mindful self-care

Mindful self-care is an iterative, embodied process that involves being aware of what the self and body need given the demands of the current situation and engaging in self-care practices to address these internal needs and external demands in a way that serves well-being (Cook-Cottone, 2015a, 2019; Cook-Cottone & Guyker, 2018). It includes physical care (e.g., nutrition, hydration), self-compassion and purpose (e.g., supportive and comforting self-talk, engaging in meaningful activities), supportive relationships (e.g., respect of boundaries), supportive structure (e.g., comfortable and pleasing living environment, manageable schedule), mindful awareness (e.g., calm awareness of thoughts and feelings), and mindful relaxation (e.g., intentional behaviors to relax) (Cook-Cottone & Guyker, 2018). For example, if a college student is studying for an exam, mindful self-care would entail studying *and* nourishing their body, receiving adequate sleep the days leading up to the exam, hearing encouraging messages from themselves and others, and engaging in practices that help them relax.

By providing a context to regularly experience embodied states and build stable embodied characteristics, yoga may help individuals remain aware of and connected to what their body needs and facilitate their engagement in embodied practices (Cook-Cottone, 2015a, 2019; Cook-Cottone & Guyker, 2018). Given the relevance of mindful self-care to well-being and the advancement of the Mindful Self-Care Scale (Cook-Cottone & Guyker, 2018), it is important that researchers explore whether embodying states and stable characteristics that are developed through yoga do indeed predict mindful self-care practices over time.

Intuitive eating

Intuitive eating involves being connected to, trusting in, and (mostly) eating according to the body's internal hunger and satiety cues (Tylka & Kroon Van Diest, 2013; Resch & Tylka, 2019). Further, it entails eating for physical rather than emotional reasons and choosing foods that help the body function well while eating in a flexible and non-restrictive manner. Much research provides evidence for intuitive eating's connection to psychological well-being and physical health among various age, gender, and cultural groups (for a review, see Resch & Tylka, 2019).

The acceptance model of intuitive eating (Augustus-Horvath & Tylka, 2011; Avalos & Tylka, 2006) suggests that when individuals feel that their bodies are accepted and they are in a body-positive environment, they will appreciate their bodies more and engage in body surveillance less, which then facilitates intuitive eating (Avalos & Tylka, 2006). Research provides evidence for the acceptance model of intuitive eating with adolescent, college, and community samples. For example, in a sample of adolescent girls, Andrew et al. (2016) found that body acceptance by others predicted increased body appreciation, and body appreciation predicted increased intuitive eating, over a 1-year period. Self-compassion (Kelly & Stephen, 2016) and body image flexibility (Schoenefeld & Webb, 2013) have also been shown to contribute to intuitive eating among college women.

The acceptance model of intuitive eating may be applied to the yoga context. The yoga environment may be a body accepting environment for yoga practitioners if, for example, individuals of various body shapes, sizes, and abilities are represented and feel welcomed and yoga instructors integrate body positive themes within the practice (Cook-Cottone & Douglass, 2017; Halliwell et al., 2019). Perceptions of body acceptance may then encourage yoga practitioners' own body appreciation and lower their body surveillance by increasing their body awareness and body responsiveness, which then may foster their intuitive eating. Indeed, in a sample of yoga practitioners, body awareness and body responsiveness were linked to higher intuitive eating (Dittmann & Freedman, 2009).

Attuned exercise

Attuned exercise involves moving the body in various ways that cultivate joy, mindful attention, self-compassion, self-acceptance, body connection, and body responsiveness (Calogero et al., 2019). It is based on a foundation of physical and psychological *safety* (i.e., movement that does not harm the body) on which people can focus on the *process* of becoming more aware, connected, and responsive to their body and come to experience *joy* through physical activity.

Calogero and Pedrotty (2004) developed and facilitated an experiential, psychoeducational exercise program for women with eating disorders during residential treatment with the purpose of replacing dysfunctional exercise with attuned exercise. Compared to those who had traditional care (i.e., no structured exercise program), those in the attuned exercise group had significant reductions in dysfunctional exercise attitudes and behaviors, and the program did not adversely impact weight restoration. Furthermore, in community samples of women and men, attuned exercise attitudes and behaviors were associated with higher body appreciation, self-compassion, mindfulness, body responsiveness, intuitive eating, and lower body surveillance (Calogero & Mensinger, 2015; Reel et al., 2016). Directing research attention to determine additional embodied experiences and stable embodied characteristics that may be cultivated during yoga and promote attuned exercise, and the factors that moderate the strength of these associations, is necessary.

Moderators

Although there is ample evidence of a positive association between yoga participation and positive embodiment (Halliwell et al., 2019; Mahlo & Tiggemann, 2016), in contemporary yoga practices, there are a number of factors that could either support or undermine this relationship. Results of a recent qualitative study with young adults revealed that the majority of participants felt yoga had a positive impact on their body image; however, 25% of participants responded that yoga had a negative impact (Neumark-Sztainer, Watts et al., 2018). Therefore, certain variables may moderate the impact of yoga practice on positive embodiment. Moderators have largely been overlooked in research exploring the impact of yoga on positive embodiment. Therefore, we do not know whether the moderators mentioned below are empirically supported. Our hope is that researchers investigate these, and other, possibilities.

Contextual variables

Variables linked to the yoga context and type of yoga practiced may moderate the connection between yoga practice and positive embodiment. Contextual variables can include characteristics of the yoga studio or environment (e.g., presence of mirrors, practicing yoga in a gym setting), the content and tone of the yoga instruction, the type of yoga practiced (e.g., Hatha, Bikram), other class participants (e.g., body diversity represented versus predominantly thin/fit bodies, loose comfortable clothing versus form-fitting clothing), and instructor characteristics (e.g., physical appearance, dress, provision of assists and touch). For example, an instructor who focuses on appearance in class (e.g., by including statements such as "planks

help define your abs") may be less effective in promoting positive embodiment than an instructor who emphasizes tuning in to physical sensations
during yoga (e.g., "notice your spine lengthen as you lift your hips").

Cook-Cottone and Douglass (2017) emphasized the importance of creating
yoga contexts that foster the acceptance and inclusion of individuals with diverse
bodies in order to support positive embodiment. Neumark-Sztainer et al. (2018)
found evidence for this assertion in their qualitative study. Specifically, they
interviewed individuals who practiced yoga who noted that the presence of
diverse body shapes supported their positive body image. Furthermore, participants were more likely to be critical of themselves when they perceived others in
the class to be more fit, thinner, or wearing form-fitting clothes. The presence of
mirrors made comparing oneself to others more likely. Consequently, both
Cook-Cottone and Douglass (2017) and Neumark-Sztainer et al. (2018) provide
recommendations: Yoga instructors can address some of these factors that can
potentially undermine positive embodiment by eliminating mirrors, avoiding
diet or appearance-related talk, and creating a climate of personal improvement
and growth (see task-involving climate) by encouraging participants to look
inward and place emphasis on their own individual path. In both articles, the
authors argue that it is important for yoga instructors to foster a diverse,
inclusive, and welcoming yoga environment by using language that is supportive
and inclusive of all regardless of experience, skill, or the shape or size of one's
body.

Indeed, recent intervention studies have provided preliminary evidence that it
is effective to emphasize particular aspects of positive embodiment in the way
that the classes are taught. For example, emphasizing self-compassion is a central
focus in Kripalu yoga, and multiple studies have demonstrated significant gains
in self-compassion after sustained yoga practice in this tradition (Braun et al.,
2012; Gard et al., 2012). As another illustration, Halliwell et al. (2019) designed
a 4-week yoga intervention that incorporated body positive themes, and participants exhibited significant gains in body appreciation and body connection at
post-test and a 4-week follow-up. Additionally, Delaney and Anthis (2010)
revealed that yoga classes with greater emphasis on the "mind" aspects of
yoga, such as meditation, breathing, mindfulness, and chanting, promoted
greater body awareness and fewer body shape concerns than yoga classes with
greater emphasis on the "body," such as postures and fitness. They discussed that
further attention should be directed to how the benefits of yoga differ across the
various forms of yoga, and we could apply this recommendation specifically to
positive embodiment.

Investigating contextual factors as moderators of the relationship between
yoga practice and positive embodiment is paramount, given that, over a 40-
year period, yoga images have become less diverse in age, race, and body size,
and more consistent with societal thin and fit appearance ideals, as well as
more adorned with objectifying attire with high body visibility (Vinoski et al.,

2017; Webb et al., 2017). Studios may reflect these images in their boutiques, creating an environment that potentially disrupts positive embodiment. Overall, studies are needed that attempt to better isolate and test the impact of various environmental, social, and instructional variables within the yoga context on positive embodiment variables.

Individual variables

In addition to contextual variables, yoga practitioners' *social identities, social and personal history*, and *personality traits and motives* could influence (i.e., moderate) the impact of yoga practice on positive embodiment. Social identities such as body size, age, physical limitations, race, social class, and/ or gender could impact how individuals interpret or react to specific instruction and certain asanas in a yoga class. For example, a yoga practitioner with arthritis of the toe, ankle, and/or knee joints may find many asanas challenging and painful instead of embodying, especially if there are no modifications offered by the instructor.

Social and personal history factors such as experiencing weight-stigma or disordered eating may impact how comfortable and accepted individuals feel in a yoga class. Having a history of trauma may impact whether impromptu instructor assists, touch, and focus on form are positively embodying versus violating (Emerson, 2015). Even if state embodying experiences such as state mindfulness, state self-compassion, and state body appreciation are activated in the yoga context, living in a chronically stressful environment may prevent these state embodying experiences from forming stable embodying characteristics (e.g., trait mindfulness, trait self-compassion, trait body appreciation), as well as interfere with embodying self-care practices. A history of an eating disorder and/or dysfunctional exercise, whereby internal bodily cues have been suppressed, may make it more difficult to experience embodied states during yoga, form embodied stable characteristics, and engage in embodied practices such as intuitive eating and attuned exercise.

Finally, yoga practitioners' personality traits and motives, such as their general tendency to engage in body comparison or personal goals for weight loss, will shape their experience in the yoga context. For instance, even within a context where practitioners are invited to go inward, focusing on one's goal to lose weight (i.e., changing the external self) and engaging in body comparison with other practitioners may prevent them from doing so, and in this way lessen yoga's positive impact on positive embodiment. There are many opportunities for researchers to 'dive in' and investigate the roles that personality traits and motives play in the yoga-embodiment connection.

Additional research directions and conclusions

In this article, we offer a conceptual model that brings together various theoretical perspectives to illustrate mechanisms that may help explain and determine the strength of the yoga-positive embodiment relationship. Grounding our model in these theoretical perspectives is essential in order to move this research forward in a systematic manner that builds knowledge incrementally, while simultaneously informing the development of yoga interventions and contexts aimed at supporting positive embodiment.

In addition to the suggestions for future research offered in the preceding sections, the use of innovative research methods and more rigorous research designs are needed. For example, using our conceptual model as a framework to determine variable selection, ecological momentary assessment or a daily diary approach could be used to capture how participants feel throughout the days that they participate in yoga compared to when they do not (e.g., Kishida et al., 2019). State assessments could be used to capture what participants are experiencing during yoga classes and how that may change over the course of sustained yoga participation. Indeed, a key shortcoming of extant research is that most studies have tested for change or differences in trait embodying characteristics while overlooking the state embodying experiences occurring in or shortly after the yoga classes. Furthermore, experimental research designs with random assignment and appropriate control groups are needed to help identify key mechanisms of change (e.g., instruction, environment) that may support or undermine positive embodiment. For example, elements such as gratitude, body appreciation, mindfulness, and self-compassion could be manipulated through the instruction that the yoga teacher provides, allowing for tests of how different instruction impacts positive embodiment. It is our hope that our model provides a foundation from which to continue to explore this relationship.

Finally, there is a need for testing moderated mediation models that include multiple mediators and moderators of the relationship between yoga practice and positive embodiment, and our conceptual model may be useful for devising such testable models. One example of a mediation model is by Cox et al. (2019), who found evidence for the mediating roles of body appreciation and body surveillance in the relationship between self-compassion and intrinsic motivation for general physical activity during 16 weeks of yoga participation. In this example, an embodiment trait (self-compassion) predicted other embodiment traits (body appreciation and body surveillance) which then predicted an embodied practice (engaging in physical activity for intrinsic reasons), although no moderators were examined. State embodying experiences could also be integrated in moderated mediation models, and state measures of body appreciation (Homan, 2016), positive and negative affect (Watson & Clark, 1994), mindfulness (Cox, Ullrich-French, French et al., 2016), self-compassion (Arch et al., 2014), and body surveillance (Breines et al., 2008) do exist for the ease of assessing these variables.

In conclusion, while yoga practice seems to be beneficial for most practitioners' embodiment, it is not beneficial for everyone (Neumark-Sztainer, Watts et al., 2018). Therefore, our research should be directed to help answer the following question, "Under what conditions can positive embodiment be fostered in yoga practice, and do these conditions depend on the personality traits, social experiences, histories, and identities of yoga practitioners?" Our conceptual model can be used as a framework for researchers to develop testable models to explore this question, which speaks to the connection between yoga practice and positive embodiment: its state experiences, its stable characteristics, and its embodied practices.

References

Albertson, E. R., Neff, K. D., & Dill-Shackleford, K. E. (2015). Self-compassion and body dissatisfaction in women: A randomized controlled trial of a brief meditation intervention. *Mindfulness, 6*(3), 444–454. https://doi.org/10.1007/s12671-014-0277-3

Alleva, J. M., Tylka, T. L., & Kroon Van Diest, D. A. M. (2017). The functionality appreciation scale (FAS): Development and psychometric evaluation in US community women and men. *Body Image, 23*, 28–44. https://doi.org/10.1016/j.bodyim.2017.07.008

Andrew, R., Tiggemann, M., & Clark, L. (2016). *Predictors* and health-related outcomes of positive body image in adolescent girls: A prospective study. *Developmental Psychology, 52* (3), 463–474. http://dx.doi.org/10.1037/dev0000095

Arch, J. J., Brown, K. W., Dean, D. J., Landy, L. N., Brown, K. D., & Laudenslager, M. L. (2014). Self-compassion training modulates alpha-amylase, heart rate variability, and subjective responses to social evaluative threat in women. *Psychoneuroendrocrinology, 42*, 49–58. https://doi.org/10.1016/j.psyneuen.2013.12.018

Augustus-Horvath, C. L., & Tylka, T. L. (2011). The acceptance model of intuitive eating: A comparison of women in emerging adulthood, early adulthood, and middle adulthood. *Journal of Counseling Psychology, 58*(1), 110–125. https://doi.org/10.1037/a0022129

Avalos, L., Tylka, T. L., & Wood-Barcalow, N. (2005). The body appreciation scale: Development and psychometric evaluation. *Body Image, 2*(3), 285–297. https://doi.org/10.1016/j.bodyim.2005.06.002

Avalos, L. C., & Tylka, T. L. (2006). Exploring a model of intuitive eating with college women. *Journal of Counseling Psychology, 53*(4), 486–497. https://doi.org/10.1037/0022-0167.53.4.486

Bershadsky, S., Trumpfheller, L., Kimble, H. B., Pipaloff, D., & Yim, I. S. (2014). The effect of prenatal hatha yoga on affect, cortisol, and depressive symptoms. *Complementary Theories in Clinical Practice, 20*(2), 106–113. https://doi.org/10.1016/j.ctcp.2014.01.002

Bishop, S. R., Lau, M., Shapiro, S., Carlson, L., Anderson, N. D., Carmody, J., & Devins, G. (2004). *Mindfulness: A proposed operational definition. Clinical Psychology: Science and Practice, 11*(3), 230–241. https://doi.org/10.1093/clipsy.bph077

Braun, T., Park, C. L., & Conboy, L. A. (2012). Psychological well-being, health behaviors, and weight loss among participants in a residential, Kripalu yoga-based weight loss program. *International Journal of Yoga Therapy, 22*(1), 9–22. Retrieved from https://doi.org/10.17761/ijyt.22.1.y47k2658674t1212

Braun, T. D., Park, C. L., & Gorin, A. (2016). Self-compassion, body image, and disordered eating: A review of the literature. *Body Image, 17*, 117–131. https://doi.org/10.1016/j.bodyim.2016.03.003

Breines, J. G., Crocker, J., & Garcia, J. A. (2008). Self-objectification and well-being in women's daily lives. *Personality and Social Psychology Bulletin, 34*(5), 583–598. https://doi.org/10.1177/0146167207313727

Calogero, R. M., & Mensinger, J. (2015, November). Development and validity of the experiential exercise scale: A new tool for measuring process vs. outcome-driven exercise. Poster presented at the Renfrew Center Foundation Annual Conference.

Calogero, R. M., & Pedrotty, K. N. (2004). The practice and process of healthy exercise: An investigation of the treatment of exercise abuse in women with eating disorders. *Eating Disorders, 12*(4), 273–291. https://doi.org/10.1080/10640260490521352

Calogero, R. M., Tylka, T. L., Hartman McGilley, B., & Pedrotty-Stump, K. N. (2019). Attunement with exercise. In T. L. Tylka & N. Piran (Eds.), *Handbook of positive body image and embodiment: Constructs, protective factors, and interventions.* Oxford University Press.

Cook-Cottone, C., & Douglass, L. L. (2017). Yoga communities and eating disorders: Creating safe space for positive embodiment. *International Journal of Yoga Therapy, 27*(1), 87–93. https://doi.org/10.17761/1531-2054-27.1.87

Cook-Cottone, C. P. (2015a). *Mindfulness and yoga for self-regulation: A primer for mental health professionals.* Springer.

Cook-Cottone, C. P. (2015b). Incorporating positive body image into the treatment of eating disorders: A model of attunement and mindful self-care. *Body Image, 14*, 158–167. https://doi.org/10.1016/j.bodyim.2015.03.004

Cook-Cottone, C. P. (2019). Mindful attunement. In T. L. Tylka & N. Piran (Eds.), *Handbook of positive body image and embodiment: Constructs, protective factors, and interventions.* Oxford University Press.

Cook-Cottone, C. P., & Guyker, W. M. (2018). The development and validation of the mindful self-care scale (MSCS): An assessment of practices that support positive embodiment. *Mindfulness, 9*(1), 161–175. https://doi.org/10.1007/s12671-017-0759-1

Cox, A. E., & McMahon, A. K. (2019). Exploring changes in mindfulness and body appreciation during yoga participation. *Body Image, 29*, 118–121. https://doi.org/10.1016/j.bodyim.2019.03.003

Cox, A. E., Ullrich-French, S., Cole, A. N., & D'Hondt-Taylor, M. (2016). The role of state mindfulness during yoga in predicting self-objectification and reasons for exercise. *Psychology of Sport and Exercise, 22*(1), 321–327. https://doi.org/10.1016/j.psychsport.2015.10.001

Cox, A. E., Ullrich-French, S., & French, B. F. (2016). Validity evidence for the state mindfulness scale for physical activity. *Measurement in Physical Education and Exercise Science, 20*(1), 38–49. https://doi.org/10.1080/1091367X.2015.1089404

Cox, A. E., Ullrich-French, S., Howe, H. S., & Cole, A. N. (2017). A pilot yoga physical education curriculum to promote positive body image. *Body Image, 23*, 1–8. https://doi.org/10.1016/j.bodyim.2017.07.007

Cox, A. E., Ullrich-French, S., Tylka, T. L., & McMahon, A. K. (2019). The roles of self-compassion, body surveillance, and body appreciation in predicting intrinsic motivation for physical activity: Cross-sectional associations, and prospective changes within a yoga context. *Body Image, 29*, 110–117. https://doi.org/10.1016/j.bodyim.2019.03.002

Crews, D. A., Stolz-Newton, M., & Grant, N. S. (2016). The use of yoga to build self-compassion as a healing method for survivors of sexual violence. *Journal of Religion and Spirituality in Social Work: Social Thought, 35*(3), 139–156. https://doi.org/10.1080/15426432.2015.1067583

Csikszentmihalyi, M., Abuhamdeh, S., & Nakamura, J. (2014). Flow. In M. Csikszentmihalyi (Ed.), *Flow and the foundations of positive psychology.* Springer.

Daubenmier, J. J. (2005). The relationship of yoga, body awareness, and body responsiveness to self-objectification and disordered eating. *Psychology of Women Quarterly*, *29*(2), 207–219. https://doi.org/10.1111/j.1471-6402.2005.00183.x

Delaney, K., & Anthis, K. (2010). Is women's participation in different types of yoga classes associated with different levels of body awareness satisfaction? *International Journal of Yoga Therapy*, *20*(1), 62–71. Retrived from https://doi.org/10.17761/ijyt.20.1. t44l6656h22735g6

Desikachar, T. K. V. (1995). *The heart of yoga. Developing a personal practice.* Inner Traditions International.

Dittmann, K. A., & Freedman, M. R. (2009). Body awareness, eating attitudes, and spiritual beliefs of women practicing yoga. *Eating Disorders*, *17*(4), 273–292. https://doi.org/10. 1080/10640260902991111

Emerson, D. (2015). *Trauma-sensitive yoga in therapy: Bringing the body into treatment.* W. W. Norton & Co.

Emmons, R. A., & McCullough, M. E. (2003). Counting blessings versus burdens: An experimental investigation of gratitude and subjective well-being in daily life. *Journal of Personality and Social Psychology*, *84*(2), 377–389. http://doi.org/10.1037/0022-3514.84.2.377

Felver, J. C., Butzer, B., Olson, K. J., Smith, I. M., & Khalsa, S. B. S. (2015). Yoga in public school improves adolescent mood and affect. *Contemporary School Psychology*, *19*(3), 184–192. http://doi.org/10.1007/s40688-014-0031-9

Fredrickson, B. L. (2001). The role of positive emotions in positive psychology: The broaden-and-build theory of positive emotions. *American Psychologist*, *56*(3), 218–226. http://doi.org/10.1037//0003-066X.56.3.218

Fredrickson, B. L., & Roberts, T.-A. (1997). Objectification theory: Toward understanding women's lived experiences and mental health risks. *Psychology of Women Quarterly*, *21*(2), 173–206. https://doi.org/10.1111/j.1471-6402.1997.tb00108.x

Gard, T., Brach, N., Hölzel, B. K., Noggle, J. J., Conboy, L. A., & Lazar, S. W. (2012). Effects of a yoga-based intervention for young adults on quality of life and perceived stress: The potential mediating roles of mindfulness and self-compassion. *Journal of Positive Psychology*, *7*(3), 165–175. https://doi.org/10.1080/17439760.2012.667144

Garland, E. L., Fredrickson, B., Kring, A. M., Johnson, D. P., Meyer, P. S., & Penn, D. L. (2010). Upward spirals of positive emotions counter downward spirals of negativity: Insights from the broaden-and-build theory and affective neuroscience on the treatment of emotion dysfunctions and deficits in psychopathology. *Clinical Psychology Review*, *30*(7), 849–864. http://doi.org/10.1016/j.cpr.2010.03.002

Hagger, M. S., & Protogerou, C. (2018). Affect in the context of self-determination theory. In D. M. Williams, R. E. Rhodes, & M. T. Conner (Eds.), *Affective determinants of health behavior.* Oxford University Press.

Halliwell, E., Dawson, K., & Burkey, S. (2019). A randomized experimental evaluation of a yoga-based body image intervention. *Body Image*, *28*, 119–127. https://doi.org/10.1016/j. bodyim.2018.12.005

Hayes, S. C., Barnes-Holmes, D., & Wilson, K. G. (2012). Contextual behavioral science: Creating a science more adequate to the challenge of the human condition. *Journal of Contextual Behavioral Science*, *1*(1–2), 1–16. https://doi.org/10.1016/j.jcbs.2012.09.004

Hewitt, J. (1977). *Yoga and meditation.* Barrie & Jenkins.

Hogue, C. M., Fry, M. D., Fry, A. C., & Pressman, S. D. (2013). The influence of a motivational climate intervention on participants' salivary cortisol and psychological responses. *Journal of Sport and Exercise Psychology*, *35*(1), 85–97. https://doi.org/10.1123/jsep.35.1.85

Homan, K. J. (2016). Factor structure and psychometric properties of a state version of the body appreciation scale-2. *Body Image*, *19*, 204–207. https://doi.org/10.1016/j.bodyim.2016.10.004

Homan, K. J., & Tylka, T. L. (2018). Development and exploration of the gratitude model of body appreciation in women. *Body Image, 25,* 14–22. https://doi.org/10.1016/j.bodyim.2018.01.008

Impett, E. A., Daubenmier, J. J., & Hirschman, A. L. (2006). Minding the body: Yoga, embodiment, and well-being. *Sexuality Research & Social Policy, 3*(4), 39–48. https://doi.org/10.1525/srsp.2006.3.4.39

Ivtzan, I., & Papantoniou, A. (2014). Yoga meets positive psychology: Examining the integration of hedonic (gratitude) and eudaimonic (meaning) wellbeing in relation to the extent of yoga practice. *Journal of Bodywork and Movement Therapies, 18*(2), 183–189. http://doi.org/10.1016/j.jbmt.2013.11.005

Kelly, A. C., & Stephen, E. (2016). A daily diary study of self-compassion, body image, and eating behavior in female college students. *Body Image, 17,* 152–160. https://doi.org/10.1016/j.bodyim.2016.03.006

Kiecolt-Glaser, J. K., Christian, L., Preston, H., Houts, C. R., Malarkey, W. B., Emery, C. F., & Glaser, R. (2010). Stress, inflammation, and yoga practice. *Psychosomatic Medicine, 72*(2), 113–121. http://doi.org/10.1097/PSY.0b013e3181cb9377

Kiken, L. G., Garland, E. L., Bluth, K., Palsson, O. S., & Gaylord, S. A. (2015). From a state to a trait: Trajectories of state mindfulness in meditation during intervention predict changes in trait mindfulness. *Personality and Individual Differences, 81,* 41–46. https://doi.org/10.1016/j.paid.2014.12.044

Kishida, M., Molenaar, P. C., & Elavsky, S. (2019). The impact of trait mindfulness on relational outcomes in novice yoga practitioners participating in an academic yoga course. *Journal of American College Health, 67*(3), 250–262. https://doi.org/10.1080/07448481.2018.1469505

Mackenzie, M. J., Carlson, L. E., Ekkekakis, P., Paskevich, D. M., & Culos-Reed, S. N. (2013). Affect and mindfulness as predictors of change in mood disturbance, stress symptoms, and quality of life in a community-based yoga program for cancer survivors. *Evidence-based Complementary and Alternative Medicine, 2013,* 419496. http://doi.org/10.1155/2013/419496

Mahlo, L., & Tiggemann, M. (2016). Yoga and positive body image: A test of the embodiment model. *Body Image, 18,* 135–142. https://doi.org/10.1016/j.bodyim.2016.06.008

McCullough, M. E., Emmons, R. A., & Tsang, J. (2002). The grateful disposition: A conceptual and empirical topography. *Journal of Personality and Social Psychology, 82*(1), 112–127. http://doi.org/10.1037//0022-3514.82.1.112

Neff, K. (2003). Self-compassion: An alternative conceptualization of a healthy attitude toward oneself. *Self and Identity, 2*(2), 85–101. https://doi.org/10.1080/15298860309032

Neumark-Sztainer, D. (2014). *Yoga and eating disorders: Is there a place for yoga in the prevention and treatment of eating disorders and disordered eating behaviours? Advances in Eating Disorders: Theory, Research, and Practice,* 22(2), 136-145. Retrieved from https://www.tandfonline.com/doi/full/10.1080/21662630.2013.862369

Neumark-Sztainer, D. (2019). The practice of yoga: Can it help in addressing body image concerns and eating disorders? In T. L. Tylka & N. Piran (Eds.), *Handbook of positive body image and embodiment: Constructs, protective factors, and interventions.* Oxford.

Neumark-Sztainer, D., Watts, A. W., & Rydell, S. (2018). Yoga and body image: How do young adults practicing yoga describe its impact on their body image? *Body Image, 27,* 156–168. https://doi.org/10.1016/j.bodyim.2018.09.001

Nicholls, J. G. (1989). *The competitive ethos and democratic education.* Harvard University Press.

Oswald, A., Chapman, J., & Wilson, C. (2017). Do interoceptive awareness and interoceptive responsiveness mediate the relationship between body appreciation and intuitive eating in young women? *Appetite, 109*, 66–72. https://doi.org/10.1016/j.appet.2016.11.019

Park, C. L., Riley, K. E., & Braun, T. D. (2016). Practitioners' perceptions of yoga's positive and negative effects: Results of a national United States survey. *Journal of Bodywork and Movement Therapies, 20*(2), 270–279. https://doi.org/10.1016/j.jbmt.2015.11.005

Patañjali & Feuerstein, G. (1989). *The yoga-sutra of Patanjali: A new translation and commentary*. Inner Traditions International.

Piran, N. (2002). Embodiment: A mosaic of inquiries in the area of body weight and shape preoccupation. In S. Abbey (Ed.), *Ways of knowing in and through the body: Diverse perspectives on embodiment*. Soleil Publishing.

Piran, N. (2016). Embodied possibilities and disruptions: The emergence of the experience of embodiment construct from qualitative studies with girls and women. *Body Image, 18*, 43–60. https://doi.org/10.1016/j.bodyim.2016.04.007

Piran, N. (2017). *Journeys of embodiment at the intersection of body and culture: The developmental theory of embodiment*. Elsevier.

Piran, N. (2019). The experience of embodiment construct: Reflecting the quality of embodied lives. In T. L. Tylka & N. Piran (Eds.), *Handbook of positive body image and embodiment: Constructs, protective factors, and interventions*. Oxford University Press.

Reel, J. J., Galli, N., Miyairi, M., Voelker, D., & Greenleaf, C. (2016). Development and validation of the intuitive exercise scale. *Eating Behaviors, 22*, 129–132. https://doi.org/10.1016/j.eatbeh.2016.06.013

Resch, E., & Tylka, T. L. (2019). Intuitive eating. In T. L. Tylka & N. Piran (Eds.), *Handbook of positive body image and embodiment: Constructs, protective factors, and interventions*. Oxford University Press.

Riley, K. E., & Park, C. L. (2015). How does yoga reduce stress? A systematic review of mechanisms of change and guide to future inquiry. *Health Psychology Review, 9*(3), 379–396. https://doi.org/10.1080/17437199.2014.981778

Roberts, T.-A., Calogero, R. M., & Gervais, S. (2018). Objectification theory: Continuing contributions to feminist psychology. In C. Travis & J. White (Eds.), *APA handbook of the psychology of women* (Vol. 1). American Psychological Association.

Rogers, C. B., Webb, J. B., & Jafari, N. (2018). A systematic review of the roles of body image flexibility as a correlate, moderator, mediator, and in intervention science (2011–2018). *Body Image, 27*, 43–60. https://doi.org/10.1016/j.bodyim.2018.08.003

Ryan, R. M., & Deci, E. L. (2017). *Self-determination theory: Basic psychological needs in motivation, development, and wellness*. Guilford Publications.

Sandoz, E. K., Webb, J. B., Rogers, C. B., & Squyres, E. (2019). Body image flexibility. In T. L. Tylka & N. Piran (Eds.), *Handbook of positive body image and embodiment: Constructs, protective factors, and interventions*. Oxford University Press.

Schoenefeld, S. J., & Webb, J. B. (2013). Self-compassion and intuitive eating in college women: Examining the contributions of distress tolerance and body image acceptance and action. *Eating Behaviors, 14*(4), 493–496. https://doi.org/10.1016/j.eatbeh.2013.09.001

Seifriz, J. J., Duda, J. L., & Chi, L. (1992). The relationship of perceived motivational climate to intrinsic motivation and beliefs about success in basketball. *Journal of Sport & Exercise Psychology, 14*(4), 375–391. https://doi.org/10.1123/jsep.14.4.375

Tanay, G., & Bernstein, A. (2013). State mindfulness scale (SMS): Development and initial validation. *Psychological Assessment, 25*(4), 1286–1299. https://doi.org/10.1037/a0034044

Teixeira, P. J., Carraça, E. V., Markland, D., Silva, M. N., & Ryan, R. M. (2012). Exercise, physical activity, and self-determination theory: A systematic review. *International Journal of Behavioral Nutrition and Physical Activity, 9*(1), 78. https://doi.org/10.1186/1479-5868-9-78

Tiggemann, M., & Hage, K. (2019). Religion and spirituality: Pathways to positive body image. *Body Image, 28*, 135–141. https://doi.org/10.1016/j.bodyim.2019.01.004

Tylka, T. L., & Iannantuono, A. C. (2016). Perceiving beauty in all women: Psychometric evaluation of the broad conceptualization of beauty scale. *Body Image, 17*, 67–81. https://doi.org/10.1016/j.bodyim.2016.02.005

Tylka, T. L., & Kroon Van Diest, D. A. M. (2013). The intuitive eating scale-2: Item refinement and psychometric evaluation with college women and men. *Journal of Counseling Psychology, 60*(1), 137–153. https://doi.org/10.1037/a0030893

Tylka, T. L., & Wood-Barcalow, N. L. (2015). The body appreciation scale-2: Item refinement and psychometric evaluation. *Body Image, 12*, 53–67. https://doi.org/10.1016/j.bodyim.2014.09.006

Vadiraja, H. S., Raghavendra Rao, M., Nagarathna, R., Nagendra, H. R., Rekha, M., Vanitha, N., Gopinath, K. S., Srinath, B. S., Vishweshwara, M. S., Madhavi, Y. S., Ajaikumar, B. S., Bilimagga, S. R., & Rao, N. (2009). Effects of yoga program on quality of life and affect in early breast cancer patients undergoing adjuvant radiotherapy: A randomized controlled trial. *Complementary Therapies in Medicine, 17*(5–6), 274–280. https://doi.org/10.1016/j.ctim.2009.06.004

Vinoski, E., Webb, J. B., Warren-Findlow, J., Brewer, K. A., & Kiffmeyer, K. A. (2017). Got yoga?: A longitudinal analysis of thematic content and models' appearance-related attributes in advertisements spanning four decades of yoga journal. *Body Image, 21*(1), 1–5. https://doi.org/10.1016/j.bodyim.2017.01.006

Wasylkiw, L., MacKinnon, A. L., & MacLellan, A. M. (2012). Exploring the link between self-compassion and body image in university women. *Body Image, 9*(2), 236–245. https://doi.org/10.1016/j.bodyim.2012.01.007

Watkins, P. C. (2014). *Gratitude and the good life: Toward a psychology of appreciation.* Springer.

Watson, D., & Clark, L. A. (1994). *The PANAS-X: Manual for the positive and negative affect scale-expanded form.* University of Iowa.

Webb, J. B., Vinoski, E. R., Warren-Findlow, J., Burrell, M. I., & Putz, D. Y. (2017). Downward dog becomes fit body, inc.: A content analysis of 40 years of female cover images of yoga journal. *Body Image, 22*, 129–135. https://doi.org/10.1016/j.bodyim.2017.07.001

West, J., Otte, C., Geher, K., Johnson, J., & Mohr, D. C. (2004). Effects of Hatha yoga and African dance on perceived stress, affect, and salivary cortisol. *Annals of Behavioral Medicine, 28*(2), 114–118. https://doi.org/10.1207/s15324796abm2802_6

Wood, A. M., Froh, J. J., & Geraghty, A. W. A. (2010). Gratitude and well-being: A review and theoretical integration. *Clinical Psychology Review, 30*(7), 890–905. https://doi.org/10.1016/j.cpr.2010.03.005

Wood-Barcalow, N. L., Tylka, T. L., & Augustus-Horvath, C. L. (2010). "But I like my body": Positive body image characteristics and a holistic model for young-adult women. *Body Image, 7*(2), 106–116. https://doi.org/10.1016/j.bodyim.2010.01.001

Research update

Yoga and eating disorder prevention and treatment: a comprehensive review and meta-analysis

Ashlye Borden and Catherine Cook-Cottone

ABSTRACT

Yoga is frequently used in conjunction with standard treatment approaches for eating disorders. However, yoga's efficacy and effectiveness in preventing and treating eating disorders has remained unclear. The aim of this comprehensive review and meta-analysis is to review the extant literature and assess the effects of yoga in the prevention and intervention of eating disorder symptoms and correlates in both clinical and non-clinical populations. Studies assessing yoga and its effect on eating disorder symptoms and/or body image as related to disordered eating, were eligible for inclusion. The comprehensive review details correlational, non-controlled, non-randomized controlled, and yoga comparison studies. For the meta-analysis, only randomized controlled trials comparing a yoga-based intervention to a non-yoga control group were included. In total, 43 studies are included in this review, with 11 trials involving 754 participants included in the meta-analysis. Results of the comprehensive review and meta-analyses results indicated yoga interventions demonstrated a small, significant effect on global eating disorder psychopathology, a moderate-to-large effect on binge eating and bulimia, and a small effect on body image concerns, as compared to the control conditions. There was no statistically significant effect on dietary restraint in either direction. Additionally, results indicated a small-to-moderate effect on a composite measure of eating disorder-related constructs. These findings suggest that yoga-based interventions may be an effective approach supporting the prevention and treatment of eating disorders.

Clinical implications

- Yoga interventions reduce global eating disorder psychopathology, binge eating and bulimia, and eating disorder-related constructs.
- Yoga interventions have a positive effect on body image concerns.
- Yoga interventions have no significant effect on dietary restraint in either direction.
- Yoga-based interventions may be an effective approach supporting the prevention and treatment of eating disorders.

Introduction

Anorexia nervosa (AN), bulimia nervosa (BN), and binge eating disorder (BED), the three primary eating disorders (EDs), are a set of complex disorders affecting how a person relates to food, eating, and the body (American Psychiatric Association, 2013; Cook-Cottone, 2020). In AN, individuals restrict food, have a distorted experience of their body and body image, demonstrate a drive for thinness, and may binge and purge (American Psychiatric Association, 2013). In BN, individuals struggle with emotional and physical dysregulation; body and body image concerns; and engage in a binge-purge cycle (American Psychiatric Association, 2013). In BED, individuals engage in frequent binges, experience emotional and physical dysregulation, and do not compensate with purging (American Psychiatric Association, 2013). For those with EDs, the body and eating become the central point of cognitive and emotional focus (Cook-Cottone, 2020). The body is the perceived source of symptoms (e.g., body dissatisfaction, felt sense of emotions) as well as the place where many of the symptoms take a toll (e.g., bone density issues, malnutrition, electrolyte imbalance, and other consequences of extreme weight loss or gain; American Psychiatric Association, 2013).

Outcomes related to treatment for EDs have shown only moderate effects with cognitive behavioral therapy, bonafide psychotherapy, and family-based interventions showing the most promise (Cook-Cottone, 2020; Grenon et al., 2019; Van den Berg et al., 2019). While comprehensive treatment programs across methodologies address cognitive and emotional symptoms, rarely do these manualized programs integrate somatic or body work. The same could be said for prevention. Ariel-Donges et al. (2019) report that, for many years, the gold standard for addressing body dissatisfaction has been cognitive dissonance and media literacy interventions, both of which are cognitive approaches. Those at risk for and struggling with EDs have little opportunity to learn and practice positive embodiment, such as learning how to be and work with their bodies in healthy ways and experiencing the body as a source for grounding, connection, breathwork, emotional experience, relaxation, and intuition (Cook-Cottone, 2020; Neumark-Sztainer et al., 2020; Perey & Cook-Cottone, 2020; Piran & Neumark-Sztainer, 2020). Perhaps in response to this gap in intervention, many treatment centers regularly include embodied practices, such as yoga, in their therapeutic offerings.

Yoga, a mind-body practice, is frequently used in conjunction with standard treatment approaches for EDs, with many treatment centers incorporating yoga classes into their schedules, and practitioners referring patients to yoga. Yoga is theorized to help support and maintain protective factors associated with wellbeing, and reduce risk for disordered eating through active practice being with and working with physical sensations, emotions, and cognitions

(Cook-Cottone, 2020). However, despite the acceptance and utilization of yoga among practitioners and the growing support for a positive embodiment model for understanding the mechanism of change, yoga's efficacy and effectiveness in preventing and treating EDs is unclear (Cook-Cottone, 2020; Klein & Cook-Cottone, 2013). In order to address this need in a comprehensive manner, this review and meta-analysis was written as one component of a special issue on yoga, embodiment, and eating disorders which includes two articles on the theoretical connection among yoga, embodiment, and disordered eating (see Perey & Cook-Cottone, 2020; Piran & Neumark-Sztainer, 2020), an article detailing a conceptual model describing mechanisms for how yoga practice may support positive embodiment (Cox & Tylka, 2020), an article on social justice and inclusion issues as related to these three constructs (Webb et al., 2020), as well as an article detailing potential future directions in research (Cox, Cook-Cottone et al., 2020). The specific aim of this review and meta-analysis, within the context of the larger special issue, is to assess the effects of yoga on ED symptoms and correlates in both clinical and non-clinical populations via a review and analysis of the extant literature.

Eating disorders, mechanisms of change, and yoga

When EDs are viewed from the perspective of being with and working with the experiences of the body, there is a clear intersection among biopsychosocial mechanisms associated with ED risk, the onset and maintenance of EDs, factors associated with wellbeing and recovery, and the mechanisms and benefits of yoga (Cook-Cottone, 2015, 2020). As the body of work exploring yoga as a prevention and treatment intervention for disordered eating grows, so does the theoretical framework for understanding its effectiveness. Yoga and ED researchers have identified several factors that appear to be related to risk and pathology that are also known to be positively affected by the practice of yoga. These include: stress reactivity (Hopkins et al., 2016), negative affect (e.g., depression and anxiety; Ariel-Donges et al., 2019; Carei et al., 2010; Halliwell et al., 2018; Pacanowski et al., 2020), emotion regulation difficulties (Brennan et al., 2020; Hopkins et al., 2016), self-objectification (Cox et al., 2016; Daubenmier, 2005; Fredrickson & Roberts, 1997; Mahlo & Tiggemann, 2016), negative body image (Ariel-Donges et al., 2019; Halliwell et al., 2019), body dissatisfaction (Halliwell et al., 2018; Pacanowski et al., 2020), body surveillance (Halliwell et al., 2019, 2018), self-criticism (Brennan et al., 2020) and loneliness and isolation (Pacanowski et al., 2020).

Going beyond the amelioration of risk and dysregulation, yogic approaches to disordered eating are also aligned with positive psychological approaches in which flourishing and positive embodiment are emphasized (Cook-Cottone, 2015, 2020). Positive embodiment is defined as a way of being in which awareness and experience is conceptualized as residing in and manifesting from the body (Cook-Cottone, 2020). In addition to shifting how individuals think about their body, theories of embodiment hold that interventions must also change how individuals inhabit and experience their bodies (Cook-Cottone, 2020; Halliwell et al., 2019, 2018; Menzel & Levine, 2011; Piran, 2016). Existing interventions addressing body image components of disordered eating have incorporated behavioral elements allowing for active practice of new ways of being; however, most are primarily cognitive and based on models of attitude change (Halliwell et al., 2019). Notably, positive embodiment practices such as yoga offer something beyond the reprieve from symptoms (Cook-Cottone, 2020). They offer skills for, and direction toward, a life that an individual wants to be present in, a life in which the body is a resource and connection with the self is the center of an unfolding experience of being each and every day (Cook-Cottone, 2020).

Yoga has been identified as a specific and accessible approach to positive embodiment (Cook-Cottone, 2015, 2020; Halliwell et al., 2019). Further, yoga is readily available and cost effective (Ariel-Donges et al., 2019). Yoga cultivates a direct experience of the body (Karlsen et al., 2018). Yoga incorporates concentration and meditation practices, physical awareness and movement, as well as breath awareness (McIver et al., 2009). Yoga is believed to be a practice in body awareness which involves attentive focus on, and awareness of, internal body sensations, which has been found to be low among persons with EDs (Karlsen et al., 2018). Yoga and ED researchers have identified several constructs that are aligned with a positive embodiment approach to prevention and recovery. These include: mindfulness (Brennan et al., 2020; Douglass, 2009), self-compassion (Brennan et al., 2020), body appreciation (Halliwell et al., 2018), positive body image (Halliwell et al., 2019; Tylka & Wood-Barcalow, 2015), body connectedness (Halliwell et al., 2019), functionality appreciation (Halliwell et al., 2018), positive affect (Pacanowski et al., 2020), and cultivating of a sense of community (Pacanowski et al., 2020).

To date there have been three comprehensive reviews, but no meta-analyses, conducted on the research related to yoga and EDs (Domingues & Carmo, 2019; Klein & Cook-Cottone, 2013; Ostermann, Vogel, Boehm et al., 2019). In 2013, Klein and Cook-Cottone reviewed the extant research which included 14 articles (40% cross sectional studies and 60% longitudinal designs) that explored the effectiveness of yoga interventions for preventing and treating EDs. Overall, findings indicated that yoga practitioners were reported to be at a decreased risk for EDs, and ED risk and symptoms were either reduced or unchanged after yoga interventions.

In 2019, Domingues and Carmo reviewed 12 cross-sectional studies and concluded that the results across studies were inconsistent. Yoga practice was reported to be associated with healthier eating behaviors, lower disordered eating symptoms, higher positive body image, and stronger body satisfaction. They also suggested that a high dosage of yoga may be associated with a higher prevalence of ED behaviors. The specific studies that reported this were unique and relative outliers in terms of the specific relevance to the larger question of yoga risk and ED recovery. For example, one of the studies combined yoga and Pilates (a physical fitness system that integrates the use of apparatus to complete strength and flexibility exercises) as a single construct, finding increased risk of binge eating and unhealthy and extreme weight control behaviors to occur only in male survey respondents (Neumark-Sztainer et al., 2011). The second study found higher rates of orthorexia (a condition involving obsessive behavior organized around the pursuit of a healthy diet) among instructors of body/mind classes (Herranz Valera et al., 2014). Note, orthorexia is not a clinical ED.

Last, Ostermann, Vogel, Boehm et al. (2019) conducted a systematic review on the effects of yoga on EDs, reviewing eight randomized controlled trials and four non-randomized controlled trials on yoga for patients with EDs and other individuals with disordered eating and/or body dissatisfaction. The authors reported that comparison of yoga to untreated control groups yielded effect sizes that were small to moderately sized and, in most cases, not significant. This report concluded that there was limited evidence on the safety and effectiveness of yoga among patients with EDs. This review included citations through July 2018. A significant limitation of the review was that it analyzed all eating-related symptoms as one construct, rather than by specific symptoms relevant to the prevention and treatment of EDs. Further, the statistical analysis was limited to the calculation of an effect size for each outcome measure within each study. Without statistically combining data across studies, the ability to meaningfully synthesize the data is limited.

To meet the need for an updated review and meta-analysis of RCTs, this study was conducted to integrate recently published studies as well as to systematically analyze constructs relevant and specific to the prevention and treatment of disordered eating. Note, 9 of the 43 articles (21%) included in this review and meta-analysis were published in 2019 and 2020. This report is detailed in two sections. The first section is a comprehensive literature review. The second section includes a series of meta-analyses of the qualifying RCTs comparing yoga to non-yoga (control) groups for ED prevention and intervention. The meta-analyses address four domains of outcomes including: global ED psychopathology; binge eating and bulimia; dietary restraint and eating concerns; and body image concerns. A fifth meta-analysis measures an overall, or summary, effect.

Comprehensive review of the literature (2005 to 2020)

This section reviews correlational, non-controlled, non-randomized controlled, and qualitative studies. Two RCTs were included in the section under non-controlled trials as they explored various conditions under which yoga was provided, rather than comparing a yoga intervention to a non-yoga control group. Papers eligible for this review were found using the search strategy and meeting the eligibility criteria detailed in the methods section below.

Study characteristics

All studies included in the systematic review were published between 2005, when research on eating disorders and yoga began, and 2020. Of the 43 included articles, 10 of them were correlational studies (Bak-Sosnowska & Urban, 2017; Daubenmier, 2005; Delaney & Anthis, 2010; Dittmann & Freedman, 2009; Flaherty, 2014; Mahlo & Tiggemann, 2016; Martin et al., 2013; Neumark-Sztainer, MacLehose, et al., 2018; Prichard & Tiggemann, 2008; Zajac & Schier, 2011), 11 were non-controlled trials (Cook-Cottone et al., 2008, 2010; Dale et al., 2009; Diers et al., 2020; Cox et al., 2016, 2019; Hall et al., 2016; Impett et al., 2006; Kramer & Cuccolo, 2019; Rani & Rao, 2005; Scime et al., 2006), 5 were non-randomized controlled trials (Cook-Cottone et al., 2017; Cox et al., 2017; Gammage et al., 2016; Norman et al., 2014; Scime & Cook-Cottone, 2008), 2 were RCTs comparing yoga conditions without a no-yoga control group (Cox, Ullrich-French, et al., 2020; Frayeh & Lewis, 2018), 6 were qualitative studies (Diers et al., 2020; Dittmann & Freedman, 2009; McIver et al., 2009; Neumark-Sztainer, Watts et al., 2018; Ostermann, Vogel, Starke et al., 2019; Pizzanello, 2016), and 11 were RCTs. Note, the Dittmann and Freedman (2009) article included two studies and was therefore assigned to both the correlational and qualitative categories. The Diers et al. (2020) study utilized a mixed-methods design and was assigned to both the non-controlled trials and qualitative categories.

Correlational studies

The 10 correlational studies varied substantially: 8 compared yoga practitioners to those who engaged in fitness exercise, and/or those who did no yoga or exercise; 1 surveyed yoga practitioners; and 1 compared different types of yoga. See Table 1 for study design, participants, and yoga-related outcomes. Overall, these studies suggest that those who practice yoga have more body awareness (Daubenmier, 2005; Dittmann & Freedman, 2009), body responsiveness (Daubenmier, 2005; Dittmann & Freedman, 2009), and body satisfaction (Daubenmier, 2005; Dittmann & Freedman, 2009; Flaherty, 2014; Neumark-Sztainer, MacLehose et al., 2018); score higher on body image and esteem measures (Bak-Sosnowska & Urban, 2017; Mahlo & Tiggemann, 2016);

Table 1. Characteristics of correlational studies included in the review.

Study	Design Notes	Participants	Yoga-Related Outcome Notes
		Yoga vs. Exercise, No-Yoga, or No-Exercise	
Bak-Sosnowska & Urban, 2017	Surveyed women participating in group yoga classes and other types of group fitness classes, and compared body image between the two groups	Group yoga class participants (n = 56) between the ages of 24 and 60 years (M = 35.10, SD = 7.94) Other group fitness class participants (n = 56) between the ages of 18 and 59 years (M = 32.51, SD = 9.55)	High levels of weekly physical activity were found in both groups. Yoga practitioners had higher body esteem across all subscales (i.e., sexual attractiveness, weight concern, physical condition) and less body dissatisfaction than other group fitness class participants.
Daubenmier, 2005	Surveyed a community sample of women, comparing yoga practitioners, aerobics class participants, and a baseline comparison group that did not participate in either yoga or aerobics classes	Community women (n = 139) between the ages of 18 and 87 years (M = 37.16, SD = 14.29)	Yoga practitioners showed higher body awareness, body responsiveness, and body satisfaction, as well as lower self-objectification than both the aerobics and baseline comparison groups. The yoga group reported lower ED symptomology than the aerobics group and similar levels of ED symptomology as the baseline comparison group. More hours spent doing yoga each week was associated with less self-objectification, and more yoga expertise was associated with greater body satisfaction. Amount of experience was not associated with ED symptomology in the yoga group, however, in the aerobics group, time spent doing aerobics each week was positively associated with ED symptomology. Body responsiveness and body awareness explained group differences in self-objectification, body satisfaction and ED symptomology.
Flaherty, 2014	Surveyed men recruited from yoga studios and fitness centers, and examined body image satisfaction among yoga beginners, experienced yoga practitioners, and non-yoga practicing aerobic and weight training exercisers	Yoga beginners (n = 26, M age = 40.3 yrs, SD = 11.6) Experienced yoga practitioners (n = 22, M age = 46.4 yrs, SD = 11.6) Non-yoga practicing aerobic and weight training exercisers (n = 34, M age = 41.2 yrs, SD = 11.9)	Body image satisfaction was significantly higher among yoga groups than among exercisers. There was no significant difference in body image satisfaction between beginner and experienced yoga practitioners.

(Continued)

Table 1. (Continued).

Study	Design Notes	Participants	Yoga-Related Outcome Notes
Mahlo & Tiggemann, 2016	Surveyed female Iyengar yoga practitioners, Bikram yoga practitioners, and university students that did not practice yoga	Iyengar practitioners ($n = 124$) between the ages of 22 and 75 years ($M = 51.16$, $SD = 12.34$) Bikram practitioners ($n = 69$) between the ages of 18 and 66 years ($M = 36.35$, $SD = 11.53$) University students ($n = 127$) between the ages of 17 and 57 years ($M = 21.37$, $SD = 7.27$)	Yoga practitioners scored higher on positive body image and embodiment, and lower on self-objectification, than non-yoga participants. The relationship between yoga participation and positive body image was serially mediated by embodiment and reduced self-objectification. Bikram practitioners endorsed appearance-related reasons for participating in yoga more than Iyengar practitioners. There were no significant differences between Iyengar and Bikram yoga practitioners on body image variables.
Martin et al., 2013	Surveyed female exercisers from fitness centers, yoga centers, and the community	Females ($n = 159$) between the ages of 18 and 80 years ($M = 41.81$, $SD = 16.43$)	Yoga participation was positively associated with mindful eating, trait mindfulness, and body awareness, and negatively associated with disordered eating. The relationship between yoga practice and disordered eating was mediated by body awareness. Cardio-based exercise participation was positively associated with disordered eating and negatively associated with trait mindfulness.
Neumark-Sztainer, MacLehose, et al., 2018	Sampled participants in Project EAT, a 15-year longitudinal study, using two waves (EAT-III and EAT-IV) collected five years apart	General population, young adults ($n = 1664$, M age $= 31.1$ yrs, $SD = 1.6$) 16.2% ($n = 268$) of the sample reported practicing yoga 30 minutes or more each week	At EAT-IV data collection, yoga practitioners had higher concurrent body satisfaction than those not practicing yoga (after controlling for EAT-III body satisfaction and body mass index). Among yoga practitioners, more time practicing yoga each week was associated with increased body satisfaction. Among those with prior low levels of body satisfaction (i.e., 1st quartile at EAT-III), EAT-IV body satisfaction was higher among yoga practitioners than other young adults.

(Continued)

Table 1. (Continued).

Study	Design Notes	Participants	Yoga-Related Outcome Notes
Prichard & Tiggemann, 2008	Surveyed fitness class participants exploring exercise type, reasons for exercise, self-objectification, body esteem, and ED behavior	Female fitness class participants (n = 571) between the ages of 18 and 71 years (M = 35.99, SD = 11.93)	Participation in yoga-based exercise classes was negatively associated with self-objectification and appearance-related reasons for exercise, and positively associated with health and fitness reasons for exercise. No relationship was found between yoga participation and disordered eating. Participation in cardio-based workouts (e.g., on cardiovascular machines) was positively associated with self-objectification, disordered eating, and appearance-related reasons for exercise, and negatively associated with body esteem. Time spent exercising within the fitness center environment was more strongly related to body image and eating disturbance, than time spent exercising outside of that environment. Appearance-related reasons for exercise mediated the relationships between exercise types and self-objectification, disordered eating, and body esteem.
Zajac & Schier, 2011	Surveyed body image dysphoria and motivation to exercise in Polish and Canadian women practicing yoga or aerobics	Canadian aerobics participants (n = 38, M age = 26.82 yrs, SD = 12.86) Canadian yoga practitioners (n = 30, M age = 24.37 yrs, SD = 10.26) Polish aerobics participants (n = 40, M age = 25.55 yrs, SD = 5.32) Polish yoga practitioners (n = 30, M age = 35.73 yrs, SD = 9.79)	Polish yoga practitioners scored significantly lower than the three other groups on measures of negative body related emotions, suggesting some interplay between specific cultural and motivational factors. Yoga practitioners (of both nationalities) scored significantly higher on positive health and stress management reasons for exercise, and significantly lower on weight management reasons for exercise, than aerobics participants.
Yoga Practitioners			

(Continued)

Table 1. (Continued).

Study	Design Notes	Participants	Yoga-Related Outcome Notes
Delaney & Anthis, 2010	Surveyed women who practice yoga, exploring the relationship between type of yoga and different aspects of body image. Classes were considered high, medium, or low mind-body, determined by how well they emphasized the "mind" aspects of yoga (e.g., meditation, breathing, mindfulness, and chanting) as much as the "body" aspects of yoga (e.g., postures and fitness)	Adult female yoga practitioners ($n = 92$) between the ages of 23 and 81 years ($M = 45.31$, $SD = 11.95$)	Participants that primarily attended high or medium mind-body yoga classes showed greater internalization of yoga principles than low mind-body yoga class participants. Medium mind-body yoga participants had significantly greater body awareness and body satisfaction than low mind-body yoga participants; high mind-body participants scored similarly to the medium mind-body participants, however, the scores between the high and low mind-body groups were not significantly different. Greater internalization of yoga principles was associated with higher body satisfaction, as well as a greater belief that the participant's weight and appearance is within her control. More yoga experience was associated with lower body surveillance. Longer duration of yoga class attendance and greater self-rated yoga expertise were both associated with higher body awareness. Greater self-rated yoga expertise was also associated with fewer body shape concerns. None of the yoga measures were associated with ED attitudes and behaviors.
Dittmann & Freedman, 2009	Surveyed women who practice yoga, exploring relationships among body satisfaction, body awareness, body responsiveness, intuitive eating, spirituality, and reasons for practicing yoga	Adult female yoga practitioners ($n = 157$) between the ages of 22 and 72 years ($M = 47.4$, $SD = 11.19$)	Yoga participants scored high on measures of body awareness, body responsiveness, intuitive eating, body satisfaction, and spiritual readiness. Higher body responsiveness was associated with higher body awareness and intuitive eating, and higher spiritual readiness was correlated with higher scores on body awareness, body responsiveness, and body satisfaction. When exploring reasons for practice (psychospiritual vs. physical), participants did not vary in regard to body awareness, body responsiveness, or body satisfaction. Psychospiritual reasons for practicing yoga was associated with increased home practice of yoga.

and show more embodiment (Mahlo & Tiggemann, 2016) and intuitive eating (Dittmann & Freedman, 2009). Further, they have less self-objectification (Daubenmier, 2005; Mahlo & Tiggemann, 2016; Prichard & Tiggemann, 2008), lower negative body-related emotions (Zajac & Schier, 2011), less exercising for weight management and appearance reasons (Prichard & Tiggemann, 2008; Zajac & Schier, 2011), and fewer ED symptoms (Daubenmier, 2005; Martin et al., 2013). Notably, internalization of yoga principles, regular yoga practice, positive body image, cultural nuances, and reasons for exercise may all play a role in these relationships, mediating or moderating yoga effects (e.g., Zajac & Schier, 2011). These studies are the building blocks for more causal research, demonstrating associations and relationships among variables. Risk of bias across all studies reported is high as samples were secured via non-probabilistic sampling, leaving risk for sampling bias high (Elfil et al., 2017). Additionally, there are no comparative control groups. Further, with the exception of Neumark-Sztainer, MacLehose et al. (2018), directionality remains unclear.

Non-controlled and non-randomized studies

In total there were 10 non-controlled trials and 5 non-randomized controlled trials. Twelve of the studies were preventative in nature and three studies explored the role of yoga in the treatment of EDs (see Table 2).

Prevention research
Overall, yoga for youth and adults may have a protective effect in terms of increasing protective factors, as well as decreasing ED risk factors, correlates, and symptoms. Five of these studies were part of a 10-year initiative assessing *Girls Growing Wellness and Balance: Yoga and Life Skills to Empower*, a yoga-based ED prevention program integrating psychoeducational, emotional regulation, and dissonance content for 5th grade, middle school girls (Cook-Cottone et al., 2013). These studies found reductions in drive for thinness (Cook-Cottone et al., 2010, 2017; Norman et al., 2014; Scime et al., 2006), body dissatisfaction (Cook-Cottone et al., 2010, 2017; Norman et al., 2014; Scime & Cook-Cottone, 2008; Scime et al., 2006), and bulimia symptoms (Cook-Cottone et al., 2010); and increased social self-concept (Cook-Cottone et al., 2010; Scime & Cook-Cottone, 2008) and self-care (Cook-Cottone et al., 2017). Note, because this series of studies combined yoga with psychoeducational content, it is difficult to ascertain if the yoga, the psychoeducational content, or the combination was what caused the positive effects (e.g., Cook-Cottone et al., 2013).

Several of the prevention studies investigated yoga classes (Cox et al., 2016; Gammage et al., 2016), yoga courses (Cox et al., 2016; Kramer & Cuccolo, 2019), yoga immersions (Impett et al., 2006), yoga trainings (Rani & Rao, 2005), or yoga physical education curriculum (Cox et al., 2017).

Table 2. Characteristics of non-controlled trials; non-randomized, controlled trials; and RCTs comparing yoga conditions included in the review.

Study	Design Notes	Participants	Yoga-Related Outcome Notes
		Prevention Trials	
Cook-Cottone et al., 2010	Non-controlled trial of a 10-week yoga-based eating disorder prevention program, Girls Growing in Wellness and Balance, using a matched sample of participants identifying as either white or non-white minority, analyzed using repeated measures MANOVA	5th grade white ($n = 25$) and non-white minority ($n = 25$) female Girls Group participants (M age = 10.2 yrs, $SD = 0.53$)	Both white and non-white minority Girls Group members showed significant decreases in drive for thinness, body dissatisfaction, and bulimia symptoms, and increases in competence, physical self-concept, social self-concept from pre-test to post-test. These improvements were similar for white and non-white minority girls. There was no change in perceived stress for either group.
Cook-Cottone et al., 2017	Non-randomized, controlled trial of a 14-week version of the yoga-based eating disorder prevention program, Girls Growing in Wellness and Balance, that examined its effect on ED risk factors and self-care, analyzed using repeated measures ANOVAs	5th grade females in Girls Group ($n = 92$, M age = 10.13 yrs, $SD = 0.5$) and waitlist control group ($n = 40$, M age = 10.8 yrs, $SD = 0.27$)	Girls Group participants showed significantly larger decreases in drive for thinness and body dissatisfaction and increases in self-care from pre-test to post-test, as compared to controls. There was no significant difference between Girls Group and control group on change in bulimia symptoms from pre-test to post-test. Participants' bulimia symptoms at pre-test were low.
Cox et al., 2016	Non-controlled, prospective study that assessed the degree to which participants' state mindfulness during yoga explained changes in self-objectification and related outcomes across an 8-week period, analyzed using repeated measures MANOVAs and regression analyses	University students enrolled in yoga classes for academic physical activity credit ($n = 148$, 80% female, 88% between the ages of 18 and 23 years)	Participants reported significant decreases in self-objectification and increases in physical self-concept, health/fitness reasons for exercise, and state mindfulness from pre-test to post-test. There was no change in body shame, mood/enjoyment reasons for exercise, or appearance reasons for exercise. Mindfulness during exercise was linked to increases in health/fitness and mood/enjoyment reasons to exercise and decreases in self-objectification over time.
Cox et al., 2017	Non-randomized, controlled trial examining the effects of a 12-week yoga-based physical education curriculum to promote positive body image, analyzed using repeated measures MANCOVA and multi-level modeling	High school students in a yoga-based PE class ($n = 20$, 90% female, M age = 16.45 yrs) and a traditional PE class ($n = 23$, 57% female, M age = 14.52 yrs)	There was a significant and moderate decrease in trait body surveillance and minimal, insignificant increase in physical self-worth for the yoga class but not the traditional PE class. There was no effect on body appreciation. For students in both yoga-based and traditional PE classes, more mindfulness of the body was associated with less body surveillance.

(Continued)

Table 2. (Continued).

Study	Design Notes	Participants	Yoga-Related Outcome Notes
Cox et al., 2019	Non-controlled, prospective study of college women taking a yoga course, analyzed using latent variable structural equation modeling and latent growth curve analyses	College women taking a yoga course ($n = 323$, M age = 20.31 yrs, $SD = 2.12$)	A change in self-compassion over time predicted positive changes in body surveillance and body appreciation. Change in body appreciation predicted intrinsic motivation for physical exercise.
Gammage et al., 2016	Prettest-posttest repeated measures design that compared a Hatha-style yoga class with a resistance exercise class in a counterbalanced order, analyzed using MANOVA	University women who exercised 2 times per week or less ($n = 46$, M age = 18.98 yrs, $SD = 1.48$)	Body satisfaction was significantly increased after the yoga class. After both classes there was a significant decrease in social physique anxiety, with the magnitude larger after the yoga class compared to the resistance class.
Impett et al., 2006	Non-controlled study of a 2-month Anusara yoga immersion program that examined the associations between yoga and well-being, embodiment, and self-objectification, analyzed using paired-sample t-tests and hierarchical linear modeling	Female ($n = 17$) and male ($n = 2$) yoga immersion participants between the ages of 23 and 57 years ($M = 34.4$, $SD = 8.6$)	Women in the study reported significantly less self-objectification post-test. No significant changes were found in participants' positive affect, negative affect, satisfaction with life, self-acceptance, body awareness, or body responsiveness from pre-immersion to post-immersion. However, practicing more yoga (than one's average) during a given week was associated with increased body awareness, positive affect, and life satisfaction, and decreased negative affect that week.
Kramer & Cuccolo, 2019	Non-controlled study of college students taking an 8-week yoga course, assessing changes in ED symptomology, body image, and related factors over time, analyzed using repeated measures ANOVAs	College students ($n = 99$; 77.8% female; female M age = 20.0 yrs, $SD = 1.46$; male M age = 20.78 yrs, $SD = 1.67$)	Following the course, students reported significantly lower body dissatisfaction and ED pathology, and increased body appreciation, self-compassion, and yoga self-efficacy. No changes in mindfulness were found. Men showed greater reductions in concern with being overweight and greater improvements in body image perception than women.
Norman et al., 2014	Non-randomized, controlled study that explored the role of interpersonal style on the outcomes of a 12-week version of the yoga-based eating disorder prevention program, Girls Growing in Wellness and Balance, analyzed using MANOVA and ANOVAs	5th grade females in Girls Group ($n = 82$) or waitlist control ($n = 37$), between the ages of 9 and 12 years ($M = 10.6$)	Drive for thinness and body dissatisfaction were significantly reduced in the yoga intervention group, compared to controls. No significant differences were found for bulimia symptoms. Symptoms of bulimia were related to a lower personal affiliation among those in the yoga intervention group.
Rani & Rao, 2005	Non-controlled trial investigating the impact of a 2-week yoga training course on body image and mood, analyzed using t-tests	Male ($n = 23$) and female ($n = 17$) young adults between the ages of 20 and 29 years	No significant improvement in body image was found. Depression scores were significantly reduced from pre-test to post-test, and body image was negatively correlated with depression.

(Continued)

Table 2. (Continued).

Study	Design Notes	Participants	Yoga-Related Outcome Notes
Scime & Cook-Cottone, 2008	Non-randomized, controlled study of a 10-week yoga-based eating disorder prevention program, Girls Growing in Wellness and Balance, analyzed using repeated measures MANOVAs and ANOVAs	5th grade females in Girls Group yoga group ($n = 75$) or waitlist control ($n = 69$)	Significant decreases in body dissatisfaction and bulimia attitudes/behaviors and increases in social self-concept were found for the yoga group. No effects were found in drive for thinness, current methods of ED behaviors, future intention to engage in ED behavior, competence, physical self-concept, or perceived stress.
Scime et al., 2006	Non-controlled, pilot study of a 10-week yoga-based eating disorder prevention program, Girls Growing in Wellness and Balance, analyzed using paired samples t-tests	5th grade females ($n = 45$) between the ages of 9 and 11 years	Significant decreases in drive for thinness, body dissatisfaction, and media influence were found from pre-test to post-test.
Treatment Trials			
Cook-Cottone et al., 2008	Non-controlled trial of a manualized, yoga-based group treatment program for females with EDs, analyzed using paired samples t-tests	Adolescent and adult females ($n = 29$) between the ages of 14 and 35 years ($M = 20$), diagnosed with AN or BN	Significant decreases in drive for thinness and body dissatisfaction were found from pre-test to post-test. There was no difference in bulimia symptoms.
Dale et al., 2009	Non-controlled pilot study of a 6-day yoga workshop for women with a history of EDs, analyzed using repeated measures ANOVAs and paired samples t-tests	Adult females ($n = 5$) between the ages of 22 and 36 years ($M = 30$)	Significant decreases in interoceptive deficits, emotion dysregulation, and affective problems were found from baseline to post-test, and maintained at one-month follow-up. There was no significant change in drive for thinness, bulimia, body dissatisfaction, self-esteem, personal alienation, interpersonal insecurity, interpersonal alienation, perfectionism, asceticism, maturity fear, eating disorder risk, ineffectiveness, interpersonal problems, over control, and general psychological adjustment.

(Continued)

Table 2. (Continued).

Study	Design Notes	Participants	Yoga-Related Outcome Notes
Diers et al., 2020	Non-controlled pilot study of a novel 8-week, group-based, therapeutic yoga and body image program for individuals in outpatient treatment for an ED, analyzed using paired samples t-tests	Adults ($n = 67$) between the ages of 18 and 66 years ($M = 38.1$, $SD = 11.1$) receiving outpatient treatment for an ED	Significant improvement in body image concerns were found from pre-test to post-test. For example, decreases were reported in: avoidance of social situations and romantic relationships, dating, or physical intimacy because of feelings about one's body; mood and self-esteem being connected to one's body; percentage of the day spent thinking about one's body; and shame or embarrassment about one's body. Increases were reported in: ability to think about or experience one's body without getting emotionally reactive; feeling confident about one's body shape and appearance; feeling [physically] connected to one's body; and being kind to one's body by one's thoughts and behaviors.
Hall et al., 2016	Non-controlled study of a yoga pilot program for individuals in outpatient treatment for an ED, analyzed using generalized estimating equations	Females ($n = 20$) between the ages of 11 and 18 years ($M = 15.9$, $SD = 1.8$) in outpatient treatment for AN, BN, ARFID, or OSFED	Significant decreases in depression, measured clinical states of anorexia nervosa, state anxiety, weight concern, and shape concern were found over time. There was no change in restraint or eating concerns.
RCTs Comparing Yoga Conditions			
Cox, Ullrich-French, et al., 2020	RCT examining the effect of teaching a single, 45-minute yoga class, comparing three different conditions of yoga instruction delivery: mindfulness-based, appearance-based, and neutral, analyzed using ANOVAs	Females ($n = 62$) between the ages of 18 and 54 years ($M = 23.89$, $SD = 6.86$)	The mindfulness condition showed a greater increase in affect from before to after the yoga class, compared to the appearance condition. The appearance condition reported lower remembered and forecasted pleasure compared to the mindfulness and neutral conditions. Body surveillance was lower in the mindfulness and neutral conditions compared to the appearance condition. There were no significant differences in state mindfulness of the body and state body appreciation across conditions.
Frayeh & Lewis, 2018	RCT examining body image and appearance comparisons, comparing the effect of a single, 60-minute yoga class, delivered in a mirrored vs. non-mirrored room, analyzed using independent samples t-tests, repeated measures MANCOVA and ANCOVAs, and regression analyses	Female university students ($n = 97$) between the ages of 18 and 25 years ($M = 20.71$)	State body satisfaction and state social physique anxiety improved from pre-test to post-test for both conditions. The non-mirrored condition reported significantly fewer appearance comparisons during yoga, and experienced a larger decrease in state social physique anxiety, than the mirrored condition. Within the mirrored condition, those who engaged in more appearance comparisons reported higher state social physique anxiety than those who engaged in fewer comparisons. No between-group differences were found on state body satisfaction and self-objectification.

These studies found yoga to be associated with decreased: body surveillance (Cox et al., 2017, 2019), body dissatisfaction (Kramer & Cuccolo, 2019), depression (Rani & Rao, 2005), negative affect (Impett et al., 2006), self-objectification (Cox et al., 2016; Impett et al., 2006), social physique anxiety (Gammage et al., 2016), and ED pathology (Kramer & Cuccolo, 2019). Among these studies, yoga was reported to increase: mindfulness (Cox et al., 2016), body awareness (Impett et al., 2006), body appreciation (Cox et al., 2019; Kramer & Cuccolo, 2019), body satisfaction (Gammage et al., 2016), positive body image (Cox et al., 2017; Gammage et al., 2016), exercising for health and fitness reasons (Cox et al., 2016), physical self-concept (Cox et al., 2016), life satisfaction (Impett et al., 2006), self-compassion (Cox et al., 2019; Kramer & Cuccolo, 2019), and yoga self-efficacy (Kramer & Cuccolo, 2019).

Among the non-controlled and non-randomized controlled studies, risk of bias is higher in those studies with smaller sample sizes (e.g., Cox et al., 2017; Gammage et al., 2016; Impett et al., 2006; Rani & Rao, 2005) and those without controls (Cook-Cottone et al., 2010; Cox et al., 2016, 2019; Kramer & Cuccolo, 2019; Scime et al., 2006). Further, although causality can be inferred in some cases, risk for bias remains a concern for non-controlled and non-randomized, controlled studies. Without randomized group allocation to a yoga or no-yoga condition, participants either self-select into a group or are placed into a group based on convenience or scheduling demands clouding efficacy inferences.

Treatment research

There are three non-controlled trials exploring the effect of yoga in adjunct to treatment (Cook-Cottone et al., 2008; Hall et al., 2016) or among those with a history of disordered eating (Dale et al., 2009). Outcomes suggest improvement in some ED symptoms and correlates in some cases and no effect in others. Overall, these studies found yoga to be associated with decreases in drive for thinness (Cook-Cottone et al., 2008), body dissatisfaction (Cook-Cottone et al., 2008), weight concern (Dale et al., 2009), shape concern (Dale et al., 2009), AN symptoms (Hall et al., 2016), interoceptive deficits (Dale et al., 2009), emotion dysregulation (Dale et al., 2009), affective problems (Dale et al., 2009), depression (Hall et al., 2016), and anxiety (Hall et al., 2016). No differences were found in these studies for bulimia symptoms (Cook-Cottone et al., 2008; Dale et al., 2009). Dale et al. (2009) found no difference in multiple outcomes, including body dissatisfaction, drive for thinness, self-esteem, perfectionism, eating disorder risk, and general psychological adjustment. Hall et al. (2016) found no change in restraint and eating concern. For all three studies, the risk of bias is high given the small sample sizes and absence of control groups. Further, Cook-Cottone et al. (2008) combined yoga and psychotherapeutic group content, making the contribution of yoga to outcomes unclear.

RCTs comparing yoga conditions

There are two RCTs that could not be included in the meta-analyses as they compared different yoga conditions and did not include a no-yoga group (see Table 2). However, these researchers are the first to take the needed, important next steps of asking questions about the best way to teach a yoga class in order to ameliorate risk for triggering or maintaining ED thoughts and behaviors (see Cook-Cottone & Douglass, 2017 for guidelines). In 2018, Frayeh and Lewis found that individuals in a mirrored yoga condition reported a significantly higher level of state social physique anxiety and more appearance comparisons when compared to the non-mirrored yoga condition. Further, the higher the state social comparisons a person reported, the higher their physique anxiety. In 2020, Cox et al. found significantly higher body surveillance and lower forecasted pleasure in the appearance-based yoga class when compared to mindfulness-based and neutral yoga instruction classes. These well-designed studies suggested that how yoga is delivered has implications for the role yoga can play in ED prevention.

Qualitative studies

Qualitative findings were generally positive across a breadth of important constructs, with two cautions related to body image and yoga being used in service of EDs. The six qualitative studies identified for this review explored the experiences of women engaged in a yoga treatment program for binge eating via data from personal journals (N = 20; McIver et al., 2009), the insights of women recovered from AN who used yoga as part of the recovery process using interviews (N = 16; Pizzanello, 2016), the impact of yoga on young adults' body image using interviews (N = 34; Neumark-Sztainer, Watts et al., 2018), answers to open-ended questions following a pilot yoga and body image intervention (N = 67; Diers et al., 2020), experience of female yoga practitioners via interviews (N = 18; Dittmann & Freedman, 2009), and the experience of a patient with AN using an interview (N = 1; Ostermann, Vogel, Starke et al., 2019). Qualitative study participants reported that their yoga practice was related to reduced ED pathology and behaviors, such as reduced quantity of food eaten as related to binge eating and decreased eating speed (McIver et al., 2009). Further, participants reported a more positive connection with food (McIver et al., 2009). Positive effects on body image were fostered through developing gratitude for one's body (Neumark-Sztainer, Watts et al., 2018), self-confidence (Diers et al., 2020; Neumark-Sztainer, Watts et al., 2018), a sense of accomplishment related to yoga practice, and the benefit of witnessing different types of bodies practicing yoga (Neumark-Sztainer, Watts et al., 2018).

In three studies, there were reports of a potentially negative influence of yoga. For example, when participants made upward comparisons with others (i.e., comparative critique) or engaged in negative self-talk (i.e., inner critique) yoga was perceived to have a negative impact on body image (Diers et al., 2020; Neumark-Sztainer, Watts et al., 2018). Among those who were recovered from AN, some participants cautioned that yoga could be used as a tool for the ED, in the form of over-exercise, or as a pathway to perfectionism, stringent self-discipline, and self-abuse (Pizzanello, 2016). Some participants reported feeling that yoga exposed emotional challenges, as they felt vulnerable or confronted feelings that they were uncomfortable with (Diers et al., 2020).

Qualitative participants also described yoga being associated with increased embodiment and connection (Diers et al., 2020; Dittmann & Freedman, 2009; McIver et al., 2009; Ostermann, Vogel, Starke et al., 2019; Pizzanello, 2016). Participants across studies reported feeling more aware of, connected to, and positive about their physical and emotional well-being and accepting of their bodies (Diers et al., 2020; Dittmann & Freedman, 2009; McIver et al., 2009). One woman with AN reported perceiving and feeling herself again and learning to utilize her body to cope with her traumatic experiences (Ostermann, Vogel, Starke et al., 2019). The practice of yoga was reported to help women shift from judging the body's appearance to appreciating its functionality; recognize the body's ability to ground and stabilize mood; and view embodiment as a pathway for introspection or spiritual growth (Dittmann & Freedman, 2009).

Some participants reported yoga helped them move toward a more authentic experience of self (Pizzanello, 2016), with less discrepancy between the real and ideal self (Dittmann & Freedman, 2009). In three studies, participants reported feeling empowered and in awe of what the body can do related to their yoga practice (Dittmann & Freedman, 2009; Neumark-Sztainer, Watts et al., 2018; Pizzanello, 2016). Other findings included: self-empowerment (McIver et al., 2009; Pizzanello, 2016), decreased perfectionism (Dittmann & Freedman, 2009), and increased present moment awareness (Dittmann & Freedman, 2009; McIver et al., 2009).

Limitations and conclusions of the comprehensive review

Despite the trend toward positive outcomes in ED risk factors, correlates, and behaviors across correlational; non-controlled; non-randomized, controlled; RCTs comparing yoga conditions; and qualitative studies, the question of efficacy of yoga for the prevention and treatment of EDs remains unanswered due to non-probabilistic sampling, study design (no controls or lack of randomization of assignment), and small samples sizes. The limitations of these studies highlight the importance of RCTs exploring the efficacy of yoga for ED prevention and treatment. The next section of this report aggregates and analyzes the RCTs and makes recommendations for future research and practice.

Method

Protocol

PRISMA guidelines were followed to complete this review. Each study is cited, summarized, and evaluated. A study protocol was not completed for this review. To conserve space, we did not include web addresses for funding sources for included studies. All other guidelines were followed and integrated into this review and meta-analysis.

Eligibility criteria

Studies were eligible for inclusion in the review and meta-analysis if they met the following criteria: (a) published in a peer-reviewed journal; (b) yoga was a primary component of intervention or target of inquiry; and (c) investigated ED symptoms and behaviors, or body image as related to disordered eating (e.g., related to risk or maintenance of EDs as indicated in text or by other measures used), as a primary outcome. Articles were excluded if EDs or disordered eating were not the target of study (e.g., body image in the context of cancer or pregnancy), the study explored mindfulness-based practices not explicitly identified as yoga, or the primary aim of the study was weight loss. Studies were also excluded if they were conference abstracts or dissertations/ theses, or were not published in English. Clinical guidelines, opinion papers, and reflection papers were excluded.

Search strategy

Studies were identified through electronic database searches of Academic Search Complete, Alt HealthWatch, CINAHL Plus, Health Source: Nursing/ Academic Edition, MEDLINE, PsycARTICLES, Psychology and Behavioral Sciences Collection, and PsycINFO. The following search terms were used with Boolean search logic: [(yoga) AND (ED OR disordered eating OR eating pathology OR anorexia OR bulimia OR dietary restraint OR binge eating OR purge OR body image OR body dissatisfaction OR body esteem OR drive for thinness OR body image disturbance OR body preoccupation OR eating attitudes OR food preoccupation)]. Searches were limited to articles written in English. The search was last conducted on January 6, 2020. Additionally, the table of contents of the *International Journal of Yoga Therapy* (through volume 29, issue 1), *International Scientific Yoga Journal SENSE* (through volume 6, number 6), and *Journal of Yoga and Physical Therapy* (through volume 9, issue 3) were searched manually. Separate searches of author names were also conducted. Finally, reference lists of previous reviews were also checked.

Study selection and data collection

The selection process for studies is displayed in Figure 1. After duplicates were removed, both authors independently screened the titles and abstracts of the identified papers for eligibility. Full-text papers were then reviewed. Disagreements were resolved through discussion between authors. All 11 RCTS included in the meta-analysis were published between 2007 and 2020 (Ariel-Donges et al., 2019; Brennan et al., 2020; Carei et al., 2010; Halliwell et al., 2019, 2018; Hopkins et al., 2016; Karlsen et al., 2018; McIver et al., 2009; Mitchell et al., 2007; Pacanowski et al., 2020, 2017). One author (AB) performed data extraction on participants (e.g., age, gender), style of yoga, yoga dosage (e.g., session duration and frequency), control type, measures, measurement time points, and outcome. Extracted data was double-checked for accuracy by author CCC.

Methods for assessing risk to internal validity

Risk of bias of individual studies was rated independently by each author using the Cochrane Collaboration's tool, which assesses risk of bias on the following criteria: random sequence generation, allocation concealment, blinding of participants and personnel, blinding of outcome assessment, incomplete outcome data, selective reporting, and other sources of bias.

Calculation of effect sizes

All analyses were performed using Comprehensive Meta-Analysis (CMA; version 3) software. CMA calculated the standardized mean difference (SMD) for individual studies, which was then converted to Hedge's g to correct for small sample sizes (Borenstein et al., 2009). Mean scores for some scales were multiplied by −1 to correct for differences in the direction of the scales. When a study included multiple measures of the same outcome, a mean effect size was computed so that only one effect size for each study was included in the meta-analysis. When a study included a waitlist control and an active comparison group, only the data from the participants in the waitlist control group were used in order to minimize study heterogeneity. A negative g indicates that those in the yoga condition had lower levels of ED behaviors and body image concerns at post-test relative to the control condition. The weight of each study was calculated using the inverse of the variance, as recommended by Borenstein et al. (2009). We conducted analyses using random effects models due to the assumed heterogeneity between studies (Borenstein et al., 2009).

Heterogeneity and subgroup analyses

Q-statistic and I^2 were used to assess heterogeneity of effect sizes between studies. The Q-statistic is used to evaluate the statistical significance of the heterogeneity of effect sizes, while the I^2 statistic measures the proportion of observed variance that is due to true heterogeneity rather than chance (Borenstein et al., 2009). The I^2 statistic ranges from 0–100%, with values of 25%, 50%, and 75% suggesting low, moderate, and high levels of heterogeneity, respectively (Higgins et al., 2003). Outcomes that had significant effect size heterogeneity across studies were further explored using subgroup analyses to identify possible sources of the heterogeneity. All subgroup analyses were conducted using random effects models with the estimate of T^2 pooled across subgroups. This approach is recommended when there are few studies within each subgroup (Borenstein et al., 2009).

Outcome variables

Between-group analyses were performed on the following outcomes:

(1) Global eating disorder psychopathology. This outcome consisted of self-report and clinical interview measures that assessed ED symptoms and behaviors.
(2) Dietary restraint and eating concerns. This outcome consisted of self-report and clinical interview measures of the cognitive and behavioral aspects of restricting food, concern about eating particular foods, drive to be thinner, and fear of gaining weight. This relates cognitive fears with the dietary restraint that is unique to ED behaviors.
(3) Binge eating and bulimia. This outcome consisted of self-report and clinical interview measures of the frequency of binge eating episodes, number of binge eating episodes, and number of days of binge eating in previous 30 days.
(4) Body image concerns. This outcome consisted of self-report and clinical interview measures that assessed body dissatisfaction, weight and shape concerns, thin-ideal internalization, and extent of investment in one's appearance.
(5) Overall summary effect. This outcome consisted of a composite measure of all ED-related constructs, including those that did not fit into one of the aforementioned categories (i.e., body surveillance).

Meta-analysis results

Characteristics of included studies

Figure 1 presents a flowchart of the literature search. Database searches yielded a total of 284 articles, and an additional 10 articles were identified through manual searches of journals, manual searches of authors, and reviewing reference lists. After duplicates were removed, the titles and abstracts of 155 articles were screened for eligibility. Of these, 77 full texts were assessed. There was a total of 11 RCTs that met criteria for inclusion in the meta-analysis.

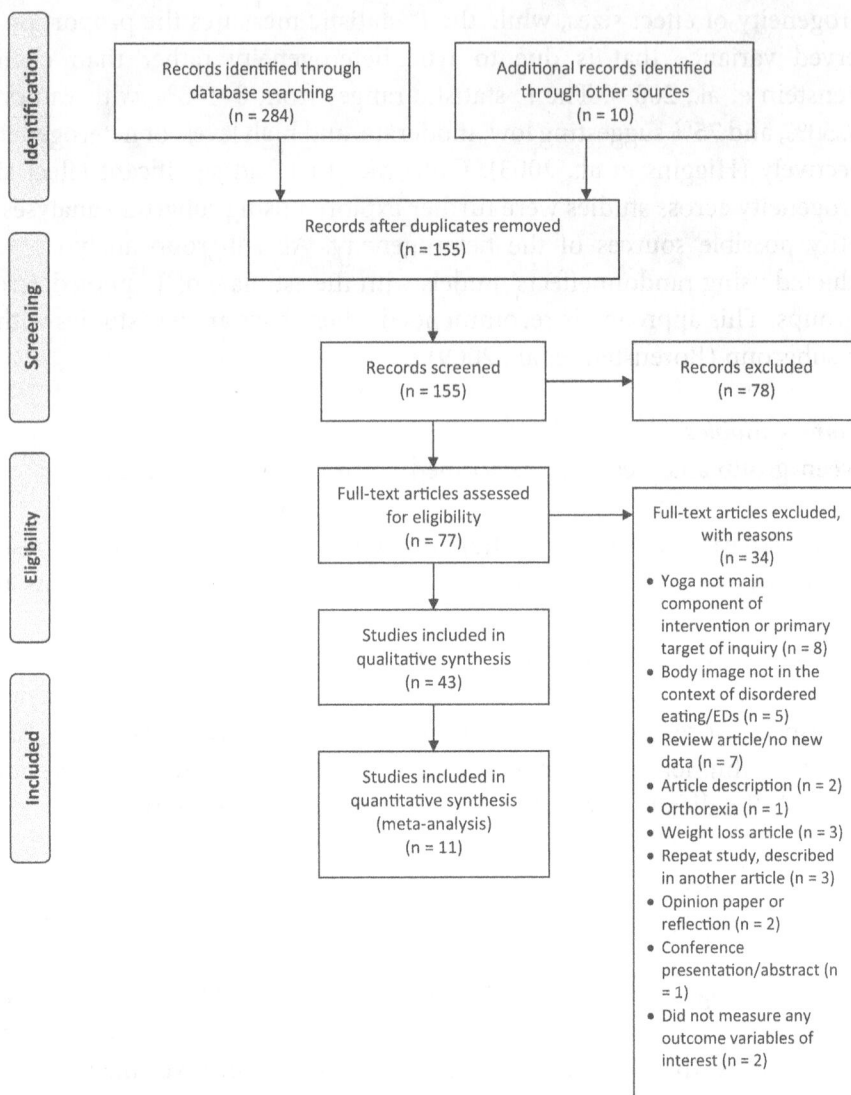

Figure 1. Flowchart of the study selection process.

Among the RCTs, sample sizes ranged from 30 to 344 with a median sample size of 52. The majority of RCTs ($k = 9$) sampled adults only, while 1 study sampled children/adolescents only, and 1 study sampled adolescents and young adults. Five studies utilized a clinical sample. Six of the RCTs were conducted in the United States. The remaining RCTs were conducted in the United Kingdom (Halliwell et al., 2019, 2018), Australia (McIver et al., 2009), Norway (Karlsen et al., 2018), and Canada (Brennan et al., 2020).

Intervention duration ranged from five consecutive days (Pacanowski et al., 2017) to 12 weeks (Ariel-Donges et al., 2019; McIver et al., 2009), with an average duration of 7.6 weeks. Each yoga session ranged from 40 minutes

(Halliwell et al., 2018) to 90 minutes (Hopkins et al., 2016; Karlsen et al., 2018) in length, with an average of about one hour. In the majority of the studies, yoga sessions were once ($k = 5$) or twice ($k = 4$) per week. Styles of yoga used in the in interventions varied widely and included Bikram, Hatha, Iyengar, and Viniyoga.

Finally, the risk of bias ratings for each study varied. Allocation conceal-ment, blinding, and selective outcome reporting were judged by the authors to be unclear in the majority of the studies ($k = 10$). Risk of bias ratings for each study are shown in Table 4.

Synthesis of results

Effect sizes for the five RCT outcomes (global ED psychopathology, dietary restraint and eating concerns, binge eating and bulimia, body image concerns, and overall effects) are displayed in Figure 2.

Global eating disorder pathology

Six of the RCTS included a measure of global ED psychopathology. The effect size for global ED psychopathology was $g = -0.237$, 95% CI [−0.466, −0.008], $p = .043$, indicating a small but statistically significant effect in favor of the yoga condition. Effect sizes did not significantly differ between studies, Q (5) = 3.231, $p = .664$.

Dietary restraint and eating concerns. Six of the RCTs included a measure of dietary restraint and eating concerns. The effect size for dietary restraint and eating concerns was non-significant, $g = -0.132$, 95% CI [−0.373, 0.109], $p = .284$.

Binge eating and bulimia

Five of the RCTs included a measure of binge eating and bulimia. The summary effect for binge eating and bulimia was moderate-to-large, $g = -0.609$, 95% CI [−1.214, −0.004], $p = .049$, with significant heterogeneity of effect sizes between studies, $Q(4) = 22.965$, $I^2 = 82.582$. We performed a subgroup analysis that compared studies with clinical samples to studies with non-clinical samples. The point estimate for clinical samples was $g = -1.280$, $se = 0.285$, $z = -4.485$, $p < .001$, indicating that there was a large, statistically significant effect of yoga on binge eating and bulimia symptoms in clinical samples. The point estimate for non-clinical samples was $g = -0.148$, $se = 0.221$, $z = -0.671$, $p = .502$, indicating that there was no significant effect of yoga interventions on binge eating and bulimia symptoms in non-clinical samples. The difference between groups was significant, $Q(1) = 9.824$, $p = .002$, indicating that the effect of yoga on binge eating and bulimia was significantly different between clinical and non-clinical samples.

Meta-analysis results

Global ED psychopathology.

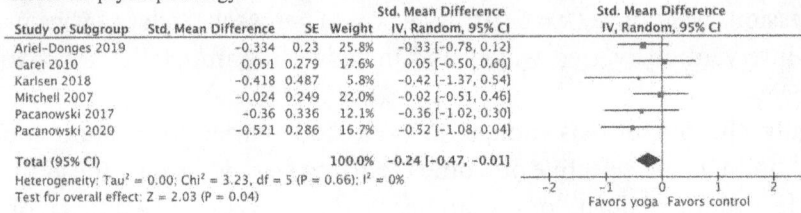

Study or Subgroup	Std. Mean Difference	SE	Weight	Std. Mean Difference IV, Random, 95% CI
Ariel-Donges 2019	-0.334	0.23	25.8%	-0.33 [-0.78, 0.12]
Carei 2010	0.051	0.279	17.6%	0.05 [-0.50, 0.60]
Karlsen 2018	-0.418	0.487	5.8%	-0.42 [-1.37, 0.54]
Mitchell 2007	-0.024	0.249	22.0%	-0.02 [-0.51, 0.46]
Pacanowski 2017	-0.36	0.336	12.1%	-0.36 [-1.02, 0.30]
Pacanowski 2020	-0.521	0.286	16.7%	-0.52 [-1.08, 0.04]
Total (95% CI)			100.0%	-0.24 [-0.47, -0.01]

Heterogeneity: Tau^2 = 0.00; Chi^2 = 3.23, df = 5 (P = 0.66); I^2 = 0%
Test for overall effect: Z = 2.03 (P = 0.04)

Binge eating and bulimia.

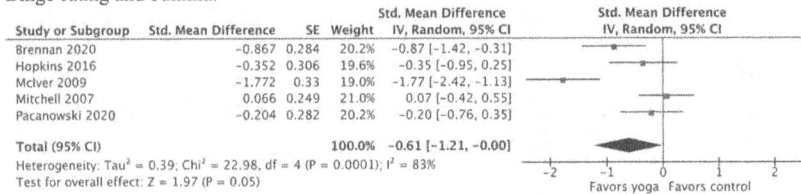

Study or Subgroup	Std. Mean Difference	SE	Weight	Std. Mean Difference IV, Random, 95% CI
Brennan 2020	-0.867	0.284	20.2%	-0.87 [-1.42, -0.31]
Hopkins 2016	-0.352	0.306	19.6%	-0.35 [-0.95, 0.25]
McIver 2009	-1.772	0.33	19.0%	-1.77 [-2.42, -1.13]
Mitchell 2007	0.066	0.249	21.0%	0.07 [-0.42, 0.55]
Pacanowski 2020	-0.204	0.282	20.2%	-0.20 [-0.76, 0.35]
Total (95% CI)			100.0%	-0.61 [-1.21, -0.00]

Heterogeneity: Tau^2 = 0.39; Chi^2 = 22.98, df = 4 (P = 0.0001); I^2 = 83%
Test for overall effect: Z = 1.97 (P = 0.05)

Body image concerns.

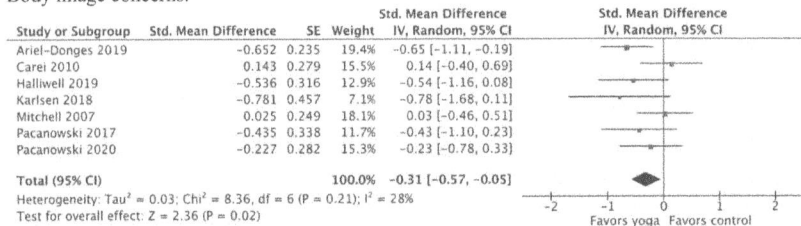

Study or Subgroup	Std. Mean Difference	SE	Weight	Std. Mean Difference IV, Random, 95% CI
Ariel-Donges 2019	-0.652	0.235	19.4%	-0.65 [-1.11, -0.19]
Carei 2010	0.143	0.279	15.5%	0.14 [-0.40, 0.69]
Halliwell 2019	-0.536	0.316	12.9%	-0.54 [-1.16, 0.08]
Karlsen 2018	-0.781	0.457	7.1%	-0.78 [-1.68, 0.11]
Mitchell 2007	0.025	0.249	18.1%	0.03 [-0.46, 0.51]
Pacanowski 2017	-0.435	0.338	11.7%	-0.43 [-1.10, 0.23]
Pacanowski 2020	-0.227	0.282	15.3%	-0.23 [-0.78, 0.33]
Total (95% CI)			100.0%	-0.31 [-0.57, -0.05]

Heterogeneity: Tau^2 = 0.03; Chi^2 = 8.36, df = 6 (P = 0.21); I^2 = 28%
Test for overall effect: Z = 2.36 (P = 0.02)

Dietary restraint and eating concerns.

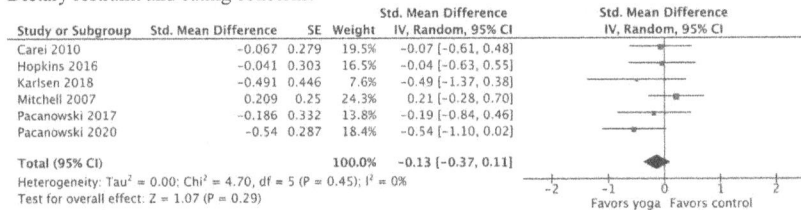

Study or Subgroup	Std. Mean Difference	SE	Weight	Std. Mean Difference IV, Random, 95% CI
Carei 2010	-0.067	0.279	19.5%	-0.07 [-0.61, 0.48]
Hopkins 2016	-0.041	0.303	16.5%	-0.04 [-0.63, 0.55]
Karlsen 2018	-0.491	0.446	7.6%	-0.49 [-1.37, 0.38]
Mitchell 2007	0.209	0.25	24.3%	0.21 [-0.28, 0.70]
Pacanowski 2017	-0.186	0.332	13.8%	-0.19 [-0.84, 0.46]
Pacanowski 2020	-0.54	0.287	18.4%	-0.54 [-1.10, 0.02]
Total (95% CI)			100.0%	-0.13 [-0.37, 0.11]

Heterogeneity: Tau^2 = 0.00; Chi^2 = 4.70, df = 5 (P = 0.45); I^2 = 0%
Test for overall effect: Z = 1.07 (P = 0.29)

Overall effects.

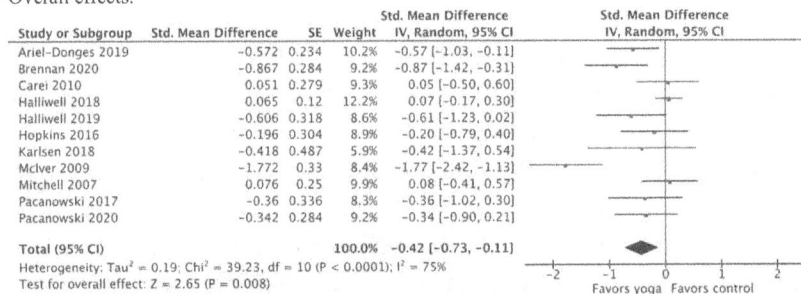

Study or Subgroup	Std. Mean Difference	SE	Weight	Std. Mean Difference IV, Random, 95% CI
Ariel-Donges 2019	-0.572	0.234	10.2%	-0.57 [-1.03, -0.11]
Brennan 2020	-0.867	0.284	9.2%	-0.87 [-1.42, -0.31]
Carei 2010	0.051	0.279	9.3%	0.05 [-0.50, 0.60]
Halliwell 2018	0.065	0.12	12.2%	0.07 [-0.17, 0.30]
Halliwell 2019	-0.606	0.318	8.6%	-0.61 [-1.23, 0.02]
Hopkins 2016	-0.196	0.304	8.9%	-0.20 [-0.79, 0.40]
Karlsen 2018	-0.418	0.487	5.9%	-0.42 [-1.37, 0.54]
McIver 2009	-1.772	0.33	8.4%	-1.77 [-2.42, -1.13]
Mitchell 2007	0.076	0.25	9.9%	0.08 [-0.41, 0.57]
Pacanowski 2017	-0.36	0.336	8.3%	-0.36 [-1.02, 0.30]
Pacanowski 2020	-0.342	0.284	9.2%	-0.34 [-0.90, 0.21]
Total (95% CI)			100.0%	-0.42 [-0.73, -0.11]

Heterogeneity: Tau^2 = 0.19; Chi^2 = 39.23, df = 10 (P < 0.0001); I^2 = 75%
Test for overall effect: Z = 2.65 (P = 0.008)

Figure 2. Meta-analysis results. Global ED psychopathology.Binge eating and bulimia.Body image concerns.Dietary restraint and eating concerns.Overall effects.

Body image concerns

Seven of the RCTs included a measure of body image concerns. On average, yoga participants reported significantly lower levels of body image concerns compared to controls. The summary effect size was small, $g = -0.311$, 95% CI [−0.568, −0.053], $p = .018$. Effect sizes did not significantly differ between studies, $Q(6) = 8.355$, $p = .213$, $I^2 = 28.185$.

Overall effect

All 11 RCTs were included in a meta-analysis examining the overall effect on ED-related measures. The summary effect size was small-to-moderate, $g = -0.422$, 95% CI [−0.734, −0.110], $p = .008$. There was significant heterogeneity between studies $Q(10) = 39.209$, $I^2 = 74.496$. Results of the subgroup analysis indicated that the point estimate for clinical samples was $g = -0.676$, $se = 0.231$, $z = -2.927$, $p = .003$. The point estimate for non-clinical samples was $g = -0.240$, $se = 0.190$, $z = -1.265$, $p = .206$. The difference between groups was not statistically significant, $Q(1) = 2.121$, $p = .145$. However, this does not necessarily indicate that the true effect sizes were the same. It is possible that the effect is either small or that there was not enough statistical power to detect an effect, particularly given the limited number of studies included in each subgroup (Borenstein et al., 2009).

Discussion

Overall, the comprehensive review and meta-analysis of the 43 qualifying articles found yoga to be generally effective for the prevention and treatment of EDs. Specifically, the comprehensive review of studies showed a trend in the reduction of ED risk, correlates and symptoms in prevention and treatment conditions among the 10 correlational, 11 non-controlled, 5 non-randomized controlled, 2 RCTS comparing yoga conditions, and 6 qualitative studies. The first on this topic, the meta-analysis of 11 RCTs comparing yoga to control conditions in the prevention and treatment of EDs found a significant reduction in global ED psychopathology, binge eating and bulimia symptoms, and body image concerns. There was no effect on dietary restraint and eating concerns.

The comprehensive review demonstrated the growing breadth of research in this area, beginning with the first studies published on yoga and EDs (2005). Correlational studies found a trend toward yoga practice being associated with increased body awareness, body responsiveness, body satisfaction, body image and esteem, embodiment, and intuitive eating, and less self-objectification, negative body-related emotions, and exercising for weight and appearance reasons, as well as fewer ED symptoms. Further, these studies showed that internalization of yoga principles, regular yoga practice, positive body image, cultural nuances, and reasons for exercise may play a role in these relationships. Non-controlled and controlled studies addressed yoga as pre-vention for and support in the treatment of EDs. Prevention studies suggested that yoga for youth and adults may have some protective effect in terms of increasing protective factors, as well as decreasing ED risk factors, correlates, and symptoms. The three noncontrolled treatment studies had mixed findings, with improvement in some ED symptoms and correlates, but no effect on others. The two RCTs with different yoga conditions showed that the condi-tions in a yoga class matter, and that some conditions (e.g., mirrors, appear-ance-related instruction) can place yoga practitioners at increased risk or attenuate positive outcomes. Qualitative studies support positive findings and echoed the potential risk of yoga in some conditions and contexts, reporting that comparative critiques, negative self-talk and use of yoga as a pathway to perfectionism, stringent self-discipline, and accomplishment may increase risk.

Meta-analytic findings

First, findings indicate that yoga is beneficial as related to the reduction in global ED psychopathology (small and significant effect). This is consistent with positive findings explicated in reviews by Klein and Cook-Cottone (2013) and Domingues and Carmo (2019), and inconsistent with Ostermann, Vogel, Boehm et al.'s (2019) finding that yoga has no effect on eating related symp-toms. It is likely that the superior methodology (i.e., meta-analysis) and addition of recent, well-designed studies contributed to our positive findings. Further, the meta-analytic portion of our study focused exclusively on ED symptoms and behaviors. To increase translational utility, separate analyses were conducted for each distinct ED symptom and behavior rather than a sole focus on general outcomes.

Next, as related to specific ED symptoms, our study found that yoga was significantly beneficial in the reduction of binge eating and bulimia symptoms (medium effect) and body image concerns (small effect). Our results on the binge eating and bulimia outcome are consistent with the findings of Klein and Cook-Cottone (2013); binge eating and bulimia symptoms were not specifi-cally reported on by Domingues and Carmo (2019) or Ostermann, Vogel, Boehm et al. (2019). The body image concerns results are consistent with findings reported by Klein and Cook-Cottone (2013) as well as Domingues and Carmo (2019), who reported that yoga was correlated with higher body image and stronger body satisfaction. Interestingly, participation in yoga did not have an effect on dietary restraint and eating concerns. It may be that yoga is able to support interoceptive/body awareness, body image, body connection, affect regulation (reduce negative affect, increase positive affect), body image other factors more specifically supportive of reductions in binge eating and purging behaviors (Dale et al., 2009; Diers et al., 2020; Hall et al., 2016; Klein &

Cook-Cottone, 2013). It is important to note that food restriction is one of the primary symptoms of anorexia nervosa, the most difficult to treat ED, with food avoidance and restriction requiring very specific treatment techniques, including food exposure and activities like family meals (Cardi et al., 2019). These behaviors appear to be more resistant to treatment in general and may take longer to address. The relative short durations of yoga trials may not be sufficient to show effect on restraint. Last, as mentioned in qualitative findings yoga can be utilized, by some and in specific circumstances, in a way that aligns with traits associated with restraint such as perfectionism, stringent self-discipline, and self-abuse (e.g., Pizzanello, 2016). Notably and importantly, these findings suggest that yoga does not appear to cause an increase in dietary restraint and eating concerns.

Limitations and future directions

This meta-analysis had several limitations. First, despite the growing body of literature on yoga and eating disorders, there were still a relatively small number of RCTs we were able to include in the meta-analysis. Second, due to the limited number of studies, we were unable to run subgroup analyses for a variety of important study characteristics, including dosage (Cook-Cottone, 2013), style of yoga, and use of active vs. waitlist control groups. Third, we were unable to conduct a meta-analysis using positive embodiment and related positive constructs as an outcome because these variables were included in only two studies. A random-effects meta-analysis with only two studies is likely to produce an inaccurate summary effect and misleading confidence interval (Borenstein et al., 2009). Finally, each meta-analysis examined the effects of the yoga interventions only at post-test; due to high variability in follow-up measurement dates, we were unable to examine the long-term effects of the interventions.

Future directions should include continued encouragement of use of best practices for RCT research (e.g., manualization, treatment integrity assessments, active control groups). Within the current body of research, there is insufficient attention paid to the factors listed in the Cochrane risk of bias tool including adequate sequence generation (related to randomization procedures), allocation concealment, blinding (participants and study personnel), selective outcome reporting, and other sources of bias (see Table 4). Further, future designs should target specific mechanisms of change (e.g., the content of instructor guidance; style of yoga; sequences and specific practices designed to manage body image, mood, stress, or trauma symptoms) and include detailed reports of protocols so that they can be replicated and extended. More detailed guidance in these areas follows.

Specific to the delivery of yoga, the authors should report the style of yoga, describe in detail the dose and delivery of yoga, manualize the components of the yoga intervention, explicate the specific class sequences for replicability and treatment integrity measures, consider the size of classes (e.g., Brennan et al., 2020 kept all class sizes under 12 to ensure individual attention), and describe how instructors will deal with modifications (Ariel-Donges et al., 2019; Sherman, 2012). The specific yoga protocol should be published as a manual and treatment integrity measures should be utilized. There are a variety of methods for conducting treatment integrity checks. For example, Ariel-Donges et al. (2019) audio recorded all sessions to allow replication by other researchers. Further, a trained research coordinator evaluated 12.5% of the yoga classes offered, using a treatment fidelity checklist based on Sherman's (2012) guidelines to assess consistency across instructors and adherence to protocols.

Exposure to yoga prior to the intervention (naivety to yoga) as well as home/studio practice during the study are critical variables to assess. Among published studies there is substantial variability in regard to yoga experience with limited or no yoga experience part of inclusion criteria for some studies (e.g., Brennan et al., 2020; Karlsen et al., 2018; Pacanowski et al., 2020), regular yoga practice part of exclusion criteria for other studies (Hopkins et al., 2016; McIver, O'Halloran, et al., 2009) and many studies do not address the issue at all. Some studies explicitly encouraged at home practice (e.g., Karlsen et al., 2018; McIver, McGartland, et al., 2009) with many studies not addressing home practice with intervention or control participants. Given the popularity of yoga, assessing this in both the treatment and control group is necessary. Further, requesting that the control group not engage in mind/body and yoga-based activities during the study may be necessary.

Yoga instructors are key to the delivery of yoga. Each author should explain their selection criteria and process for choosing instructors. Instructors should be certified and trained and their certification and training specifically detailed (Ariel-Donges et al., 2019). To avoid biases introduced by within-class inter-actions, follow the exemplar detailed by Ariel-Donges et al. (2019). These researchers balanced the exposure to individual instructors by requiring the participants to attend classes taught by at least two of the three instructors. Using one instructor is not a sufficient way to address this issue. For example, Carei et al. (2010) used the same instructor for all individual sessions, making it impossible to parse out interventionist and intervention effects.

Overall, the studies included in this meta-analysis used waitlist controls or treatment/school as usual (e.g., Ariel-Donges et al., 2019; Brennan et al., 2020; Carei et al., 2010; Halliwell et al., 2018). Mitchell et al. (2007) and Halliwell et al. (2019) used active controls. Mitchell et al. (2007) found that a dissonance induction intervention worked more effectively than yoga when offered over 6 weeks at a low dose of 45 minutes per week, with no differences found between the yoga and assessment-only control groups. Karlsen et al. (2018) used an active control (i.e., two 90-minute educational meetings) to account for the group effect. Halliwell et al. (2019) used pamphlets on yoga, finding positive effects for the yoga vs. control group. Future studies should consider using dissonance-based and exercise-only control groups for prevention yoga interventions, and exercise-only control groups for treatment-based yoga interventions.

More research on the possible contraindications, safety, and conditions under which yoga may be detrimental should be conducted (see Cook-Cottone & Douglass, 2017 for guidelines). Certain conditions may be less helpful, harmful, or more helpful than others (e.g., mirrors; Frayeh & Lewis, 2018; mindfulness vs weight and shape focused instruction; Cox, Ullrich-French, et al., 2020). Qualitatively, some participants cautioned that yoga could be used as tool for the ED as a form of over-exercise or a pathway to perfectionism, stringent self-discipline, and self-abuse (Pizzanello, 2016). How might a yoga intervention counter such phenomena and what approach is most effective?

A specific concern for those with AN is that participation in yoga may be associated with weight loss. In three studies that assessed BMI at pre and posttest, there were mixed findings. Carei et al. (2010) reported no change in BMI among participants that included those diagnosed with AN as well as those with other clinical EDs. McIver et al. (2009) found that those who participated in yoga did have a significant decrease in BMI. However, the participants were adult females diagnosed with BED; it is understandable that a reduction in bingeing would correspond with a reduction in BMI. Hopkins et al. (2016) also measured BMI at pre—and post-test in their study with a community sample of participants. Although there was evidence of a decrease in BMI in the yoga group, it was not statistically significant. Despite evidence suggesting that yoga is likely safe in the prevention and treatment of EDs, more research is needed to better understand the nuances, contexts, and unique risks that yoga participation may pose for some.

Although there are trends emerging in the data, the current body of research is not comprehensive enough to offer specific prescriptions for age, gender, or risk/psychopathology level. In terms of age, correlational, non-controlled, and non-randomized controlled, studies have focused primarily college students and adults with the exception of the series of studies completed by Cook-Cottone's team focusing on 5th grade females (i.e., Cook-Cottone et al., 2010, 2017; Norman et al., 2014; Scime et al., 2006; Scime & Cook-Cottone, 2008) and the study completed by Cox studying adolescents (Cox et al., 2017) suggesting yoga has protective benefits related to ED risk and symptoms (see Tables 1 and 2). Most of the more rigorous studies have been conducted on college age or older participants with only two RCTs assessing outcomes among youth (Carei et al., 2010; Halliwell et al., 2018; Table 3). Overall studies have included mostly females. About a third of correlational studies included males (Table 1) and among the non-controlled, non-randomized controlled studies 33% included males (Table 2). Nearly all the RCTs have been conducted with girls and women with only two RCTs also including boys and young men (Carei et al., 2010; Halliwell et al., 2018; Table 3). Therefore, despite the growing body of evidence, we cannot readily generalize these findings to males or those under college age.

Potential differential efficacy for clinical and non-clinical populations should be further explored. More research is needed to fully understand the best approaches and research protocols for impact among those at risk and those who are already struggling. All of the correlational studies were conducted among non-clinical populations (see Table 1). Twenty percent of the non-controlled and non-randomized controlled studies were conducted among clinical populations (Table 2). The RCT studies were split about equally between clinical and non-clinical populations (Table 3). Currently, most of the intervention studies focus on reducing psychopathology and ED correlates, whereas prevention studies integrate more positive psychology and embodiment variables.

Finally, in terms of exploring mechanisms of change, specific mechanisms associated with the delivery of the yoga class need to be specifically explored such as the nature and extent of mindfulness teachings (Ariel-Donges et al., 2019; Brennan et al., 2020) and the effect of specific poses, breathing exercises, and relaxation techniques (Ariel-Donges et al., 2019). Further, there is currently insufficient data to know if yoga should be offered individually or within the group context and for whom one or the other might be best (Norman et al., 2014). Moreover, studies should continue to look at outcomes related to ED risk, etiology, and maintenance as well as integrate positive psychology constructs and assessments that can effectively explore positive embodiment.

Practice implications and conclusions

Yoga is an affordable and relatively accessible practice for those both in and out of treatment (Ariel-Donges et al., 2019). Overall, these findings suggest that there appears to be a benefit in participation in yoga sessions for those at-risk for and struggling with disordered eating. Findings suggest that yoga may be helpful in reducing global ED psychopathology, binge eating and bulimia symptoms, and body image concerns. Further, there appears to be no effect on dietary restraint and eating concern, neither increasing nor decreasing restriction behaviors. Last, with no studies reporting safety issues, there is no indication that yoga is not safe for those with EDs. However, specific research asking safety-related questions is needed. Additionally, Halliwell et al. (2019) warn that there has been an increase in yoga classes being offered that focus on appearance ideals (e.g., Beach Body Yoga) with less focus on important mindfulness constructs

Table 3. Characteristics of randomized controlled trials included in the review.

Study	Participants	Type of yoga	Dosage	Control type(s)	Outcomes meta-analyzed	Country
Ariel-Donges et al., 2019	75 college females, ages 18 to 30, with body image dissatisfaction and normal eating behaviors	Vinyasa, Ashtanga	60 mins, 2x/week for 12 weeks	Waitlist control	Global ED (EAT-26) Body image concern (MBSRQ-AS)	United States
Brennan et al., 2020	53 adult females, community sample, met diagnostic criteria for BN or BED	Kripalu	90 minutes, 1x/week for 8 weeks	Waitlist control	Binge eating/bulimia (two EDE-Q items on binge eating)	Canada
Carei et al., 2010	53 adolescents, ages 11 to 21, in outpatient treatment for AN, BN, or EDNOS	Private, Viniyoga	60 minutes, 2x/week for 8 weeks	Received standard medical care	Global ED (EDE) Restraint/eating concerns (EDE-R, EDE-EC) Body image concern (EDE-WC, EDE-SC)	United States
Halliwell et al., 2018	344 British children, ages 9 to 11, recruited from four schools	Hatha	40 minutes, 1x/week for 4 weeks	Assessment-only control, attended PE as usual	OBCS-Y-BS [a]	United Kingdom
Halliwell et al., 2019	44 undergraduate females, mean age 20.21	Anusara, Iyengar, Vinyasa	60 minutes, 1x/week for 4 weeks	Reviewed and rated 2 articles about yoga	Body image concern (MBSRQ-BASS) OBCS-BS [a]	United Kingdom
Hopkins et al., 2016	52 females, ages 25 to 45, with elevated levels of perceived stress, dietary restraint, and emotional eating	Bikram	90 minutes, 2x/week for 8 weeks	Waitlist control	Binge eating/bulimia (EDDS item 8) Restraint/eating concerns (DRES)	United States

(Continued)

Table 3. (Continued).

Study	Participants	Type of yoga	Dosage	Control type(s)	Outcomes meta-analyzed	Country
Karlsen et al., 2018	30 adult females, mean age 32.4, with BN or EDNOS	Hatha	90 minutes, 2x/week for 11 weeks	Received two 90 minute group meetings. Topics included nutrition, physical activity, and eating disorders	Global ED (EDE, EDI-2) Restraint/eating concerns (EDE-R, EDE-EC) Body image concern (EDE-WC, EDE-SC)	Norway
McIver, O'Halloran, et al., 2009	50 females, ages 25 to 63, met diagnostic criteria for BED, BMI > 25	Hatha yoga, yoga nidra	60 minutes, 1x/week for 12 weeks	Waitlist control	Binge eating/bulimia (BES)	Australia
Mitchell et al., 2007	93 female undergraduate psychology students, mean age 19.56	Integral	45 minutes, 1x/week for 6 weeks	Dissonance-based intervention group; assessment-only control	Global ED (EDDS) Binge eating/bulimia (BES) Restraint/eating concerns (EDI-DT, TFEQ-R) Body image concern (BSQ-R-10, EDI-BD, IBSS-R)	United States
Pacanowski et al., 2017	38 patients at a residential eating disorder treatment facility, mean age 26.8	Modified Viniyoga	50 minutes/day for 5 consecutive days	Treatment as usual	Global ED (EDE-Q) Restraint/eating concerns (EDE-Q-R, EDE-Q-EC) Body image concern (EDE-Q-WC, EDE-Q-SC)	United States

(Continued)

Table 3. (Continued).

Study	Participants	Type of yoga	Dosage	Control type(s)	Outcomes meta-analyzed	Country
Pacanowski et al., 2020 United States	51 female undergraduate students, ages 18 to 26, mean age 19.6	Modified Viniyoga	50 minutes, 3x/week for 10 weeks	Assessment-only control	Global ED (EAT-26) Binge eating/bulimia (BES, EAT-26-B) Restraint/eating concerns (EAT-26-OC, EAT-26-D, MBSRQ-OWP) Body image concern (MBSRQ)	

Note. BES, Binge Eating Scale; BSQ-R-10, Body Shape Questionnaire-Revised-10; DRES, Dutch Restrained Eating Scale; EAT-26, Eating Attitudes Test-26;—B, Bulimia and Food Preoccupation subscale,—D, Dieting subscale,—OC, Oral Control subscale; EDI, Eating Disorder Inventory:—BD, Body Dissatisfaction subscale,—DT, Drive for Thinness subscale; EDDS, Eating Disorder Diagnostic Scale; EDE/EDE-Q, Eating Disorder Examination/Eating Disorder Examination-Questionnaire:—R, Restraint subscale,—EC, Eating Concern subscale,—WC, Weight Concern subscale,—SC, Shape Concern subscale; IBSS-R, Ideal Body Stereotype Scale-Revised; MBSRQ, Multidimensional Body-Self Relations Questionnaire:—AS, Appearance Scales,—BASS, Body Areas Satisfaction Scale,—OWP, Overweight Preoccupation subscale; OBCS-BS, Objectified Body Consciousness Scale—Body Surveillance subscale; OBCS-Y-BS, Objectified Body Consciousness Scale-Youth Body Surveillance subscale; TFEQ Restraint, Three-Factor Eating Questionnaire Restraint subscale.
[a]This measure was included only in the meta-analysis for overall effects.

such as mindfulness, body appreciation, self-compassion, and acceptance. They assert that these developments in the yoga industry make it difficult to simply recommend yoga as a pathway to wellbeing. Therefore, offering referrals to vetted classes, styles, and instructors may be important. Given the right referral, yoga may be a place of reprieve from risk and struggle, as described by this participant with a clinical ED after participating in yoga classes as part of the intervention, "*This is the only hour in my week when I don't think about my weight.*" (Carei et al., 2010, p. 350).

References

References marked with an asterisk indicate studies included in the meta-analysis, 0000.

American Psychiatric Association. (2013). *Diagnostic and statistical manual of mental disorders* (5th ed.). Washington, DC. https://doi.org/10.1176/appi.books.9780890425596

*Ariel-Donges, A. H., Gordon, E. L., Bauman, V., & Perri, M. G. (2019). Does yoga help college-aged women with body-image dissatisfaction feel better about their bodies? *Sex Roles, 80*(1–2), 41–51.

Bak-Sosnowska, M., & Urban, A. (2017). Body image in women practicing yoga or other forms of fitness. *Archives of Psychiatry and Psychotherapy, 19*(3), 58–68. https://doi.org/10.12740/APP/76338

Borenstein, M., Hedges, L. V., Higgins, J. P., & Rothstein, H. R. (2009). *Introduction to meta-analysis.* John Wiley & Sons.

*Brennan, M. A., Whelton, W. J., & Sharpe, D. (2020). Benefits of yoga in the treatment of eating disorders: Results of a randomized controlled trial. *Eating Disorders: The Journal of Treatment and Prevention, XX*(X), XX–XX. https://doi.org/10.1080/10640266.2020.1731921

Cardi, V., Leppanen, J., Mataix-Cols, D., Campbell, I. C., & Treasure, J. (2019). A case series to investigate food-related fear learning and extinction using in vivo food exposure in anorexia nervosa: A clinical application of the inhibitory learning framework. *European Eating Disorders Review, 27*(2), 173–181. https://doi.org/10.1002/erv.2639

*Carei, T. R., Fyfe-Johnson, A. L., Breuner, C. C., & Brown, M. A. (2010). Randomized controlled clinical trial of yoga in the treatment of eating disorders. *Journal of Adolescent Health, 46*(4), 346–351. https://doi.org/10.1016/j.jadohealth.2009.08.007

Cook-Cottone, C. (2013). Dosage as a critical variable in yoga therapy research. *International Journal of Yoga Therapy, 23*(2), 11–12. https://doi.org/10.17761/ijyt.23.2.g3787hvr118l823p

Cook-Cottone, C., Beck, M., & Kane, L. (2008). Manualized-group treatment of eating disorders: Attunement in mind, body, and relationship (AMBR). *The Journal for Specialists in Group Work, 33*(1), 61–83. https://doi.org/10.1080/01933920701798570

Cook-Cottone, C., & Douglass, L. L. (2017). Yoga communities and eating disorders: Creating safe space for positive embodiment. *International Journal of Yoga Therapy, 27*(1), 87–93.

Cook-Cottone, C., Jones, L. A., & Haugli, S. (2010). Prevention of eating disorders among minority youth: A matched-sample repeated measures study. *Eating Disorders: The Journal of Treatment and Prevention, 18*(5), 361–376. https://doi.org/10.1080/10640266.2010.511894

Cook-Cottone, C., Talebkhah, K., Guyker, W., & Keddie, E. (2017). A controlled trial of a yoga-based prevention program targeting eating disorder risk factors among middle school females. *Eating Disorders: The Journal of Treatment and Prevention, 25*(5), 392–405. https://doi.org/10.1080/10640266.2017.1365562

Cook-Cottone, C. P. (2015). *Mindfulness and yoga for self-regulation: A primer for mental health professionals.* Springer.

Cook-Cottone, C. P. (2020). *Embodiment and the treatment of eating disorders: The body as a resource in recovery.* W. W. Norton.

Cook-Cottone, C. P., Kane, L., Keddie, E., & Haugli, S. (2013). *Girls growing in wellness and balance: Yoga and life skills to empower.* Schoolhouse Educational Services.

Cox, A. E., Cook-Cottone, C. P., Tylka, T. T., & Neumark-Sztainer, D. (2020). Future directions for research on yoga and positive embodiment. *Eating Disorders: The Journal of Treatment and Prevention, XX*(X), XX–XX.

Cox, A. E., & Tylka, T. L. (2020). A conceptual model describing mechanisms for how yoga practice may support positive embodiment. *Eating Disorders: The Journal of Treatment and Prevention, XX*(X), XX–XX. https://doi.org/10.1080/10640266.2020.1740911

Cox, A. E., Ullrich-French, S., Cole, A., & D'Hondt-Taylor, M. (2016). The role of state mindfulness during yoga in predicting self-objectification and reasons for exercise. *Psychology of Sport and Exercise, 22,* 321–327. https://doi.org/10.1016/j. psychsport.2015.10.001

Cox, A. E., Ullrich-French, S., Cook-Cottone, C., Tylka, T. L., & Neumark-Sztainer, D. (2020). Examining the effects of mindfulness-based yoga instruction on positive embodiment and affective responses.*Eating Disorders: The Journal of Treatment and Prevention, XX*(X), XX–XX. https://doi.org/10.1080/10640266.2020.1738909

Cox, A. E., Ullrich-French, S., Howe, H. S., & Cole, A. N. (2017). A pilot yoga physical educational curriculum to promote positive body image. *Body Image, 23,* 1–8. https://doi. org/10.1016/j.bodyim.2017.07.007

Cox, A. E., Ullrich-French, S., Tylka, T., & McMahon, A. K. (2019). The roles of self-compassion, body surveillance, and body appreciation in predicting intrinsic motivation for physical activity: Cross-sectional associations, and prospective changes within a yoga context. *Body Image, 29,* 110–117. https://doi.org/10.1016/j.bodyim.2019.03.002

Dale, L. P., Mattison, A. M., Greening, K., Galen, G., Neace, W. P., & Matacin, M. I. (2009). Yoga workshop impacts psychological functioning and mood of women with self-reported history of eating disorders. *Eating Disorders: The Journal of Treatment and Prevention, 17*(5), 422–434. https://doi.org/10.1080/10640260903210222

Daubenmier, J. J. (2005). The relationship of yoga, body awareness, and body responsiveness to self-objectification and disordered eating. *Psychology of Women Quarterly, 29*(2), 207–219.

Delaney, K., & Anthis, K. (2010). Is women's participation in different types of yoga classes associated with different levels of body awareness satisfaction? *International Journal of Yoga Therapy, 20*(1), 62–71.

Diers, L., Rydell, S. A., Watts, A., & Neumark-Sztainer, D. (2020). A yoga-based therapy program designed to improve body image among an outpatient eating disorder population: Program description and results from a mixed methods pilot study. *Eating Disorders: The Journal of Treatment and Prevention, XX*(X), XX–XX. https://doi.org/10.1080/10640266. 2020.1740912

Dittmann, K. A., & Freedman, M. R. (2009). Body awareness, eating attitudes, and spiritual beliefs of women practicing yoga. *Eating Disorders: The Journal of Treatment and Prevention, 17*(4), 273–292. https://doi.org/10.1080/10640260902991111

Domingues, R. B., & Carmo, C. (2019). Disordered eating behaviours and correlates in yoga practitioners: A systematic review. *Eating and Weight Disorders 24,* 1015–1024. https://doi. org/10.1007/s40519-019-00692-x

Douglass, L. (2009). Yoga as an intervention in the treatment of eating disorders: Does it help? *Eating Disorders: The Journal of Treatment and Prevention, 17*(2), 126–139. https://doi.org/ 10.1080/10640260802714555

Elfil, M., Negida, A., Sheikh, H., Vahedi, M., & Momeni, M. (2017). Sampling methods in clinical research; an educational review. *Emergency, 5*(1), e52. https://www.ncbi.nlm.nih.gov/pmc/articles/PMC5325924/

Flaherty, M. (2014). Influence of yoga on body image satisfaction in men. *Perceptual and Motor Skills, 119*(1), 201–214. https://doi.org/10.2466/27.50.PMS.119c17z1

Frayeh, A., & Lewis, B. (2018). The effect of mirrors on women's state body image response to yoga. *Psychology of Sport Exercise, 35*, 47–54. https://doi.org/10.1016/j.psychsport.2017.11.002

Fredrickson, B. L., & Roberts, T. A. (1997). Objectification theory: Toward understanding women's lived experiences and mental health risks. *Psychology of Women Quarterly, 21*(2), 173–206. https://doi.org/10.1111/j.1471-6402.1997.tb00108.x

Gammage, L., Drouin, B., & Lamarche, L. (2016). Comparing a yoga class with a resistance exercise class: Effects on body satisfaction and social physique anxiety among university women. *Journal of Physical Activity & Health, 13*(11), 1202–1209. https://doi.org/10.1123/jpah.2015-0642

Grenon, R., Carlucci, S., Brugnera, A., Schwartze, D., Hammond, N., Ivanova, I., Mcquaid, N., Proulx, G., & Tasca, G. A. (2019). Psychotherapy for eating disorders: A meta-analysis of direct comparisons. *Psychotherapy Research, 29*(7), 833–845. https://doi.org/10.1080/10503307.2018.1489162

Hall, A., Ofei-Tenkorang, N. A., Machan, J. T., & Gordon, C. M. (2016). Use of yoga in outpatient eating disorder treatment: A pilot study. *Journal of Eating Disorders, 4*(Article), 38. https://doi.org/10.1186/s40337-016-0130-2

*Halliwell, E., Jarman, H., Tylka, T. L., & Slater, A. (2018). Evaluating the impact of a brief yoga intervention on preadolescents' body image and mood. *Body Image, 27*, 196–201. https://doi.org/10.1016/j.bodyim.2018.10.003

*Halliwell, E., Dawson, K., & Burkey, S. (2019). A randomized experimental evaluation of a yoga-based body image intervention. *Body Image, 28*, 119–127. https://doi.org/10.1016/j.bodyim.2018.12.005

Herranz Valera, J., Acuña Ruiz, P., Romero Valdespino, B., & Visioli, F. (2014). Prevalence of orthorexia nervosa among ashtanga yoga practitioners: A pilot study. *Eating and Weight Disorders, 19*(4), 469–472. https://doi.org/10.1007/s40519-014-0131-6

Higgins, J. P., Thompson, S. G., Deeks, J. J., & Altman, D. G. (2003). Measuring inconsistency in meta-analyses. *BMJ, 327*(7414), 557–560. https://doi.org/10.1136/bmj.327.7414.557

*Hopkins, L. B., Medina, J. L., Baird, S. O., Rosenfield, D., Powers, M. B., & Smits, J. A. J. (2016). Heated hatha yoga to target cortisol reactivity to stress and affective eating in women at risk for obesity-related illnesses: A randomized controlled trial. *Journal of Consulting and Clinical Psychology, 84*(6), 558–564. https://doi.org/10.1037/ccp0000091

Impett, E. A., Daubenmier, J. J., & Hirschman, A. L. (2006). Minding the body: Yoga, embodiment, and well-being. *Sexuality Research & Social Policy, 3*(4), 39–48.

*Karlsen, K. E., Vrabel, K., Bratland-Sanda, S., Ulleberg, P., & Benum, K. (2018). Effect of yoga in the treatment of eating disorders: A single-blinded randomized controlled trial with 6-months follow-up. *International Journal of Yoga, 11*(2), 166–169. https://doi.org/10.4103/ijoy.IJOY_3_17

Klein, J., & Cook-Cottone, C. (2013). The effects of yoga on eating disorder symptoms and correlates: A review. *International Journal of Yoga Therapy, 23*(2), 41–50. https://doi.org/10.17761/ijyt.23.2.2718421234k31854

Kramer, R., & Cuccolo, K. (2019). Yoga practice in a college sample: Associated changes in eating disorder, body image, and related factors over time. *Eating Disorders: The Journal of Treatment and Prevention, XX*(X), XX–XX. https://doi.org/10.1080/10640266.2019.1688007

Mahlo, L., & Tiggemann, M. (2016). Yoga and positive body image: A test of the embodiment model. *Body Image, 18*, 135–142. https://doi.org/10.1016/j.bodyim.2016.06.008

Martin, R., Prichard, I., Hutchinson, A. D., & Wilson, C. (2013). The role of body awareness and mindfulness in the relationship between exercise and eating behavior. *The Journal of Sport and Exercise Psychology, 35*(6), 655–660. https://doi.org/10.1123/jsep.35.6.655

*McIver, S., O'Halloran, P., & McGartland, M. (2009). Yoga as a treatment for binge eating disorder: A preliminary study. *Complementary Therapies in Medicine, 17*(4), 196–202. https://doi.org/10.1016/j.ctim.2009.05.002

McIver, S., McGartland, M., & O'Halloran, P. (2009). "Overeating is not about the food:" Women describe their experience of a yoga treatment program for binge eating. *Qualitative Health Research, 19*(9), 1234–1245.

Menzel, J. E., & Levine, M. P. (2011). Embodying experiences and the promotion of positive body image: The example of competitive athletics. In R. M. Calogero, S. Tantleff-Dunn, & J. K. Thompson (Eds.), *Self-objectification in women: Causes, consequences, and counter-actions* (pp. 163–186). American Psychological Association. https://doi.org/10.1037/12304-008

*Mitchell, K. S., Mazzeo, S. E., Rausch, S. M., & Cooke, K. L. (2007). Innovative interventions for disordered eating: Evaluating dissonance-based and yoga interventions. *International Journal of Eating Disorders, 40*(2), 120–128. https://doi.org/10.1002/eat.20282

Neumark-Sztainer, D., Cook-Cottone, C. P., Tylka, T. L., & Cox, A. E. (2020). Introduction to the special edition on yoga and positive embodiment: A note from the editors on how we got here. *Eating Disorders: The Journal of Treatment and Prevention, XX*(X), XX–XX.

Neumark-Sztainer, D., Eisenberg, M. E., Wall, M., & Loth, K. A. (2011). Yoga and pilates: Associated with body image and disordered-eating behaviors in a population-based sample of young adults. *International Journal of Eating Disorders, 44*(3), 276–280. https://doi.org/10.1002/eat.20858

Neumark-Sztainer, D., MacLehose, R. F., Watts, A. W., Pacanowski, C. R., & Eisenberg, M. E. (2018). Yoga and body image: Findings from a large population-based study of young adults. *Body Image, 24*, 69–75. https://doi.org/10.1016/j.bodyim.2017.12.003

Neumark-Sztainer, D., Watts, A. W., & Rydell, S. (2018). Yoga and body image: How do young adults practicing yoga describe its impact on their body image? *Body Image, 27*, 156–168. https://doi.org/10.1016/j.bodyim.2018.09.001

Norman, K., Sodano, S. M., & Cook-Cottone, C. (2014). An exploratory analysis of the role of interpersonal styles in eating disorder prevention outcomes. *The Journal for Specialists in Group Work, 39*(4), 301–315.

Ostermann, T., Vogel, H., Boehm, K., & Cramer, H. (2019). Effects of yoga on eating disorders– A systematic review. *Complementary Therapies in Medicine, 46*, 73–80.

Ostermann, T., Vogel, H., Starke, C., & Cramer, H. (2019). Effectiveness of yoga in eating disorders- A case report. *Complementary Therapies in Medicine, 42*, 145–148. https://doi.org/10.1016/j.ctim.2018.11.014

*Pacanowski, C. R., Diers, L., Crosby, R. D., Mackenzie, M., & Neumark-Sztainer, D. (2020). Yoga's impact on risk and protective factors for disordered eating: A primary prevention pilot trial. *Eating Disorders: The Journal of Treatment and Prevention, XX*(X), XX–XX.

Pacanowski, C. R., Diers, L., Crosby, R. D., & Neumark-Sztainer, D. (2017). *Yoga in the treatment of eating disorders within a residential program: A randomized controlled trial. *Eating Disorders: The Journal of Treatment and Prevention, 25*(1), 37–51. https://doi.org/10.1080/10640266.2016.1237810

Perey, I., & Cook-Cottone, C. P. (2020). Eating disorders, embodiment, and yoga: A conceptual overview. *Eating Disorders: The Journal of Treatment and Prevention, XX*(X), XX–XX.

Piran, N. (2016). Embodied possibilities and disruptions: The emergence of the experience of embodiment construct from qualitative studies with girls and women. *Body Image, 18*, 43–60. https://doi.org/10.1016/j.bodyim.2016.04.007

Piran, N., & Neumark-Sztainer, D. (2020). Yoga and the experience of embodiment: A discussion of possible links. *Eating Disorders: The Journal of Treatment and Prevention, XX*(X), XX–XX. https://doi.org/10.1080/10640266.2019.1701350

Pizzanello, H. D. (2016). Evolving from an illusionary self destructive quest for power to a state of empowerment: The curative potential yoga may hold as a vehicle to reclaiming the bodily empowerment for women with anorexia. *Journal of Sociology and Social Welfare, 43*(4), 37–60. http://scholarworks.wmich.edu/jssw/vol43/iss4/4

Prichard, I., & Tiggemann, M. (2008). Relations among exercise type, self-objectification, and body image in the fitness centre environment: The role of reason for exercise. *Psychology of Sport and Exercise, 9*(6), 855–866. https://doi.org/10.1016/j.psychsport.2007.10.005

Rani, N. J., & Rao, P. V. K. (2005). Impact of yoga training on body image and depression. *Psychological Studies, 50*(1), 98–100. https://psycnet.apa.org/record/2006-00679-014

Scime, M., & Cook-Cottone, C. (2008). Primary prevention of eating disorders: A constructivist integration of mind and body strategies. *International Journal of Eating Disorders, 41*(2), 134–142. https://doi.org/10.1002/eat.20480

Scime, M., Cook-Cottone, C., Kane, L., & Watson, T. (2006). Group prevention of eating disorders with fifth-grade females: Impact on body dissatisfaction, drive for thinness, and media influence. *Eating Disorders: The Journal of Treatment and Prevention, 14*(2), 143–155. https://doi.org/10.1080/10640260500403881

Sherman, K. J. (2012). Guidelines for developing yoga interventions for randomized trials. *Evidence-Based Complementary and Alternative Medicine*, 143271. Article. https://doi.org/10.1155/2012/143271

Tylka, T. L., & Wood-Barcalow, N. L. (2015). What is and what is not positive body image? Conceptual foundations and construct definition. *Body Image, 14*, 118–129. https://doi.org/10.1016/j.bodyim.2015.04.001

van den Berg, E., Houtzager, L., de Vos, J., Daemen, I., Katsaragaki, G., Karyotaki, E., Cuijpers, P., & Dekker, J. (2019). Meta-analysis on the efficacy of psychological treatments for anorexia nervosa. *European Eating Disorders Review, 27*(4), 331–351. https://doi.org/10.1002/erv.2683

Webb, J. B., Rogers, C. B., & Thomas, E. V. (2020). Realizing yoga's all-access pass: A social justice critique of westernized yoga and inclusive embodiment. *Eating Disorders: The Journal of Treatment and Prevention, XX*(X), XX–XX. https://doi.org/10.1080/10640266.2020.1712636

Zajac, A. U., & Schier, K. (2011). Body image dysphoria and motivation to exercise: A study of Canadian and Polish women participating in yoga or aerobics. *Archives of Psychiatry and Psychotherapy, 4*, 67–72. http://www.archivespp.pl/uploads/images/2011_13_4/Zajac67_APP_4_2011.pdf

Benefits of yoga in the treatment of eating disorders: results of a randomized controlled trial

Margaret A. Brennan ⓘ, William J. Whelton, and Donald Sharpe

ABSTRACT

Yoga has begun to be incorporated into the treatment of eating disorders despite limited empirical support for this practice. The purpose of this study was to investigate the efficacy of incorporating Yoga into the treatment of eating disorders. This preliminary randomized controlled trial investigated the benefits of participating in an eight-week Kripalu Yoga program for 53 women with symptoms of bulimia nervosa and binge eating disorder. Compared to waitlist controls, Yoga participants experienced decreases in binge eating frequency, emotional regulation difficulties and self-criticism, and increases in self-compassion. Yoga participants also experienced increases in state mindfulness skills across the eight weeks of the Yoga program. While these results are encouraging and suggest Yoga may have a valuable role to play in the treatment of eating disorders, it is important to stress their tentative nature. Further research, adopting a more rigorous design, is needed to address the limitations of the present study and expand on these findings.

Clinical implications

- Yoga may aid in the treatment of binge eating disorder and bulimia nervosa.
- Binge eating frequency decreased following participation in an 8-week Yoga program.
- Participants experienced decreases in emotion dysregulation and self-criticism.
- Participants also experienced gains in self-compassion and mindfulness skills.
- These results support continued study of Yoga in eating disorder treatment.

Bulimia nervosa (BN) and binge eating disorder (BED) pose serious physical and psychological consequences. Alarmingly, the majority of women with these disorders do not seek treatment from a mental health professional

(Mond, Hay, Rodgers, & Owen, 2007), less than half receive treatment (National Eating Disorder Association [NEDA], 2013), and standard psychological treatments are ineffective for up to half of those seeking help (Wilson, Grilo, & Vitousek, 2007). While the more recent enhanced version of cognitive behavioral therapy (CBT-E) has improved treatment results, it is only effective for anywhere from 52–67% of individuals with BN and 54–73% of individuals with eating disorders not otherwise specified (EDNOS; Fairburn et al., 2009). Therefore, it is essential to find treatment approaches for individuals with BN and BED that are effective for those not helped by standard treatments.

Traditional treatments for eating disorders suffered from a lack of attention to issues of emotional regulation (Stice, 2002). This lack of attention has diminished considerably over the past twenty years. Research has begun to identify struggles with the processing of affect and the regulating of emotions as central to the development and treatment of eating disorders (e.g., Leehr et al., 2015; Telch, Agras, & Linehan, 2001; Treasure, Corfield, & Cardi, 2012). From an emotional regulation perspective, binge eating can be viewed as a means of managing negative affect (Dolhanty & Greenberg, 2007). One contributor to negative affect is self-criticism (Gilbert, 2009). Self-critical individuals are not only hard on themselves but also perceive others as critical and judgmental, making them susceptible to feelings of dysphoria (Dunkley, Zuroff, & Blankenstein, 2003) and shame (Whelton & Greenberg, 2005). Not surprisingly, individuals with eating disorders are often highly self-critical (Fennig et al., 2008), rendering them vulnerable to shame and other unpleasant emotions. Without effective emotion regulation skills, individuals with BN and BED rely on eating disordered behaviors in order to manage their emotions. While these behaviors may ameliorate difficult feelings temporarily, these behaviors are viewed as evidence of one's deficiency, further perpetuating self-critical thoughts and feelings of shame (Goss & Allan, 2009).

A recent trend in the treatment of eating disorders is the incorporation of mindfulness-based practices. Mindfulness appears well-suited to the treatment of BN and BED, having been shown to increase emotion regulation capabilities (Teper, Segal, & Inzlicht, 2013). Dialectical behavior therapy (DBT) is one therapeutic approach incorporating mindfulness that has been adapted for eating disorders and specifically targets emotion dysregulation (Safer, Telch, & Agras, 2001). DBT may help reduce binge eating, though further research is needed, but it does not improve emotion regulation as intended (Safer & Jo, 2010; Safer et al., 2001; Telch et al., 2001). What many forms of CBT, IPT, and DBT have tended to lack is a well-developed focus on self-compassion as a systematic and structured intervention, although this has begun to change. Gilbert and Procter (2006) described Compassionate Mind Training (CMT) as a structured and systematic intervention to engage in self-soothing and self-reassurance as antidotes to feelings of shame, self-criticism, and inferiority. Since that time, self-compassion has been studied on its own and as a transdiagnostic adjunct to other treatments like CBT and DBT in the treatment of eating disorders (e.g., Kelly, Carter, & Borairi, 2014; Steindl, Buchanan, Goss, & Allan, 2017). Self-compassion helps to counteract the effects of self-criticism and enhance emotion regulation, and is starting to be seen as a component of emotion regulation in its own right (Diedrich, Grant, Hoffman, Hiller, & Berking, 2014). Self-compassion has also been shown to predict better eating disorder treatment outcomes (Kelly, Carter, Zuroff, & Borairi, 2013).

The growing acceptance of mindfulness and other contemplative practices has seen the introduction of Yoga into the treatment of eating disorders. Yoga is a mindfulness-based practice and a holistic approach to wellness (Feuerstein, 2002). A brief presentation of open trials of Yoga will be outlined next, followed by an overview of RCTs investigating Yoga as an eating disorder treatment.

Giles (1985) was the first to propose incorporating Yoga practice into a multi-faceted treatment approach for eating disorders, believing that Yoga delivered before or after meals could help to reduce food preoccupation. Subsequently, Yoga has been shown to increase body satisfaction and decrease self-objectification (Impett, Daubenmier, & Hirschman, 2006), both of which are linked to eating disorder pathology. While Yoga is increasingly being incorporated into the treatment of eating disorders, research into its effectiveness is limited. Cook-Cottone, Beck, and Kane (2008) administered an eight-week eating disorder treatment consisting of interactive discourse/psychoeducation, Yoga, and meditation. The participants, 24 women between the ages of 14 to 35, experienced decreases pre- to post-treatment in drive for thinness and body dissatisfaction, but no changes in the frequency of binge eating or purging. Clarke (2008) explored the effects of a ten-week Yoga group emphasizing mindfulness for 17 women and men with BED. Participants in Clarke's study experienced decreases in the number of binge episodes per week, and eating, shape, and weight concerns. More recently, adolescent females from an eating disorder clinic participated in six to 12 weekly Yoga classes, and experienced decreases in anxiety, depression, and body image disturbance (Hall, Ofei-Tenkorang, Machan, & Gordon, 2016).

McIver, O'Halloran, and McGartland (2009) conducted one of the first RCTs in which they compared the effects of a 12-week Yoga program to a waitlist control amongst 50 women self-identifying with a binge eating problem. Compared to waitlist controls, Yoga participants experienced decreased binge eating frequency that was maintained at a three-month follow-up. In the first RCT investigating the effects of Yoga on individuals meeting diagnostic criteria for an eating disorder (Carei, Fyfe-Johnson, Breuner, & Brown, 2010), 54 adolescents attending a hospital outpatient eating disorder treatment program were assigned to an eight-week Yoga program or a waitlist control. Compared to controls, Yoga group participants experienced larger decreases in eating disorder psychopathology and lower levels of food preoccupation. Another RCT (Pacanowski, Diers, Crosby, & Neumark-Sztainer, 2017) examined 38 individuals (overwhelmingly female) from a residential eating disorder treatment program who took part in pre-meal Yoga for a five day intervention period. Pre-meal negative affect and anxiety were reduced for Yoga group members compared to controls, but these differences were not exhibited post-meal. No reductions in eating disorder measures were found, attributed by the authors to the brief intervention period. More recently, an RCT investigated the differences between 30 adult females diagnosed with BN or EDNOS assigned to an eleven week Yoga program or a control group, consisting of two 90-minute presentations (Karlsen, Vrabel, & Benum, 2018). Relative to the control group, the Yoga group showed declines on the Eating Disorder Examination—Interview global, restraint, and eating concern subscales at posttest and six-month follow-up.

The present study is one of only a few RCTs investigating the use of Yoga in eating disorder treatment and to the best of our knowledge it is the first RCT to investigate the impact of Yoga on self-compassion, self-criticism, and emotion regulation in individuals meeting diagnostic criteria for an eating disorder. It is also the first RCT to investigate the effects of Kripalu Yoga on individuals with BN or BED. Kripalu Yoga appears particularly well-suited to address the self-criticism and emotion dysregulation that serve to perpetuate eating disorders because of its emphasis on *witness consciousness* and compassion for self and others (Faulds, 2005). Witness consciousness, essentially mindfulness, is defined as "the ability to closely observe what is occurring without reactivity" (Faulds, 2005, p. 291). Compared to control participants, Yoga group participants were anticipated to show (a) a reduction in binge eating frequency, (b) a reduction in emotion regulation difficulties, (c) a reduction in self-criticism, and (d) an increase in self-compassion. It was also hypothesized that Yoga participants would experience increased ability to invoke a mindfulness state.

Method

Participants

Participants were recruited through advertisements posted at local universities, gyms, coffee shops, supermarkets, and mental health centers, as well as social media sites (e.g., Facebook). To be eligible for inclusion in the study, participants had to be 18 years of age or older, meet DSM-5 criteria for BN or BED, and have no or limited Yoga experience (defined as having practiced less than six times per year in the past five years). Exclusion criteria included active suicidal ideation, psychosis, or substance abuse, or a pre-existing diagnosis of borderline personality disorder (BPD). Those with BPD were thought to be better suited to a longer, slower treatment with more support such as DBT. The final sample consisted of 53 women (26 treatment and 27 control subjects). Demographic characteristics of the sample can be seen in Table 1.

Measures

Eating disorder diagnostic scale (EDDS)

The EDDS (Stice, Telch, & Rizvi, 2000) is a 22-item self-report measure used to diagnose AN, BN, and BED. The EDDS has demonstrated high internal consistency ($α = .89$), high test-retest reliability ($r = .87$), and good convergent validity with other measures of eating pathology (Krabbenborg et al., 2011). The criteria for frequency and duration of binge eating and compensatory behaviors were adjusted to meet DSM-5 criteria as the EDDS uses DSM-IV-TR diagnostic criteria.

Table 1. Sample demographics.

	n	%
Ethnicity		
Caucasian	38	71.7
Asian Canadian	4	7.5
Aboriginal/Metis	3	5.7
East Indian	2	3.8
Hispanic	1	1.9
Chinese	1	1.9
South East Asian	1	1.9
Other	3	5.7
Education		
High School	24	45.3
College Diploma	6	11.3
Undergraduate Degree	16	30.2
Graduate Degree	7	13.2
Employment		
Unemployed	4	7.5
Employed	22	41.5
Student	27	50.9
BMI		
Normal Weight	28	52.8
Overweight	8	15.1
Obese	17	32.1
Diagnosis		
Bulimia Nervosa	40	75.5
Binge Eating Disorder	13	24.5
Previous Therapy		
Yes	42	79.2
No	11	20.8
Psychotropic Medication		
Yes	16	30.19
No	37	69.81

Eating disorder examination questionnaire (EDE-Q)

Two items from the EDE-Q 6.0 (Fairburn & Beglin, 2008) assessed binge eating frequency over the past 28 days: number of times binge eating (TB) and number of binge days (BD). These two items were administered with the instruction sheet developed by Goldfein, Devlin, and Kamenetz (2005).

Difficulties in emotion regulation scale (DERS)

The DERS (Gratz & Roemer, 2004) is a 36-item self-report scale designed to measure emotional processing. Items are rated on a five-point Likert scale ranging from one (almost never) to five (almost always). The DERS has demonstrated test-retest reliability ($r = .88$), high internal consistency ($\alpha = .93$), and associations with other measures of emotion dysregulation (Gratz & Roemer, 2004).

The forms of self-criticizing/attacking and self-reassuring scale (FSCRS)

The FSCRS (Gilbert, Clark, Hempel, Miles, & Irons, 2004) is a 22-item self-report measure of self-criticism and self-reassurance that has demonstrated good internal consistency. The items are rated on a five-point Likert scale ranging from zero (not at all like me) to four (extremely like me). Two subscales of the FSCRS assess self-criticism characterized by a sense of personal inadequacy (IS) and self-criticism characterized by self-hatred (HS).

Self-compassion scale–short form (SCS-SF)

The SCS-SF (Raes, Pommier, Neff, & Van Gucht, 2011) is a self-report measure of self-compassion. The SCS-SF consists of twelve items rated on a five-point Likert scale ranging from one (almost never) to five (almost always). The SCS-SF provides a total self-compassion score that has demonstrated good internal consistency ($\alpha = .87$).

Toronto mindfulness scale (TMS)

The TMS (Lau et al., 2006) is a self-report measure of an individual's ability to invoke a mindfulness state. Responses yield two subscale scores. The curiosity subscale measures whether an individual brings an attitude of curiosity, openness, and acceptance to his or her present moment experience. The decentering subscale measures an individual's ability to be aware of his or her present moment experience without overly identifying with this experience.

Attitudes toward seeking professional psychological help–short form (ATSPPH-SF)

The ATSPPH-SF (Fischer & Farina, 1995) is a ten-item self-report measure of attitudes toward seeking help. A coefficient alpha of .84 and a one-month test-retest reliability coefficient of .80 provide evidence of reliability. High correlations with help-seeking behaviors provide evidence of criterion-related validity (Fischer & Farina, 1995).

Procedure

Individuals interested in participating were directed to an online screening questionnaire. The primary investigator telephoned individuals when further information was needed to ascertain participant eligibility. Eligible participants were asked to attend one of several information sessions where they completed the dependent measures. Participants were then randomly assigned to either the Yoga group (n = 36) or the waitlist control group (n = 36). All participants completed the same assessment battery again after eight weeks, during which time the treatment group completed the eight-week Yoga program, and then again one month later. Individuals assigned to the waitlist control group were provided with the opportunity to participate in the eight-week Yoga program following the completion of the study.

Participants assigned to the Yoga condition were expected to attend eight 90-minute weekly Yoga sessions held on a university campus. Class sizes were capped at twelve in order to ensure participants would receive proper and personalized instruction. Participants were assigned to a class time based on their availability and preferences. The first author, a Registered Yoga Teacher trained in the Kripalu Yoga tradition, led all of the Yoga classes. Participants completed the TMS immediately following the first, third, sixth and eighth Yoga classes. Yoga classes followed a pre-determined, structured format, consisting of pranayama (breathing), asana (postures), and meditation practices. New postures and breathing practices were gradually introduced, progressing toward more advanced practices. Mindfulness and self-compassion were emphasized throughout the Yoga classes. The Kripalu Yoga program trained participants to be aware of their internal experiences (i.e., physical sensations, emotions, thoughts) whether pleasant, unpleasant, or neutral, with curiosity, kindness, openness, non-reactivity and acceptance. Participants were also frequently reminded to listen to their bodies, and to respect their physical and psychological limitations. Self-compassion was encouraged through the compassionate and gentle language of the Yoga teacher, respect for differing physical capabilities among students and verbal reminders to bring compassionate attention to one's self and one's internal experiences.

Results

Data were analyzed using the Statistical Package for Social Sciences (IBM SPSS 22.0). Violations of the assumption of sphericity for mixed-model ANOVAs were corrected using the Huynh-Feldt adjustment when epsilon values were greater than .75. Effect sizes were evaluated using Cohen's (1988) guidelines for partial eta squared: .01 indicates a small effect, .06 indicates a medium effect, and .14 indicates a large effect. Statistically significant main effects of time were further examined through simple main effect contrasts.

Interaction contrasts were conducted for statistically significant interactions between time and group (see Jaccard & Guilamo-Ramos, 2002). As suggested by Jaccard and Guilamo-Ramos (2002), each family of contrasts was assessed both with and without a Holm-based modified Bonferroni correction. In almost all cases, the same results were found with and without the correction. Thus, statistical significance levels in all the tables was set at $p < .05$.

Preliminary analyses

A total of 72 individuals participated with an attrition rate of 26% ($n = 19$). Participants who did not complete the study (i.e., failing to complete the assessment battery at all three time periods) had their data removed from the dataset. Participants assigned to the Yoga group needed to attend a minimum of five Yoga classes to be included in the analyses. Yoga participants attended between five and eight Yoga classes, with a modal number of eight classes attended. Randomization was successful as there were no statistically significant differences between groups on any of the demographic variables or pretest scores on the dependent variables. No statistically significant differences between groups were observed for the number of therapy sessions attended by week eight or week twelve.

Ten participants withdrew from the treatment group and nine withdrew from the control group. Only a few participants provided reasons for their decision to withdraw. Two cited shame about their body size (both with BMI scores in the obese range) and one participant disclosed feeling triggered knowing that everyone in the class had an eating disorder which increased her body dissatisfaction as she compared herself to the other participants. The only difference found between study completers and non-completers was the finding that completers scored lower on the ATSPPH-SF ($M = 20.49$, $SD = 6.07$) than non-completers ($M = 23.11$, $SD = 3.90$), suggesting participants who withdrew had more positive attitudes toward seeking professional psychological help, t (49.79) $= 2.14$, $p = .037$. Of the 27 control group participants, 24 began the Yoga program after serving as controls, fifteen of whom completed the Yoga program.

Cronbach's alpha was calculated for each measure at each time period. Reliability was found to be acceptable for all measures (see Table 2). One participant failed to answer one of 36 items on the DERS on the first administration of the scale. The group mean for that item was substituted in place of the missing score. Over the three administrations of the question asking about number of binge days, fourteen participants (seven in the treatment group and seven in the control group) provided erroneous answers (e.g., binge eating on 31 days over the past 28 days). These participants were dropped from analyses involving number of binge days. All measures were scored by a registered psychologist.

Table 2. Cronbach's alpha for dependent measures.

Measures	Time	Alpha	Items
Difficulties in Emotion Regulation	Week 0	.94	36
	Week 8	.95	
	Week 12	.95	
Self-Compassion Scale	Week 0	.82	12
	Week 8	.93	
	Week 12	.89	
Inadequate Self subscale of the FSCRS	Week 0	.87	9
	Week 8	.90	
	Week 12	.90	
Hated Self subscale of the FSCRS	Week 0	.77	5
	Week 8	.80	
	Week 12	.79	
Decentering subscale of the TMS	Week 1	.73	7
	Week 3	.81	
	Week 6	.84	
	Week 8	.88	
Curiosity subscale of the TMS	Week 1	.90	6
	Week 3	.89	
	Week 6	.88	
	Week 8	.88	

FSCRS = Forms of Self-Criticizing/Attacking and Self-Reassuring Scale; TMS = Toronto Mindfulness Scale.

Primary analyses

Descriptive statistics are presented in Table 3. Results from the mixed model ANOVAs are presented in Table 4. For all dependent measures—binge eating frequency, emotional regulation difficulties, self-criticism, and self-compassion—the interaction of group by time was statistically significant.

These statistically significant interactions were followed up first by simple main effect contrasts examining the change between week zero and week eight, and between week zero and week twelve, for the Yoga and control groups separately. The results from those simple main effect analyses appear in Table 5. For all variables, the Yoga group improved from week zero to week eight and from week zero to week twelve, whereas the control group did not improve over those time periods.

To formally test if the change scores differed between Yoga and control groups, two interaction contrasts were evaluated. The first interaction contrast compared the week zero and week eight mean differences for Yoga participants with that of controls (the first column of Table 6). The second interaction contrast compared the week zero and week twelve mean differences between the two groups (the second column of Table 6). All of these interaction contrasts were statistically significant except for the inadequate self (IS) subscale of the FSCRS comparing week zero to week eight.

Thus, we found support for the first hypothesis that there would be a greater reduction in the frequency of binge eating episodes, the second

Table 3. Descriptive statistics for treatment and control groups.

Time	Outcome Measure	Treatment Group			Control Group		
		M	SD	Range	M	SD	Range
Week 0	IS	26.38	6.24	25	26.67	6.41	24
	HS	7.96	5.08	19	8.52	4.27	16
	SCS-SF	2.20	0.50	2.25	2.16	0.57	2.25
	DERS	108.11	24.88	89	109.51	27.43	103
	TB	11.46	7.45	27	12.92	7.79	27
	BD	11.63	6.90	27	11.70	7.70	27
Week 8	IS	22.88	7.15	25	26.30	8.20	27
	HS	6.04	3.98	13	9.59	5.33	17
	SCS-SF	2.75	0.67	2.42	2.17	0.82	3.09
	DERS	92.50	20.66	70	110.44	27.32	101
	TB	5.11	5.45	20	12.11	10.22	40
	BD	4.58	5.20	20	10.60	8.58	28
Week 12	IS	21.5	7.65	26	25.96	8.06	28
	HS	5.50	4.20	16	8.74	4.90	17
	SCS-SF	2.67	0.78	2.5	2.26	0.74	3.16
	DERS	92.54	20.72	79	112.15	27.99	109
	TB	5.15	7.79	28	13.26	11.96	40
	BD	5.63	8.55	28	11.50	10.46	28

IS = Inadequate Self; HS = Hated Self; SCS-SF = Self-Compassion Scale-Short Form; DERS = Difficulties in Emotion Regulation Scale; TB = number of times binge eating; BD = number of binge days.

Table 4. Results from mixed model ANOVAs.

Variable	Effect	df	F	p	η^2
TB[a]	Group	1,51	8.59	.005*	.14
	Time	2,102	18.61	.001*	.27
	Group*Time	2,102	11.44	.001*	.18
BD[a]	Group	1,37	3.60	.066	.09
	Time	2,74	20.17	.001*	.35
	Group*Time	2,74	9.86	.001*	.21
DERS	Group	1,51	4.19	.046*	.08
	Time	1.849,94.312	4.63	.014*	.08
	Group*Time	1.849,94.312	10.19	.001*	.17
IS	Group	1,51	2.17	.147	.04
	Time	1.608,82.018	8.49	.001*	.14
	Group*Time	1.608,82.018	4.90	.015*	.09
HS	Group	1,51	4.31	.043*	.08
	Time	1.538,78.446	3.46	.048*	.06
	Group*Time	1.538,78.446	7.35	.003*	.13
SCS-SF	Group	1,51	4.25	.044*	.08
	Time	2,102	9.25	.001*	.15
	Group*Time	2,102	6.71	.002*	.12

TB = times binge eating; BD = binge days; DERS = Difficulties with Emotion Regulation Scale; IS = Inadequate Self; HS = Hated Self; SCS-SF = Self-Compassion Scale-Short Form.
[a]These variables have been square root transformed
* $p < .05$.

hypothesis that there would be a greater reduction in emotional regulation difficulties, the third hypothesis that there would be a greater reduction in self-criticism, and the fourth hypothesis that there would be a greater increase in self-compassion across time for participants in the Yoga group in comparison to control participants.

Table 5. Single main effect contrast analyses.

| | Week 0 vs. Week 8 | | | | Week 0 vs. Week 12 | | | |
| | Yoga | | Control | | Yoga | | Control | |
Variable	$t(25)$	p	$t(26)$	p	$t(25)$	p	$t(26)$	p
TB[a]	5.54	.001*	1.33	.195	5.90	.001*	.58	.568
BD[ab]	5.66	.001*	1.82	.083	5.34	.001*	1.09	.291
DERS	3.67	.001*	0.65	.523	3.85	.001*	1.42	.167
IS	2.62	.015*	0.39	.703	3.82	.001*	0.90	.376
HS	2.43	.022*	1.77	.088	2.78	.010*	0.53	.600
SCS-SF	4.16	.001*	0.07	.946	3.56	.002*	1.36	.185

TB = times binge eating; BD = binge days; DERS = Difficulties with Emotion Regulation Scale; IS = Inadequate Self; HS = Hated Self; SCS-SF = Self-Compassion Scale-Short Form.
[a]These variables have been square root transformed.
[b]t tests for Binge Days had 37 degrees of freedom.
* $p < .05$.

Table 6. Follow-up interaction contrasts.

| | Yoga vs. Controls Week 0 vs. Week 8 | | Yoga vs. Controls Week 0 vs. Week 12 | |
Variable	$t(51)$	p	$t(51)$	p
TB[a]	3.44	.001*	4.29	.001*
BD[ab]	4.02	.001*	3.51	.001*
DERS	3.26	.002*	4.01	.001*
IS	1.91	.062	2.82	.007*
HS	3.02	.004*	2.77	.008*
SCS-SF	3.31	.002*	2.47	.017*

TB = times binge eating; BD = binge days; DERS = Difficulties with Emotion Regulation Scale; IS = Inadequate Self; HS = Hated Self; SCS-SF = Self-Compassion Scale-Short Form.
[a]These variables have been square root transformed.
[b]t tests for Binge Days had 37 degrees of freedom.
* $p < .05$

The fifth hypothesis predicted that Yoga participants would experience an increase in their ability to invoke a mindfulness state across time and was assessed at four different times (weeks one, three, six, and eight). Participants experienced increases in mindfulness skills as measured by both subscales of the TMS. There was a statistically significant effect of time for the curiosity dimension of mindfulness, $F(3, 75) = 10.31$, $p = .001$, partial $\eta^2 = .29$. One degree of freedom contrasts revealed Yoga group participants experienced increases in their curiosity skills between week one ($M = 12.88$, $SD = 5.72$), week three ($M = 15.15$, $SD = 5.19$), week six ($M = 17.04$, $SD = 4.25$) and week eight ($M = 16.50$, $SD = 5.01$). There was also a statistically significant effect of time for participants' decentering subscale scores, $F(3, 75) = 15.45$, $p = .001$, partial $\eta^2 = .38$. One degree of freedom contrasts revealed Yoga participants experienced changes in their decentering skills between week one ($M = 15.85$, $SD = 4.18$), week three ($M = 16.96$, $SD = 5.10$), week six ($M = 19.92$, $SD = 4.16$), and week eight ($M = 19.92$, $SD = 5.21$).

Discussion

The aim of this study was to evaluate the efficacy of using Yoga in the treatment of eating disorders. Completion of our eight-week Kripalu Yoga program was associated with several positive outcomes.

Binge eating frequency

As hypothesized, individuals who completed the Yoga program experienced decreases in binge eating frequency. This finding is consistent with the conclusions of two meta-analyses investigating the use of mindfulness-based interventions in the treatment of binge eating (Godfrey, Gallo, & Afari, 2015; Katterman, Kleinman, Hood, Nackers, & Corsica, 2014). The decrease in binge eating episodes experienced by the Yoga participants is also consistent with existing research exploring the use of Yoga in the treatment of BED (Clarke, 2008) and women reporting problematic binge eating behavior (McIver et al., 2009). It is important to note that similar to the present study, the Clarke (2008) and McIver et al. (2009) studies did not involve an active control condition. Participants in a waitlist control condition are not systematically engaged in efforts to change while waiting, increasing the likelihood that any intervention will stand out as highly effective by comparison.

Emotion regulation difficulties

Another promising result of this study was the improvement in emotion regulation abilities following completion of the Yoga program. This finding is consistent with other studies investigating the effects of Yoga (e.g., Gard, Noggle, Park, Vago, & Wilson, 2014). Despite widespread acknowledgement of the role of emotion regulation deficits in individuals with eating disorders (e.g., Telch et al., 2001), standard treatments have traditionally failed to sufficiently address these deficits. Recently, enhanced CBT (CBT-E), has begun to attend to emotional deficits, however few studies have investigated the impact of CBT-E on emotion regulation. Surprisingly, while DBT for eating disorders specifically targets emotion dysregulation it has not been shown to lead to improvements in this area (Safer & Jo, 2010; Safer et al., 2001; Telch et al., 2001). The benefits observed in emotion regulation skills among Yoga participants following completion of our eight-week Kripalu Yoga program offer support for the continued use of Yoga in the treatment of eating disorders. It is possible that the impact of the Yoga program on emotion regulation skills was mediated by improvements in both mindfulness and self-compassion. Although so-called mechanisms of change are infrequently tested in psychological therapies

(Petrik & Cronin, 2014), an interesting direction for future research will be to investigate whether the Yoga program's impact on emotion regulation is mediated by self-compassion and mindfulness skills. This future research could be done by administering measures of self-compassion and mindfulness to all participants and employing scores from those as mediating variables in path or structural equation models between Yoga and emotion regulation outcomes.

Self-Criticism

Individuals with eating disorders are known to be highly self-critical, a trait that predicts poor psychotherapy outcomes (Whelton, Paulson, & Marusiak, 2007). The finding that the Yoga participants experienced decreases in self-criticism after completing the Kripalu Yoga program is significant because self-criticism is known to perpetuate eating disorder behaviors and most eating disorder treatments do not adequately address self-criticism (Fennig et al., 2008). The program's emphasis on self-compassion may have been responsible for participants' decreases in self-criticism. This speculation is consistent with Gilbert and Procter's (2006) finding that short-term therapy focusing on the development of self-compassion led to decreases in self-criticism. It is also possible that the program's positive impact on self-criticism was due to the modality of the program. Jopling (2000) asserts that "the somatic sense of self is developmentally prior to explicitly worked-out self-understandings, and normally forms the unnoticed background of thought and action" (p. 55). In other words, subtle shifts in the somatic sense of self may be an important precursor to changing one's view of self.

The relationship between bodily processes and the experience of self implied by the phrase somatic sense of self is sufficiently challenging to render rigorous research in this area difficult. Empirical investigation of the polyvagal theory (Porges, 2001) sheds some preliminary light on the complex interplay of somatic experiences, emotions, and cognitive processes. While more rigorous research is needed, an overview of the literature suggests that Yoga practice may positively impact autonomic regulation and heart rate variability (Tyagi & Cohen, 2016). Researchers have also demonstrated that self-criticism is associated with lower vagally mediated heart rate variability (vmHRV) whereas self-compassion is associated with higher vmHRV (Svendsen et al., 2016) and has been shown to activate greater vagal activity (Stellar, Cohen, Oveis, & Keltner, 2015). Interoception of internal and external safety is believed to result in the ventral vagal system orienting the individual toward social engagement and prosocial interactions (Sullivan et al., 2018), possibly with the self as well.

Interestingly, the Yoga participants experienced greater decreases in *hated self* subscale scores of the FCSRS than controls between both week zero and week eight, and between week zero and week twelve, whereas they only experienced greater decreases in *inadequate self* subscale scores between week zero and week twelve. One possible explanation is that the Yoga program more effectively targeted the hated self element of self-criticism than it did a sense of personal inadequacy because of its emphasis on mindful self-compassion, rather than any emphasis on self-correction or self-improvement. Yoga may be well-suited to those struggling with an eating disorder as self-hatred is more predictive of psychopathology than feelings of personal inadequacy (Baião, Gilbert, McEwan, & Carvalho, 2015).

Self-compassion

The Yoga participants experienced increased levels of self-compassion following completion of our Yoga program that were maintained one month later. The value of self-compassion in the treatment of eating disorders has increasingly been recognized. Low levels of self-compassion and high fear of self-compassion are predictive of poor treatment outcomes (Kelly et al., 2013). Self-compassion counteracts the effects of self-criticism, improves emotion regulation (Jazaieri et al., 2014) and is starting to be seen as a component of emotion regulation in its own right (Diedrich et al., 2014). Neff and Dahm (2014) posit that people suffering from severe shame or self-criticism "might need to first cultivate self-compassion in order to have the sense of emotional safety needed to fully turn toward their pain with mindfulness" (p. 28).

Mindfulness

As expected, the Yoga participants developed a greater ability to induce a mindfulness state across the eight-week Yoga program. Yoga is itself a mindfulness practice and thus it follows naturally that repeated Yoga practice would result in increased mindfulness. The present study is among the first to investigate the impact of a Yoga intervention on mindfulness skills in individuals meeting diagnostic criteria for an eating disorder.

The increase in mindfulness skills experienced by the Yoga group participants is consistent with Clarke's (2008) findings that women with BED experienced increases in mindfulness skills following completion of a ten-week Yoga program. An important distinction between the present study and Clarke's (2008) study is the investigation of Yoga on state versus trait mindfulness skills. The present study was the first to examine changes in state mindfulness among the eating disorder population following a Yoga intervention. While this improves our understanding of the immediate effects of Yoga practice, it will be important to examine whether the short-term effects of the eight-week Kripalu Yoga program transfer into longer-term changes.

The results of this study also shed light on possible mechanisms of change. The Kripalu Yoga program trained participants to be aware of their internal experiences with non-reactivity and acceptance. As the eight-week program progressed, participants were instructed to hold poses for longer periods of time while paying attention to their arising thoughts, emotions, and sensations with mindfulness and self-compassion. These practices directly countered the tendency to escape from unpleasant experiences that is known to lead to disordered eating. Future research could explore these possible mechanisms of change using path or structural equation models to investigate the impact of mindfulness, self-compassion, and emotion regulation skills or other potential mediators on eating disorder behaviors.

Limitations

Despite the promising results of this study, there are limitations that need to be acknowledged. First, a significant limitation is the study's reliance on a waitlist control condition. Lack of an active control condition makes it difficult to ascertain if the benefits experienced by the Yoga participants were due to the Yoga program itself or to other confounding factors, such as participant expectations or attempts at change, the positive attention of the Yoga teacher, or competition between participants. Participants in a waitlist control condition are not systematically engaged in efforts to change while waiting for treatment and may actually be less motivated to change during this time, thereby increasing the likelihood that any intervention will stand out as highly effective by comparison, resulting in over-estimated effect sizes (Furukawa et al., 2014). Second, the follow-up period of one-month was inadequate to determine if there were any lasting effects of the Yoga program. Third, the attrition rate in this study was 26%, which while high is on par with attrition rates observed in eating disorder outpatient treatments (29%–73%; Fassino, Pierò, Tomba, & Abbate-Daga, 2009) and RCTs of CBT for eating disorders (24%; Linardon, Hindle, & Brennan, 2018). Questions remain about what differentiated study completers from non-completers and this is an important area for future investigation. Fourth, participants self-selected to participate, raising the possibility of self-selection bias. The higher representation of individuals with BN than BED suggests Yoga may be more appealing to those with BN. This suggestion was supported by feedback from two participants with BMI scores in the obese range who disclosed withdrawing from the study because of shame around their body sizes. Body shame may have been a deterrent for others with high BMIs, and existing research suggests obese individuals are less likely to adhere to a Yoga intervention (Baird et al., 2016). Fifth, self-report forms were used, introducing the possibility for response bias and less definitive diagnoses than would have been achieved through a structured clinical interview. Sixth, the results of this study cannot be generalized to adolescents, males, or those with other eating disorder diagnoses, and nor can they be generalized to Yoga classes in general. While the Yoga program in this study emphasized mindfulness and self-compassion, this emphasis may or may not be true of classes offered elsewhere. Additionally, all of the students attending the classes were known to have an eating disorder, which would not be the case in a community setting.

Because of the limitations to this study, future studies are needed both to tease out the relative contributions of various therapeutic factors and to make more robust comparisons by strengthening the quality of the controls. Future studies would also benefit from including a larger sample size, employing a much longer follow-up period, incorporating where possible a mix of observational methods along with self-report, and using a structured clinical interview in order to determine more definitive diagnoses. While the results of this study support the continued study of Yoga in eating disorder treatment, it remains to be determined if different styles of Yoga or Yoga offered in a less controlled setting would have similar benefits. Additionally, further research is needed to determine the best format for offering Yoga to those with eating disorders (i.e., would offering classes specifically for individuals with larger bodies make it more appealing to those with BED or higher BMIs?).

Conclusion

The results from this study, though preliminary, support continued investigation of the use of Yoga in eating disorder treatment. The findings suggest that forms of Yoga that emphasize self-compassion and mindfulness may help to increase self-compassion and mindfulness skills in women with BN or BED. Both self-compassion and mindfulness skills have been linked to improved treatment outcomes, and may help to decrease emotion regulation difficulties and self-criticism, both of which serve to perpetuate eating disorder symptoms. The results of this study also suggest Yoga may help to decrease binge eating frequency in women with BED or BN. These results are preliminary and further studies using active control conditions, a mix of observational measures, and rigorous techniques to refine and distinguish the precise mechanisms of change, are needed.

ORCID

Margaret A. Brennan ⓘ http://orcid.org/0000-0002-7242-6612

References

Baião, R., Gilbert, P., McEwan, K., & Carvalho, S. (2015). Forms of self-criticising/attacking & self-reassuring scale: Psychometric properties and normative study. *Psychology and Psychotherapy*, *88*, 438–452. doi:10.1111/papt.12049

Baird, S. O., Hopkins, L. B., Medina, J. L., Rosenfield, D., Powers, M. B., & Smits, J. A. J. (2016). Distress tolerance as a predictor of adherence to a Yoga intervention: Moderating roles of BMI and body image. *Behavior Modification, 40*(1–2), 199–217. doi:10.1177/0145445515612401

Carei, T. R., Fyfe-Johnson, A. L., Breuner, C. C., & Brown, M. A. (2010). Randomized controlled clinical trial of Yoga in the treatment of eating disorders. *Journal of Adolescent Health, 46*, 346–351. doi:10.1080/10640266.2016.1237810

Clarke, D. P. (2008). Assessing finding Om: A Yoga and discussion-based treatment for binge eating disorder. Unpublished doctoral dissertation. (UMI Number: 3329948)

Cohen, J. (1988). *Statistical power analysis for the behavioral sciences* (2nd ed.). Hillsdale, NJ: Erlbaum.

Cook-Cottone, C., Beck, M., & Kane, L. (2008). Manualized-group treatment of eating disorders: Attunement in mind, body, and relationship (AMBR). *The Journal for Specialists in Group Work, 33*, 61–83. doi:10.1080/01933920701798570

Diedrich, A., Grant, M., Hoffman, S. G., Hiller, W., & Berking, M. (2014). Self-compassion as an emotion regulation strategy in major depressive disorder. *Behaviour Research and Therapy, 58*, 43–51. doi:10.1016/j.brat.2014.05.006

Dolhanty, D., & Greenberg, L. (2007). Emotion-focused therapy in the treatment of eating disorders. *European Psychotherapy, 7*, 97–116.

Dunkley, D. M., Zuroff, D. C., & Blankenstein, K. R. (2003). Self-critical perfectionism and daily affect: Dispositional and situational influences on stress and coping. *Journal of Personality and Social Psychology, 84*, 234–252. doi:10.1037//0022-3514.84.1.234

Fairburn, C. G., & Beglin, S. J. (2008). Eating disorder examination questionnaire (EDE-Q 6.0). In C. G. Fairburn (Ed.), *Cognitive behavior therapy and eating disorders* (pp. 309–314). New York, NY: Guilford Press.

Fairburn, C. G., Cooper, Z., Doll, H. A., O'Connor, M. E., Bohn, K., Hawker, D. M., … Palmer, R. L. (2009). Transdiagnostic cognitive-behavioural therapy for patients with eating disorders: A two-site trial with 60-week follow-up. *American Journal of Psychiatry, 166*, 311–319. doi:10.1176/appi.ajp.2008.08040608

Fassino, S., Pierò, A., Tomba, E., & Abbate-Daga, G. (2009). Factors associated with dropout from treatment for eating disorders: A comprehensive literature review. *BMC Psychiatry, 9*, 9–67. doi:10.1186/1471-244x-9-67

Faulds, R. (2005). *Kripalu Yoga*. New York, NY: Bantam Books.

Fennig, S., Hadas, A., Itzhaky, L., Roe, D., Apter, A., & Shahar, G. (2008). Self-criticism is a key predictor of eating disorder dimensions among inpatient adolescent females. *International Journal of Eating Disorders, 41*, 762–765. doi:10.1002/eat.20573

Feuerstein, G. (2002). *The Yoga tradition: Its history, literature, philosophy and practice*. New Dehli, India: Bhavana Books & Print.

Fischer, E. H., & Farina, A. (1995). Attitudes toward seeking professional psychological help: A shortened form and considerations for research. *Journal of College Student Development, 36*, 368–373. doi:10.1037/t05375-000

Furukawa, T. A., Noma, H., Caldwell, D. M., Honyashiki, M., Shinohara, K., Imai, H., … Churchill, R. (2014). Waiting list may be a nocebo condition in psychotherapy trials: A contribution from network meta-analysis. *Acta Psychiatrica Scandinavica, 13*, 181–192. doi:10.1111/acps.12275

Gard, T., Noggle, J. J., Park, C. L., Vago, D. R., & Wilson, A. (2014). Potential self-regulatory mechanisms of yoga for psychological health. *Frontiers in Human Neuroscience, 8*(770). doi:10.3389/fnhum.2014.00770

Gilbert, P. (2009). Introducing compassion-focused therapy. *Advances in Psychiatric Treatment, 15*, 199–208. doi:10.1192/apt.bp.107.005264

Gilbert, P., Clark, M., Hempel, S., Miles, J. N. V., & Irons, C. (2004). Criticizing and reassuring oneself: An exploration of forms, styles and reasons in female students. *British Journal of Clinical Psychology, 43*, 31–50. doi:10.1348/014466504772812959

Gilbert, P., & Procter, S. (2006). Compassionate mind training for people with high shame and self-criticism: Overview and pilot study. *Clinical Psychology and Psychotherapy, 13*, 353–379. doi:10.1002/cpp.507

Giles, G. (1985). Anorexia nervosa and bulimia: An activity-oriented approach. *The American Journal of Occupational Therapy, 39*, 510–517. doi:10.5014/ajot.39.8.510

Godfrey, K. M., Gallo, L., & Afari, N. (2015). Mindfulness-based interventions for binge eating: A systematic review and meta-analysis. *Journal of Behavioral Medicine, 38*, 348–362. doi:10.1007/s10865-014-9610-5

Goldfein, J. A., Devlin, M. J., & Kamenetz, C. (2005). Eating disorder examination- questionnaire with and without instruction to assess binge eating in patients with binge eating disorder. *International Journal of Eating Disorders, 37*, 107–111. doi:10.1002/eat.20075

Goss, K., & Allan, S. (2009). Shame, pride and eating disorders. *Clinical Psychology & Psychotherapy, 16*, 303–316. doi:10.1002/cpp.627

Gratz, K. L., & Roemer, L. (2004). Multidimensional assessment of emotion regulation and dysregulation: Development, factor structure, and initial validation of the difficulties in emotion regulation scale. *Journal of Psychopathology & Behavioral Assessment, 26*, 41–54. doi:10.1023/b:joba.0000007455.08539.94

Hall, A., Ofei-Tenkorang, N. A., Machan, J. T., & Gordon, C. M. (2016). Use of Yoga in outpatient eating disorder treatment: A pilot study. *Journal of Eating Disorders, 4*(1). doi:10.1186/s40337-016-0130-2

Impett, E. A., Daubenmier, J. J., & Hirschman, A. L. (2006). Minding the body: Yoga, embodiment and well-being. *Sexuality Research and Social Policy, 3*, 39–48. doi:10.1525/srsp.2006.3.4.39

Jaccard, J., & Guilamo-Ramos, V. (2002). Analysis of variance frameworks in clinical child and adolescent psychology: Advanced issues and recommendations. *Journal of Clinical Child and Adolescent Psychology, 31*, 278–294. doi:10.1207/153744202753604557

Jazaieri, H., McGonigal, K., Jinpa, T., Doty, J. R., Gross, J. J., & Goldin, P. R. (2014). A randomized controlled trial of compassion cultivation training: Effects on mindfulness, affect, and emotion regulation. *Motivation and Emotion, 38*, 23–35. doi:10.1007/s11031-013-9368-z

Jopling, D. A. (2000). *Self-knowledge and the self.* New York, NY: Routledge.

Karlsen, K. E., Vrabel, K., & Benum, K. (2018). Effect of Yoga in the treatment of eating disorders: A single-blinded randomized controlled trial with 6-month follow-up. *International Journal of Yoga, 11*, 166. doi:10.4103/ijoy.ijoy_3_17

Katterman, S. N., Kleinman, B. M., Hood, M. M., Nackers, L. M., & Corsica, J. A. (2014). Mindfulness meditation as an intervention for binge eating, emotional eating, and weight loss: A systematic review. *Eating Behaviors, 15*, 197–204. doi:10.1016/j.eatbeh.2014.01.005

Kelly, A. C., Carter, J. C., & Borairi, S. (2014). Are improvements in shame and self-compassion early in eating disorder treatment associated with better patient outcomes? *International Journal of Eating Disorders, 47*, 54–64. doi:10.1002/eat.22196

Kelly, A. C., Carter, J. C., Zuroff, D. C., & Borairi, S. (2013). Self-compassion and fear of self-compassion interact to predict response to eating disorders treatment: A preliminary investigation. *Psychotherapy Research, 23*, 252–264. doi:10.1080/10503307.2012.717310

Krabbenborg, M. A. M., Danner, U. N., Larsen, J. K., van der Veer, N., van Elburg, A. A., de Ridder, D. T. D., … Engels, R. C. M. E. (2011). The eating disorder diagnostic scale: Psychometric features within a clinical population and a cut-off point to differentiate clinical patients from healthy controls. *European Eating Disorders Review, 20*, 315–320. doi:10.1002/erv.1144

Lau, M. A., Bishop, S. R., Segal, Z. V., Buis, T., Anderson, N. D., Carlson, L., ... Carmody, J. (2006). The Toronto mindfulness scale: Development and validation. *Journal of Clinical Psychology*, *62*, 1445–1467. doi:10.1002/jclp.20326

Leehr, E. J., Krohmer, K., Schag, K., Dresler, T., Zipfel, S., & Giel, K. E. (2015). Emotion regulation model in binge eating disorder and obesity—-A systematic review. *Neuroscience and Behavioral Reviews*, *49*, 5–134. doi:10.1016/j.neubiorev.2014.12.008

Linardon, J., Hindle, A., & Brennan, L. (2018). Dropout from cognitive-behavioral therapy for eating disorders: A meta-analysis of randomized, controlled trials. *International Journal of Eating Disorders*, *5*, 381–389. doi:10.1002/eat.22850

McIver, S., O'Halloran, P., & McGartland, M. (2009). Yoga as a treatment for binge eating disorder: A preliminary study. *Complementary Therapies in Medicine*, *17*, 196–202. doi:10.1016/j.ctim.2009.05.002

Mond, J. M., Hay, P. J., Rodgers, B., & Owen, C. (2007). Health service utilization for eating disorders: Findings from a community-based study. *International Journal of Eating Disorders*, *40*, 399–409. doi:10.1002/eat.20382

National Eating Disorder Association. (2013). Binge eating disorder: A new diagnosis in the diagnostic and statistical manual of mental disorders. Retrieved from https://www.nationa leatingdisorders.org/sites/default/files/ResourceHandouts/MultiPageRGB.pdf

Neff, K. D., & Dahm, K. A. (2014). Self-compassion: What it is, what it does, and how it relates to mindfulness. In M. Robinson, B. Meier, & B. Ostafin (Eds.), *Mindfulness and self-regulation* (pp. 121–140). New York, NY: Springer.

Pacanowski, C. R., Diers, L., Crosby, R. D., & Neumark-Sztainer, D. (2017). Yoga in the treatment of eating disorders within a residential program: A randomized controlled trial. *Eating Disorders*, *25*, 37–51. doi:10.1080/10640266.2016.1237810

Petrik, A. M., & Cronin, T. J. (2014). Defining and measuring mechanisms of change in psychological therapies: The path not taken. *Australian Psychologist*, *49*, 283–286. doi:10.1111/ap.12073

Porges, S. W. (2001). The polyvagal theory: Phylogenetic substrates of a social nervous system. *International Journal of Psychophysiology*, *42*, 123–146. doi:10.1016/s0167-8760(01)00162-3

Raes, F., Pommier, E., Neff, K. D., & Van Gucht, D. (2011). Construction and factorial validation of a short form of the self-compassion scale. *Clinical Psychology and Psychotherapy*, *18*, 250–255. doi:10.1002/cpp.702

Safer, D. L., & Jo, B. (2010). Outcome from a randomized controlled trial of group therapy for binge eating disorder: Comparing dialectical behavior therapy adapted for binge eating to an active comparison group. *Behavior Therapy*, *41*, 106–120. doi:10.1016/j.beth.2009.01.006

Safer, D. L., Telch, C. F., & Agras, W. S. (2001). Dialectical behavior therapy for bulimia nervosa. *American Journal of Psychiatry*, *158*, 632–634. doi:10.1176/appi.ajp.158.4.632

Steindl, S. R., Buchanan, K., Goss, K., & Allan, S. (2017). Compassion focused therapy for eating disorders: A qualitative review and recommendations for further applications. *Clinical Psychologist*, *21*, 62–73. doi:10.1111/cp.12126

Stellar, J. E., Cohen, A., Oveis, C., & Keltner, D. (2015). Affective and physiological responses to the suffering of others: Compassion and vagal activity. *Journal of Personality and Social Psychology*, *108*, 572–585. doi:10.1037/pspi0000010

Stice, E. (2002). Risk and maintenance factors for eating pathology: A meta-analytic review. *Psychological Bulletin*, *128*, 825–848. doi:10.1037//0033-2909.128.5.825

Stice, E., Telch, C. F., & Rizvi, S. L. (2000). Development and validation of the eating disorder diagnostic scale: A brief self-report measure of anorexia, bulimia, and binge-eating disorder. *Psychological Assessment*, *12*, 123–131. doi:10.1037//1040-3590.12.2.123

Sullivan, M. B., Erb, M., Schmalzl, L., Moonaz, S., Taylor, J. N., & Porges, S. W. (2018). Yoga therapy and polyvagal theory: The convergence of traditional wisdom and contemporary neuroscience for self-regulation and resilience. *Frontiers in Human Neuroscience, 12*. doi:10.3389/fnhum.2018.00067

Svendsen, J. L., Osnes, B., Binder, P-E., Dundas, I., Visted, E., Nordby, H., … Sørensen, L. (2016). Trait self-compassion reflects emotional flexibility through an association with high vaguely mediated heart rate variability. *Mindfulness, 7*, 1103–1113. doi:10.1007/s12671-016-0549-1

Telch, C. F., Agras, W. S., & Linehan, M. M. (2001). Dialectical behavior therapy for binge eating disorder. *Journal of Consulting and Clinical Psychology, 69*, 1061–1065. doi:10.1037//0022-006x.69.6.1061

Teper, R., Segal, Z. V., & Inzlicht. (2013). Inside the mindful mind: How mindfulness enhances emotion regulation through improvements in executive control. *Current Directions in Psychological Science, 22*, 449–454. doi:10.1177/0963721413495869

Treasure, J., Corfield, F., & Cardi, V. (2012). A three-phase model of the social emotional functioning in eating disorders. *European Eating Disorders Review, 20*, 431–438. doi:10.1002/erv.2181

Tyagi, A., & Cohen, M. (2016). Yoga and heart rate variability: A comprehensive review of the literature. *International Journal of Yoga, 9*, 97–113. doi:10.4103/0973-6131.183712

Whelton, W. J., & Greenberg, L. S. (2005). Emotion in self-criticism. *Personality and Individual Differences, 38*, 1583–1595. doi:10.1016/j.paid.2004.09.024

Whelton, W. J., Paulson, B. L., & Marusiak, C. (2007). Self-criticism and the therapeutic relationship. *Counselling Psychology Quarterly, 20*, 135–148. doi:10.1080/09515070701412423

Wilson, G. T., Grilo, C. M., & Vitousek, K. M. (2007). Psychological treatment of eating disorders. *American Psychologist, 62*, 199–216. doi:10.1037/0003-066x.62.3.199

Examining the effects of mindfulness-based yoga instruction on positive embodiment and affective responses

Anne E. Cox, Sarah Ullrich-French, Catherine Cook-Cottone, Tracy L. Tylka, and Dianne Neumark-Sztainer

ABSTRACT

Empirical evidence provides support for the inclusion of yoga as part of eating disorder prevention efforts through its positive impact on positive embodiment and experience of positive core affect. However, there is a need to identify the specific instructional strategies that will more consistently support positive embodiment and positive affect. We examined the effect of teaching a single yoga class using mindfulness-based instruction compared to appearance-based and neutral instruction alternatives on embodiment (i.e., state body surveillance, state body appreciation, pleasure during yoga) and changes in affect from before to after class. Female participants ($N = 62$; $M_{age} = 23.89$, $SD = 6.86$) were randomly assigned to a yoga class that emphasized: being mindfully present in one's body, changing one's appearance, or just getting into yoga poses. ANOVAs revealed significantly higher body surveillance ($\eta_p^2 = .10$) and lower forecasted pleasure ($\eta_p^2 = .21$) in the appearance class compared to the other two classes. Participants in the mindfulness class experienced greater improvement in affect ($\eta_p^2 = .08$) from before to after class and higher remembered pleasure during the yoga class ($\eta_p^2 = .19$) compared to those in the appearance class. Emphasizing changes to appearance in yoga instruction may place participants at risk for less positive affect and less positive experiences of embodiment compared to mindfulness-based or even neutral yoga instruction.

Clinical Implications

- Participating in a mindfulness-infused or neutrally instructed yoga class may confer greater experiences of pleasure and embodiment compared to appearance-focused instruction.

- Emphasizing changes to appearance in yoga instructions puts participants at risk for less positive experiences of embodiment.

Introduction

Yoga has become increasingly recommended as a practice that may aid in the prevention of eating disorders (Klein & Cook-Cottone, 2013; Osterman et al., 2019). In their systematic review, Klein and Cook-Cottone found that yoga was associated with either lower or no change in eating disorder symptoms and reduced eating disorder risk factors (e.g., negative body image). Understanding how characteristics such as the type, or amount of yoga practiced or how instructors use language to deliver yoga influence core mechanisms of risk will lead to the development of more effective eating disorder prevention interventions. Two likely mechanisms include the cultivation of better emotion regulation and increased positive embodiment as suggested by research findings among yoga practitioners in general (Mahlo & Tiggemann, 2016), yoga practitioners with trauma-histories (Rhodes, 2015), and individuals diagnosed with disordered eating assigned to a yoga intervention (Carei et al., 2010). Eating disorder prevention research suggests that positive embodiment (Levine & Smolak, 2016; Tylka & Kroon Van Diest, 2015) and positive affect (Fredrickson, 2013) may serve as protective factors that serve to disrupt the development of negative body image and emotional dysregulation that are characteristic of eating disorders. Whereas, negative body image and negative affect are consistently associated with the clinical presentation of eating disorders (e.g., Kitsantas et al., 2003; Stice, 2002; Stice & Shaw, 2002).

In practice, yoga may help cultivate these protective factors by providing repeated opportunities to experience the body from an internal, subjective perspective, appreciate one's unique physical characteristics, and notice body sensations and emotional experiences as they come and go (Cook-Cottone, 2020). These experiences are thought to be facilitated by using breath and mindful awareness to simply be with the body and feelings rather than reacting to or attempting to suppress or avoid experience (Cook-Cottone, 2020). Examining how the characteristics of yoga instruction optimize increases in positive embodiment and positive affect may inform the development of more effective interventions aimed at preventing eating disorders in the general population.

Positive embodiment

Embodiment is a complex and multi-faceted construct. Piran (2016, 2017) has developed the Developmental Theory of Embodiment (DTE) to describe five dimensions of positive embodiment: (1) body connection and comfort, (2) agency and functionality, (3) experience and expression of desire, (4) attuned self-care, and (5) inhabiting the body subjectively rather than objectively. We focus on two dimensions that have received empirical support in the yoga context (e.g., Mahlo & Tiggemann, 2016): *inhabiting the body subjectively* and *body connection/comfort*. The DTE also describes both risks and protective processes that impact one's experience of embodiment (Piran, 2016, 2017, 2019). Physical activity participation that is characterized by being joyfully immersed and not engaging for the purpose of changing the shape or appearance of the body represents one such process (Calogero et al., 2019). Therefore, we also explore the pleasure participants experience during yoga participation as an indicator of positive embodiment.

Inhabiting the body subjectively refers to paying attention to one's internal experience of their body including a range of physical sensations while resisting the pressure to view one's body as an object from an external perspective (Piran, 2016, 2017). There is evidence that supports the relationship between yoga participation and inhabiting the body subjectively. For example, those who participate in yoga (vs. those who do not) have higher body awareness, stronger mind-body connection, and lower self-objectification/body surveillance (i.e., concern about the appearance of one's body; Daubenmier, 2005; Mahlo & Tiggemann, 2016). Body surveillance also declines over the course of sustained yoga participation (Cox, Ullrich-French, Cole, et al., 2016; Cox et al., 2017, 2019; Impett et al., 2006). *Body connection and comfort* means that one feels comfortable, connected, and positive towards their body as they move through the world (Piran, 2016, 2017). Body appreciation is one indicator of this dimension and refers to having respect, appreciation, and acceptance for the unique characteristics of the body (Avalos et al., 2005; Tylka & Wood-Barcalow, 2015). Higher body appreciation was observed in those who practice yoga compared to those who do not (Mahlo & Tiggemann, 2016), and significant increases in body appreciation were observed over the course of 16 weeks of yoga participation (Cox et al., 2019).

Finally, positive embodiment may be enhanced by joyful immersion, or experiencing pleasure during physical activity (Calogero et al., 2019; Piran, 2016, 2017, 2019). There is evidence that yoga practice supports the experience of pleasure while engaged in this form of physical activity. For example, Mackenzie et al. (2014) found that the experience of pleasure in female cancer survivors increased linearly across the duration of an 80-minute yoga class. The extent to which participants are joyfully immersed in the yoga context can be assessed by the degree of pleasure they remember experiencing during yoga participation and the degree to which they expect to experience pleasure during yoga in the future (i.e., forecasted pleasure; Kahneman et al., 1997). Remembered and forecasted pleasure are also critical for supporting future positive embodied experiences since they are predictive of physical activity behavior intentions and behavior generally (Conner et al., 2015; Kwan et al., 2017). Thus, more positive remembered and forecasted pleasure may increase the probability that individuals will seek out future yoga experiences.

Change in affect

Another pathway by which yoga may help reduce eating disorder risk is through better regulation of stress-response systems (Pascoe & Bauer, 2015), which can lead to improvements in affect. Enhanced self-regulation leads to improvements in core affect or the most basic, fundamental assessment of the degree of pleasantness or unpleasantness that one is experiencing (Ekkekakis & Petruzzello, 2000) and is one of the features underlying specific emotions such as anxiety or sadness (Russell & Barrett, 1999). Empirical evidence supports improvements in affect associated with yoga participation. For example, adults participating in a week-long yoga camp demonstrated a 13% increase in positive affect and 47% decrease in negative affect from the first to last day of the camp (Narasimhan et al., 2011). In a randomized controlled trial in a residential eating disorder treatment program, patients demonstrated lower negative affect immediately following participation in a single yoga class session compared to a control group (Pacanowski et al., 2017).

The yoga context

The research on positive embodiment and affective responses in the yoga context all point to the potential for yoga to play a role in supporting pathways to eating disorder prevention and recovery. While a majority of yoga participants have discussed the positive impacts of yoga on their body image and embodiment, a minority also voiced that practicing yoga actually prompted social comparison and negative self-talk about their body (Neumark-Sztainer et al., 2018). The variability in yoga participants' experiences underscores the importance of identifying the elements of the yoga context, such as the instruction provided, that support or undermine positive embodiment and improvement in affect. For instance, a yoga instructor may make comments regarding weight loss, body change, and body shape throughout the class (e.g., "Engage those glutes to burn the fat"). Such comments could detract from participants' ability to immerse themselves fully and joyfully in the practice, experience the body subjectively, and appreciate one's body.

Accordingly, many recommendations for supporting positive embodiment in the yoga context center on the nature of the yoga instruction participants receive (Cook-Cottone & Douglass, 2017; Piran & Neumark-Sztainer, 2020). Consistent with the DTE (Piran, 2019) and research findings (e.g., Neumark-Sztainer et al., 2018), researchers have suggested that positive embodiment can be facilitated by encouraging participants to be present in the moment and focus on the way their body feels (i.e., interoceptive cues), emphasizing a connection with the body (e.g., through the use of breath), and making references to noticing one's experience rather than changing or fixing it as well as refraining from negative body talk, fat talk, and weight loss or fitness references (Cook-Cottone, 2020; Cook-Cottone & Douglass, 2017). Despite these theoretically grounded recommendations on how to create yoga settings that support positive embodiment, tests of the effectiveness of implementing such approaches are rare. Examining potential mechanisms that explain why or how yoga facilitates improvements in positive embodiment and affective responses is a critical step towards the development of effective yoga interventions or programs that support the prevention or treatment of eating disorders.

A potential unifying theme for the practical recommendations for facilitating embodiment in yoga is mindfulness. Mindfulness refers to open, accepting, nonjudgmental attention and awareness to what is occurring in the present moment (Bishop et al., 2004; Tanay & Bernstein, 2013). Mindful attention to the body during yoga participation has shown particular relevance to embodiment variables. For example, body surveillance and state mindfulness of the body during yoga participation are inversely related (Cox, Ullrich-French, & French, 2016; Cox et al., 2017). The results of a latent growth curve analysis illustrated a positive association between growth in trait mindfulness and growth in body appreciation during 16 weeks of yoga participation in a university sample (Cox & McMahon, 2019). More rigorous experimental designs are needed to build on these observational findings to determine if manipulating mindfulness-based yoga instruction impacts participants' experiences of embodiment and affect.

The purpose of this study was to experimentally test the effect of different instructional cues in a single yoga class on positive embodiment variables and change in affect among women. Dependent variables included core affect before and after the yoga class and post-class assessments of state mindfulness, state body surveillance, state body appreciation, remembered pleasure experienced during the yoga class, and forecasted pleasure during a future yoga class. Participants were randomly assigned to one of three experimentally manipulated yoga classes: (a) mindfulness-based, (b) appearance-based, or (c) neutral. The appearance-based class was selected as a comparison class since thinking about one's outward physical appearance represents a state of low mindfulness and has been theorized to undermine positive embodiment (Cook-Cottone, 2020; Cook-Cottone & Douglass, 2017; Piran, 2016, 2017). Including a neutral class in which participants were simply instructed into the poses provided a strong test of the potential added benefit of including specific mindfulness-based instruction. We hypothesized that state mindfulness during the yoga class, positive embodiment variables, and changes in core affect would be most adaptive in the mindfulness-based class, followed by the neutral condition, and least adaptive in the appearance-based class.

Method

Participant recruitment

Participants were recruited from large representative undergraduate classes and sororities at a mid-sized university in the Northwest region of the United States. Flyers were also posted around campus and on social media.

Measures

Descriptive variables

Participants were asked to report their race, age, and whether or not they were a student. They were also asked if they were a regular exerciser (i.e., at least three times per week for at least 20 minutes at a time; yes/no), regular meditator (yes/no), or were regularly engaging in a yoga practice (yes/no). They reported their level of yoga proficiency on a scale from 1–5, with higher scores indicating greater proficiency (see Daubenmier, 2005).

Baseline variables

Key variables that were relevant to the outcome variables were assessed in order to test for baseline differences. These included trait mindfulness, physical activity motivation, and indicators of positive (i.e., body appreciation) and negative body image (i.e., body preoccupation). These variables were assessed with the Short Inventory for Mindfulness Capabilities (SIM-C; Duan & Li, 2016), the Behavioral Regulation in Exercise Questionnaire-3 (BREQ-3; Markland & Tobin, 2004), the Body Appreciation Scale-2 (BAS-2; Tylka & Wood-Barcalow, 2015), and the Body Shape Questionnaire-R-10 (BSQ-R-10; Mazzeo, 1999), respectively.

State mindfulness

The body subscale (6 items) from the State Mindfulness Scale for Physical Activity (SMS-PA; Cox, Ullrich-French, & French, 2016) assessed how mindful participants were of their physical sensations (mindfulness of the body; e.g., "I focused on the movement of my body") throughout the yoga class. Participants respond to each of the items using a response scale ranging from 0 *(not at all)* to 4 *(very much)*. Items are averaged and higher scores represent higher mindfulness of the body. There is evidence of the internal consistency reliability (current study α = .79) and construct validity of the SMS-PA with college samples (e.g., Cox, Ullrich-French, & French, 2016).

Affective responses

The Feeling Scale (FS; Hardy & Rejeski, 1989) was used to assess basic affective valence immediately before and after the yoga class. The single item scale ranges from 5 *(very good)* to −5 *(very bad)* with additional scale descriptors at 3 *(good)*, 1 *(fairly good)*, 0 *(neutral)*, −1 *(fairly bad)*, and −3 (*bad*). Studies provide concurrent validity evidence of the FS (Hardy & Rejeski, 1989; Van Landuyt et al., 2000).

Remembered and forecasted pleasure during yoga participation

Participants' memory of how pleasant the yoga class had been was assessed with a visual analogue scale (see Zenko et al., 2016). They were asked, "Using the scale below please CIRCLE the ONE number that best represents the overall amount of pleasantness or unpleasantness that you felt during the yoga class today." They responded on a 21-point scale from −10 (*Very unpleasant experience*) to 10 (*Very pleasant experience*) with 0 in the middle representing *neutral*. Zenko et al. provided evidence of construct validity using a similar scale in their study on responses to exercise. The Empirical Valence Scale (EVS; Lishner et al., 2008) was used to assess participants' forecasted pleasure. Participants were asked, "If you repeated this yoga session again (in the future), how do you think it would make you feel?" They responded by circling one descriptor on a scale from *most unpleasant imaginable* (−100) *to most pleasant imaginable* (100), with 13 additional descriptors in between. There is evidence of construct validity for the use of this scale within the context of exercise (Zenko et al., 2016).

State body appreciation

The degree to which participants experienced body appreciation immediately following the yoga class was assessed with the state version of the Body Appreciation Scale-2 (Homan, 2016). This measure captures acceptance of, opinions towards, and respect of one's body in the present moment. Participants answer nine items about how they feel at "this very moment" (e.g., "Right now, I respect my body," "At this moment, I feel good about my body") on a 5-point scale ranging from 1 (*strongly disagree*) to 5 (*strongly agree*). Items were averaged to represent a score for state body appreciation in the main analyses. There is evidence of internal consistency reliability (current study $\alpha = .93$) and construct validity in adult samples (e.g., Homan, 2016).

State body surveillance

State body surveillance was assessed using the Body Surveillance subscale of the Objectified Body Consciousness Scale (OBC; McKinley & Hyde, 1996). Participants responded to seven items that were modified to refer to their experience in the yoga class (e.g., "I rarely thought about how I looked," "I thought more about how my body felt than how my body looked") on a scale from 1 (*strongly disagree*) to 7 (*strongly agree*). One item from the original scale was not included because it was not relevant or easily modified to the state experience (i.e., "I think it is more important that my clothes are comfortable than whether they look good on me"). So that higher scores reflect higher body surveillance, five items are reverse coded and then all are averaged. Empirical evidence supports the use of this state version in physical activity settings (e.g., Cox, Ullrich-French, & French, 2016; current study α = .82).

Manipulation check items

Two manipulation check items were used to assess the degree to which the participants perceived a class focus on appearance or on being in one's body (i.e., mindfulness of the body). Participants responded on a 5-point scale (1 = *very slightly or not at all*; 2 = *a little*; 3 = *moderately*; 4 = *quite a bit*; 5 = *extremely*): 1. "The teacher in the yoga class I just completed focused on changing one's physical appearance through yoga"; 2. "The teacher in the yoga class I just completed focused on the way our body felt during the yoga class."

Procedures

A between-subjects randomized experimental design was used for this study. IRB approval was obtained from the participating university. Participants provided informed consent and then completed baseline measures via an online survey. Only those participants who identified as female, reported no more than moderate yoga proficiency (i.e., '3' on a scale from 1–5), and who answered 'no' to currently engaging in a "regular" yoga practice were invited to participate in the yoga class portion of the study. We specifically recruited less experienced participants so that they were less likely to have been influenced by previous yoga instruction which could have carry-over effects into the manipulation.

Participants were randomly assigned to one of three yoga class conditions: mindfulness-based, appearance-based, or neutral. A 45-minute yoga sequence was created for an all-levels class. The physical postures or asanas as well as the basic language used to get participants into the poses were held constant across all three conditions. A script was created for each condition and used by the yoga instructor to teach the class. The mindfulness-based and appearance-based conditions contained language for each pose that helped them be present in their body or focus on how the yoga practice would change the appearance of their body, respectively. Table 1 includes examples from each condition. To enhance the ecological validity, we allowed for some variability in the exact wording of the yoga instruction rather than having the instructor read verbatim from the script. To assess the internal validity of each condition, two research assistants independently rated the frequency of cues related to mindfulness or appearance in each class and the average number of cues was calculated by condition. The same yoga instructor taught all classes and had 200-hour certifications in Anusara Yoga and from the Yandara Institute.

On the day of their assigned yoga class, upon arrival participants completed a consent form and the Physical Activity Readiness Questionnaire

Table 1. Examples of yoga poses and instruction for the three conditions.

Pose	Mindful Instruction	Appearance Instruction	Neutral Instruction
Child's Pose	Shift your pelvis back over your feet and reach your torso and arms forward for child's pose. Soak in the feeling of being grounded and held in this restful pose.	Shift the pelvis back over the feet and reach the torso and arms forward for child's pose. Here, you can tone those arms towards one another on the mat … working on slimming the upper arms.	Shift the pelvis back over the feet and reach the torso and arms forward for child's pose.
Downward Facing Dog	Press through your feet, lift your tail into downward dog pose. Alternate bending your knees and pressing your heels into the ground to warm up your legs. Notice the feeling of strength in your shoulders and back. Allow thoughts that arise to come and go …. Breathe.	Press through the feet, lift the tail into downward dog pose. Alternate bending the knees and pressing the heels into the ground to warm up the legs. Downward dog is great for getting that muscular definition in the shoulders and back and losing excess fat there.	Press through the feet, lift the tail into downward dog pose. Alternate bending the knees and pressing the heels into the ground to warm up the legs.
Side Angle	Plug your elbow into the stability of your knee and feel the connection in side angle. From your foundation of strength, what do you notice along the right side of your body?	Lower the front elbow to knee for side angle. To increase the calorie burn, engage the legs and firm the core.	Lower the front elbow to the knee for side angle.

(PAR-Q; Warburton et al., 2014), which includes questions about one's general health and is used to determine if participants are healthy enough to safely participate in physical activity. If they answered 'yes' to any questions on the PAR-Q, it indicates that they have a health risk that may make physical activity unsafe and they were excluded. Participants were then given a survey packet to take with them and directed to sit on a mat and wait for the class to begin. Just prior to the start of class, a research assistant asked participants to complete the FS for current affective valence from the survey packet. Then the yoga instructor taught for 38 to 45 minutes in the assigned condition. At the end of the class, participants immediately completed measures of affect, state body appreciation, state mindfulness of the mind and body, state body surveillance, remembered and forecasted pleasure, and a subsample completed additional manipulation check items. Participants then turned in their survey packets and received a 5.00 USD gift card for their participation. When participants did not show up for their assigned yoga class (0–5 per session), research assistants were standing by to serve as confederates to make the class environment more realistic. Up to three confederates participated in each class session and classes. There were a total of five mindfulness-based ($n = 19$), five appearance-based ($n = 23$), and seven neutral ($n = 20$) yoga class sessions with two to eight participants per session for a total of 62 participants.

Data analyses

We first tested for assumptions of normality, homogeneity of variance, and outliers followed by a series of one-way ANOVAs and chi-square tests to test for differences in baseline variables. In order to test for differences in the primary dependent variables across the three conditions a series of one-way ANOVAs was conducted. For affective valence from the FS, change scores were created by subtracting the baseline affect scores from the post-class affect scores and used in the analysis. When the results of an ANOVA were significant, pairwise comparisons using least significant difference (equal variance assumed) were examined to determine which groups differed.

Results

Participants

There were 62 female participants ages 18–54 (M_{age} = 23.89, SD = 6.86). They mostly self-reported as Caucasian (74.2%), and 51 were students (11 graduate students). Thirty-two self-reported being at a beginner level of yoga, 25 at a beginning-intermediate level, and five at an intermediate level. Six reported having a regular meditation or mindfulness practice.

Preliminary analyses

Manipulation checks

One-way ANOVAs examining the observed frequency of cues related to mindfulness and appearance across the three conditions illustrated clear patterns that support the intended condition content. The mindfulness condition had the highest number of mindfulness cues (M = 87.1) compared to the appearance (M = 16.75) and neutral (M = 8.92) conditions, $F(2)$ = 94.07, $p < .001$, η_p^2 = .86). The appearance condition had the highest number of appearance cues (M = 21.42) compared to the mindfulness (M = 0.00) and neutral (M = 6.42) conditions, $F(2)$ = 6.24, p = .005, η_p^2 = .29). The neutral condition did not differ from the mindfulness condition on appearance cues and did not differ from the appearance condition on mindfulness cues. A subsample of participants (n = 4 from neutral, n = 6 from appearance, n = 7 from mindfulness) completed the participant manipulation check items. One-way ANOVAs revealed significant ($p < .05$) differences. For the degree of focus on changing one's appearance, $F(2)$ = 241.10, $p < .001$, η_p^2 = .97, the appearance condition participants reported a significantly ($p < .001$) higher emphasis (M = 4.83) compared to both neutral (M = 1.25) and mindfulness conditions (M = 1.00). For the degree of focus on the way their body felt, $F(2)$ = 5.64, p = .016, η_p^2 = .45, the mindfulness condition participants reported significantly (p = .013) greater emphasis (M = 5.00) compared to the appearance condition (M = 3.33) and was higher but was not significantly different from the neutral condition (M = 4.00).

Testing assumptions

There was one outlier ($z > |3.5|$) in the appearance condition on forecasted pleasure. The analysis for forecasted pleasure was conducted with and without this outlier and the interpretation of results did not change. Therefore, all participants were retained in all main analyses. In addition, several of the dependent variables violated assumptions related to normality (i.e., core affect, remembered and forecasted pleasure, state mindfulness of the body) and homogeneity of variance (i.e., remembered and forecasted pleasure, body appreciation). In these cases, appropriate robust analyses (e.g., for normality: Welsh, Brown-Forsyth; for homogeneity: Kruskal Wallis; for follow ups Man-Whitney U and Games Howell[1]) were performed to address the specific violations. In most cases, these additional analyses confirmed the traditional ANOVA results. However, we have noted the instances where this is not the case.

Hypothesis testing

There were no baseline differences in positive or negative body image, physical activity motivation, yoga proficiency or trait mindfulness across the three groups of participants ($p > .05$). Nor were there differences in meditation or mindfulness practice. These findings suggest that random assignment was successful in establishing group equivalency on these variables. Descriptive statistics and main results for all dependent variables appear in Table 2.

Table 2. Descriptive statistics for the neutral, appearance, and mindfulness yoga conditions.

	Total Range	Neutral (n = 20) M (SD) Range	Appearance (n = 23) M (SD) Range	Mindfulness (n = 19) M (SD) Range
1. Mindfulness of Body	0 to 4	3.52[a] (0.46) 2.67–4.00	3.57[a] (0.48) 2.33–4.00	3.46[a] (0.53) 2.17–4.00
2. Pre Affect	−5 to 5	2.30 (1.03) 1.00–4.00	2.17 (1.72) −1.00–5.00	2.16 (1.68) −2.00–5.00
3. Post Affect	−5 to 5	3.40 (0.75) 2.00–5.00	2.83 (2.01) −2.00–5.00	3.74 (1.33) 1.00–5.00
4. Change in Affect	−10 to 10	1.10[ab] (0.97) −1.00–3.00	0.65[a] (1.77) −4.00–4.00	1.58[b] (1.07).00–3.00
5. Remembered Pleasure	−10 to 10	6.60[a] (2.64) −2–10	3.87[b] (5.49) −8–10	8.11[c] (4.12) 5–10
6. Forecasted Pleasure	−100 to 100	58.10[a] (16.90) 24.00–70.00	33.57[b] (40.58) −70.00–70.00	66.33[a] (13.89) 38.00–85.00
7. Body Surveillance	1 to 7	2.86[a] (1.05) 1.00–5.14	3.70[b] (1.36) 1.43–6.29	2.92[a] (1.18) 1.00–5.86
8. Body Appreciation	1 to 5	3.98[a] (0.39) 3.22–5.00	3.80 [a] (0.85) 2.00–5.00	3.98 [a] (0.72) 2.00–5.00

Different superscripts indicate significant (p <.05) differences between groups.

State mindfulness

There were no significant differences in state mindfulness of the body, $F(2) = 0.26$, $p = .78$, $\eta_p^2 = .01$.

Change in affect

The ANOVA showed a modest effect size for change in affect from before to after the yoga class, $F(2) = 2.45$, $p = .10$, $\eta_p^2 = .08$. Participants in the mindfulness condition reported a greater increase in affect (i.e., more positive; $p = .03$, $d = 0.63$) compared to participants in the appearance condition. The non-parametric Kruskal Wallas test showed similar results to the ANOVA ($p = .11$), with follow-up Mann-Whitney U test confirming a significant difference between mindfulness and appearance conditions ($p = .049$).

Remembered and forecasted pleasure

The ANOVA was significant for remembered pleasure, $F(2) = 6.86$, $p = .002$, $\eta_p^2 = .19$. Participants in the appearance condition reported lower remembered pleasure compared to participants in the neutral ($p = .02$, $d = 0.62$) and mindfulness ($p = .001$, $d = 1.01$) conditions. Due to violation of homogeneity of variance and normality, non-parametric robust tests were run and confirmed condition differences. Follow-up robust tests showed the mindfulness condition was higher (Games-Howell, $p = .004$) than the appearance condition and differences based on Mann-Whitney U were found for mindfulness and neutral ($p = .032$) and mindfulness and appearance ($p = .004$) conditions.

The ANOVA was significant for forecasted pleasure, $F(2) = 7.89$, $p = .001$, $\eta_p^2 = .21$. Participants in the appearance condition reported lower forecasted pleasure compared to participants in the neutral ($p = .006$, $d = 0.77$) and mindfulness ($p < .001$, $d = 1.04$) conditions. Non-parametric robust tests were run and confirmed the condition differences.

State body surveillance and body appreciation

The ANOVA for state body surveillance was significant, $F(2) = 3.27$, $p = .045$, $\eta_p^2 = .10$. Participants in the appearance condition reported higher body surveillance compared to participants in the neutral ($p = .03$, $d = 0.70$) and mindfulness ($p = .04$, $d = 0.61$) conditions. There were no significant differences in state body appreciation, $F(2) = 0.47$, $p = .63$, $\eta_p^2 = .02$.

Discussion

In this experiment, the content of yoga instruction was investigated as a potential explanation for the effect of yoga on positive embodiment and affect, thus playing a role in eating disorder prevention. In three distinct conditions, yoga instruction was delivered in a mindful manner that encouraged an open and receptive attention to bodily sensations and experiences, an appearance-focused approach that focused on altering one's physical appearance, or in a neutral style that simply instructed participants into the poses. Overall, results suggest that appearance-based instruction may place participants at greater risk of less positive embodiment and lower positive affect compared to mindfulness-based and neutral instruction.

Consistent with hypotheses, participants in the mindfulness condition exhibited greater improvements in core affect and reported greater remembered pleasure compared to participants in the appearance condition and neutral condition (only remembered pleasure). Forecasted pleasure was higher and body surveillance lower in participants in both the mindfulness and neutral conditions compared to those in the appearance-focused condition. Consistent with the DTE (Piran, 2019) and practice guidelines (Cook-Cottone & Douglass, 2017), the data indicate that participants in the mindfulness condition had the most positive experiences during the yoga class and those in the appearance-focused class had the least positive experiences, with medium to large effect sizes. In some cases, experiences in the mindful and neutral conditions were similar (e.g., forecasted pleasure, body surveillance) indicating no specific added benefits of adding mindfulness-based instruction over and above simply moving participants through the yoga poses (i.e., the neutral condition). There was, however, some evidence of the specific protective effects of intentional mindfulness-based instruction over neutral instruction (e.g., change in affect) and no indication of risk associated with adding mindful instruction.

These findings are highly consistent with the DTE (Piran, 2019) in that physical activity experiences that are experienced as joyful and support complete immersion in the movement can be protective of positive embodiment, whereas those that are objectifying or emphasize appearance or weight can undermine positive embodiment (Calogero et al., 2019). There were apparent benefits to positive embodiment variables in both the mindfulness and neutral class compared to the appearance class. Generally, these findings are consistent with the increases documented in positive embodiment that occur with yoga participation (e.g., Cox et al., 2019; Halliwell et al., 2019) as well as the general health benefits of a traditional Asana practice throughout its long history (Salmon et al., 2009). However, there are differences across studies in terms of which embodiment variables change, indicating the need for further investigation of different types of yoga. The results also echo studies showing the negative impact of exercise settings that emphasize appearance (e.g., mirrors, instruction) on body image variables and affect (Frayeh & Lewis, 2018; Raedeke et al., 2007).

There were no differences in how mindful participants were of the physical sensations across the three conditions. Regardless of how the yoga condition was instructed, they were equally aware of the experience of being in their body. This is certainly plausible given that in the appearance condition, there were cues directing participants to think about various parts of their body (e.g., abs). The measure of state mindfulness may not be sensitive enough to detect the difference between paying attention to bodily sensations and being open and accepting of whatever sensations might arise. Therefore, future measurement development is needed to better capture these different components of mindfulness.

This initial investigation into the effects of mindfulness-based yoga instruction on participants' affective responses and experiences of embodiment provides preliminary data on how it might differ from appearance-focused instruction. However, this study was limited by a relatively small, homogenous sample and expanding to samples that are more diverse in terms of age, race, yoga experience, or body size are important future directions. In addition, larger samples would provide the opportunity to test for a number of potential moderating variables that could influence the relationship between different types of yoga instruction and affective/embodiment variables. We also included individuals who were mostly at a beginning to beginning-intermediate level of yoga proficiency. It is possible that differences in yoga skill (or even yoga experience or frequency of practice) moderated the effect of the yoga instruction and this will be important to test in future studies. Finally, although we used an experimental design with random assignment, it is important not to overstate results with absolute certainty and more studies are needed to replicate these findings. Building upon the current experimental study by testing longer yoga interventions would enable the examination of how mindfulness-focused yoga instruction may impact more trait-like variables (e.g., body appreciation, distress tolerance) and actual eating behavior over time.

Implications for practice

When it comes to protection or risk, it appears to matter how yoga is delivered. Consistent with the guidance provided by Cook-Cottone and Douglass (2017), therapists and community members interested in utilizing yoga as a pathway to positive embodiment and affect, reduction of eating disorder risk, or potentially, as an adjunct to treatment for disordered eating, should carefully vet the delivery of yoga before offering a referral. Approaches to yoga instruction that emphasize using yoga to change the appearance of the body may increase risk in the form of reinforcing an objectified or external experience of the body. The results of this study show how such an orientation can interfere with experiencing the protective aspects of yoga. More research is needed to further explore yoga instruction and other contextual influences (e.g., mirrors, images of notably thin/fit men and women doing advanced yoga poses on the walls, and the size and shape of the yoga instructor and students in the class; Cook-Cottone & Douglass, 2017). However, for now, careful referral to yoga instructors who are aware of the benefits of a mindful, embodied approach and the risk inherent to an objectifying approach is encouraged.

References

Avalos, L., Tylka, T. L., & Wood-Barcalow, N. (2005). The body appreciation scale: Development and psychometric evaluation. *Body Image, 2*, 285–297. https://doi.org/10.1016/j.bodyim.2005.06.002

Bishop, S. R., Lau, M., Shapiro, S., Carlson, L., Anderson, N. D., Carmody, J., Segal, Z. V., Abbey, S., Speca, M., Velting, D. & Devins, G. (2004). Mindfulness: A proposed operational definition. *Clinical Psychology: Science and Practice, 11(3)*, 230–241. https://doi.org/10.1093/clipsy.bph077

Calogero, R. M., Tylka, T. L., McGilley, B. H., & Pedrotty-Stump, K. N. (2019). Attunement with exercise (AWE). In T. L. Tylka & N. Piran (Eds.), *Handbook of positive body image and embodiment: Constructs, protective factors, and interventions* (pp. 80–90). Oxford University Press.

Carei, T. R, Fyfe-Johnson, A. L, Breuner, C. C, & Brown, M. A. (2010). Randomized controlled clinical trial of yoga in the treatment of eating disorders. *Journal Of Adolescent Health, 46*(4), 346-351. doi:10.1016/j.jadohealth.2009.08.007

Conner, M., McEachan, R., Taylor, N., O'Hara, J., & Lawton, R. (2015). Role of affective attitudes and anticipated affective reactions in predicting health behaviors. *Health Psychology, 34*(6), 642–652. https://doi.org/10.1037/hea0000143

Cook-Cottone, C., & Douglass, L. L. (2017). Yoga communities and eating disorders: Creating safe space for positive embodiment. *International Journal of Yoga Therapy, 27*(1), 87–93. https://doi.org/10.17761/1531-2054-27.1.87

Cook-Cottone, C. P. (2020). *Embodiment and the treatment of eating disorders: The body as a resource in recovery.* Norton.

Cox, A. E., & McMahon, A. K. (2019). Exploring changes in mindfulness and body appreciation during yoga participation. *Body Image, 29*, 118–121. https://doi.org/10.1016/j.bodyim.2019.03.003

Cox, A. E., Ullrich-French, S., Cole, A. N., & D'Hondt-Taylor, M. (2016). The role of state mindfulness during yoga in predicting self-objectification and reasons for exercise. *Psychology of Sport and Exercise, 22*, 321–327. https:/doi.org/10.1016/j.psychsport.2015.10.001

Cox, A. E., Ullrich-French, S., & French, B. F. (2016). Validity evidence for the state mindfulness scale for physical activity. *Measurement in Physical Education and Exercise Science, 20*(1), 38–49. https://doi.org/10.1080/1091367X.2015.108940

Cox, A. E., Ullrich-French, S., Howe, H. S., & Cole, A. N. (2017). A pilot yoga physical education curriculum to promote positive body image. *Body Image, 23*, 1–8. https://doi.org/10.1016/j.bodyim.2017.07.007

Cox, A. E., Ullrich-French, S., Tylka, T. L., & McMahon, A. K. (2019). The roles of self-compassion, body surveillance, and body appreciation in predicting intrinsic motivation for physical activity: Cross-sectional associations, and prospective changes within a yoga context. *Body Image, 29*, 110–117. https://doi.org/10.1016/j.bodyim.2019.03.00

Daubenmier, J. J. (2005). The relationship of yoga, body awareness, and body responsiveness to self- objectification and disordered eating. *Psychology of Women Quarterly, 29*(2), 207–219. https://doi.org/10.1111/j.1471-6402-2005.00183.x

Duan, W., & Li, J. (2016). Distinguishing dispositional and cultivated forms of mindfulness: Item-level factor analysis of five-facet mindfulness questionnaire and construction of short inventory of mindfulness capability. *Frontiers in Psychology, 7*, 1348. https://doi.org/10.3389/fpsyg.2016.01348

Ekkekakis, P., & Petruzzello, S. J. (2000). Analysis of the affect measurement conundrum in exercise psychology: I. Fundamental issues. *Psychology of Sport and Exercise*, *1*(2), 71–88. https://doi.org/10.1016/S1469-0292(00)00010-8

Frayeh, A. L., & Lewis, B. A. (2018). The effect of mirrors on women's state body image responses to yoga. *Psychology of Sport and Exercise*, *35*, 47–54. https://doi.org/10.1016/j.psychosport.2017.11.002

Fredrickson, B. L. (2013). Positive emotions broaden and build. In P. Devine & A. Plant (Eds.), *Advances in experimental social psychology* (Vol. 47, pp. 1–53). Elsevier Academic Press.

Halliwell, E., Dawson, K., & Burkey, S. (2019). A randomized experimental evaluation of a yoga-based body image intervention. *Body Image*, *28*, 119–127. https://doi.org/10.1016/j.bodyim.2018.12.005

Hardy, C. J., & Rejeski, W. J. (1989). Not what, but how one feels: The measurement of affect during exercise. *Journal of Sport and Exercise Psychology*, *11(3)*, 304–317. https://doi.org/10.1123/jsep.13.1.65

Homan, K. J. (2016). Factor structure and psychometric properties of a state version of the body appreciation scale-2. *Body Image*, *19*, 204–207. https://doi.org/10.1016/j.bodyim.2016.10.004

Impett, E. A., Daubenmier, J. J., & Hirschman, A. L. (2006). Minding the body: Yoga, embodiment, and well-being. *Sexuality Research & Social Policy*, *3*(4), 39–48. https://doi.org/10.1525/srsp.2006.3.4.39

Kahneman, D., Wakker, P. P., & Sarin, R. (1997). Back to Bentham? Explorations of experienced utility. *The Quarterly Journal of Economics*, *112*(2), 375–406. https://doi.org/10.1162/003355397555235

Kitsantas, A., Gilligan, T. D., & Kamata, A. (2003). College women with eating disorders: Self-regulation, life satisfaction, and positive/negative affect. *The Journal of Psychology*, *137* (4), 381–395. https://doi.org/10.1080/00223980309600622

Klein, J., & Cook-Cottone, C. (2013). The effects of yoga on eating disorder symptoms and correlates: A review. *International Journal of Yoga Therapy*, *23(2)*, 41–50. https://doi.org/10.17761/ijyt.23.2.2718421234k31854

Kwan, B. M., Stevens, C. J., & Bryan, A. D. (2017). What to expect when you're exercising: An experimental test of the anticipated affect–exercise relationship. *Health Psychology*, *36*(4), 309–319. https://doi.org/10.1037/hea0000453

Levine, M. P., & Smolak, L. (2016). The role of protective factors in the prevention of negative body image and disordered eating. *Eating Disorders*, *24*(1), 39–46. https://doi.org/10.1080/10640266.2015.1113826

Lishner, D. A., Cooter, A. B., & Zald, D. H. (2008). Addressing measurement limitations in affective rating scales: Development of an empirical valence scale. *Cognition and Emotion*, *22*(1), 180–192. https://doi.org/10.1080/026999930701319139

Mackenzie, M. J., Carlson, L. E., Paskevich, D. M., Ekkekakis, P., Wurz, A. J., Wytsma, K., Krenz, K. A., McAuley, E., & Culos-Reed, S. N. (2014). Associations between attention, affect and cardiac activity in a single yoga session for female cancer survivors: An enactive neurophenomenology-based approach. *Consciousness and Cognition*, *27*, 129–146. https://doi.org/10.1016/j.concog.2014.04.005

Mahlo, L., & Tiggemann, M. (2016). Yoga and positive body image: A test of the embodiment model. *Body Image*, *18*, 135–142. https://doi.org/10.1016/j.bodyim.2016.06.008

Markland, D., & Tobin, V. (2004). A modification to the behavioral regulation in exercise questionnaire to include an assessment of amotivation. *Journal of Sport and Exercise Psychology*, *26*(2), 191–196. https://doi.org/10.1123/jsep.26.2.191

Mazzeo, S. E. (1999). Modification of an existing measure of body image preoccupation and its relationship to disordered eating in female college students. *Journal of Counseling Psychology, 46*(1), 42–50. https://doi.org/10.1037/0022-0167.46.1.42

McKinley, N. M., & Hyde, J. S. (1996). The objectified body consciousness scale: Development and validation. *Psychology of Women Quarterly, 20*(2), 181–215. https://doi.org/10.1111/j.1471-6402.1996.tb00467.x

Narasimhan, L., Nagarathna, R., & Nagendra, H. R. (2011). Effect of integrated yogic practices on positive and negative emotions in healthy adults. *International Journal of Yoga, 4*(1), 13–19. https://doi.org/10.4103/0973-6131.78174

Neumark-Sztainer, D., Watts, A. W., & Rydell, S. (2018). Yoga and body image: How do young adults practicing yoga describe its impact on their body image? *Body Image, 27,* 156–168. https://doi.org/10.1016/j.bodyim.2018.09.001

Ostermann, T, Vogel, H, Boehm, K, & Cramer, H. (2019). Effects of yoga on eating disorders–a systematic review. *Complementary Therapies in Medicine, 46*. doi: 10.1016/j.ctim.2019.07.021

Pacanowski, C. R., Diers, L., Crosby, R. D., & Neumark-Sztainer, D. (2017). Yoga in the treatment of eating disorders within a residential program: A randomized controlled trial. *Eating Disorders, 25*(1), 37–51. https://doi.org/10.1080/10640266.2016.1237810

Pascoe, M. C., & Bauer, I. E. (2015). A systematic review of randomized control trials on the effects of yoga on stress measures and mood. *Journal of Psychiatric Research, 68,* 270–282. https://doi.org/10.1016/j.jpsychires.2015.07.013

Piran, N. (2016). Embodied possibilities and disruptions: The emergence of the experience of embodiment construct from qualitative studies with girls and women. *Body Image, 18,* 43–60. https://doi.org/10.1016/j.bodyim.2016.04.007

Piran, N. (2017). *Journeys of embodiment at the intersection of body and culture: The developmental theory of embodiment.* Elsevier.

Piran, N. (2019). The experience of embodiment construct: Reflecting the quality of embodied lives. In T. L. Tylka & N. Piran (Eds.), *Handbook of positive body image and embodiment: Constructs, protective factors, and interventions* (pp. 11–21). Oxford University Press.

Piran, N., & Neumark-Sztainer, D. (2020). Yoga and the experience of embodiment: A discussion of possible links. *Eating Disorders,* 1–19. https://doi.org/10.1080/10640266.2019.1701350

Raedeke, T. D., Focht, B. C., & Scales, D. (2007). Social environmental factors and psychological responses to acute exercise for socially physique anxious females. *Psychology of Sport and Exercise, 8*(4), 463–476. https://doi.org/10.1016/j.psychsport.2006.10.005

Rhodes, A. M. (2015). Claiming peaceful embodiment through yoga in the aftermath of trauma. *Complementary Therapies in Clinical Practice, 21*(4), 247–256. https://doi.org/10.1016/j.ctcp.2015.09.004

Russell, J. A., & Barrett, L. F. (1999). Core affect, prototypical emotional episodes, and other things called emotion: Dissecting the elephant. *Journal of Personality and Social Psychology, 76*(5), 805–819. https://doi.org/10.1037/0022-3514.76.5.805

Salmon, P., Lush, E., Jablonski, M., & Sephton, S. E. (2009). Yoga and mindfulness: Clinical aspects of an ancient mind/body practice. *Cognitive and Behavioral Practice, 16*(1), 59–72. https://doi.org/10.1016/j.cbpra.2008.07.002

Stice, E. (2002). Risk and maintenance factors for eating pathology: A meta-analytic review. *Psychological Bulletin, 128*(5), 825–848. https://doi.org/10.1037/0033-2909.128.5.825

Stice, E., & Shaw, H. E. (2002). Role of body dissatisfaction in the onset and maintenance of eating pathology: A synthesis of research findings. *Journal of Psychosomatic Research, 53*(5), 985–993. https://doi.org/10.1016/s0022-3999(02)00488-9

Tanay, G., & Bernstein, A. (2013). State mindfulness scale (SMS): Development and initial validation. *Psychological Assessment, 25*(4), 1286–1299. https://doi.org/10.1037/a0034044

Tylka, T. L., & Kroon Van Diest, A. M. (2015). Protective factors. In L. Smolak & M. P. Levine (Eds.), *The Wiley handbook of eating disorders* (Vol. 1, pp. 430–444). John Wiley & Sons.

Tylka, T. L., & Wood-Barcalow, N. L. (2015). The body appreciation scale-2: Item refinement and psychometric evaluation. *Body Image, 12*, 53–67. https://doi.org/10.1016/j.bodyim.2014.09.006

Van Landuyt, L. M., Ekkekakis, P., Hall, E. E., & Petruzzello, S. J. (2000). Throwing the mountains into the lakes: On the perils of nomothetic conceptions of the exercise-affect relationship. *Journal of Sport and Exercise Psychology, 22*(3), 208–234. https://doi.org/10.1123/jsep.22.3.208

Warburton, D., Jamnik, V., Bredin, S. S., & Gledhill, N. (2014). The ePARmed-X+ physician clearance follow-up. *The Health and Fitness Journal of Canada, 7*(2), 35–38. https://doi.org/10.14288/hfjc.v7i2.183

Zenko, Z., Ekkekakis, P., & Ariely, D. (2016). Can you have your vigorous exercise and enjoy it too? Ramping intensity down increases postexercise, remembered, and forecasted pleasure. *Journal of Sport and Exercise Psychology, 38*(2), 149–159. https://doi.org/10.1123/jsep.2015-0286

A yoga-based therapy program designed to improve body image among an outpatient eating disordered population: program description and results from a mixed-methods pilot study

Lisa Diers, Sarah A. Rydell ⓘ, Allison Watts, and Dianne Neumark-Sztainer

ABSTRACT

Poor body image is a critical barrier to eating disorder recovery. This pilot project was designed as a feasibility study to examine a novel group-based, therapeutic yoga and body image program (YBI) for addressing negative body image in those clinically diagnosed with an eating disorder (anorexia, bulimia nervosa, and other specified feeding or eating disorder) receiving outpatient level treatment at an eating disorder treatment center located in Minneapolis–St. Paul, Minnesota. Self-administered questionnaires were completed by 67 participants at the beginning and end of the 8-week series, to better understand the acceptability of the YBI program and its potential effects on body image and self-worth during outpatient eating disorder treatment. Quantitative survey questions assessed participants' body image concerns, while open-ended questions probed participants' experiences and the perceived impact of the yoga program on their body image. After completion of the yoga program, mean item scores on the body image concern survey improved: increases ranged from 0.3 to 0.8 points on a 5-point scale. In open-ended questions, participants described many positive changes to their body image. Participants reported that the yoga program improved their self-acceptance, self-awareness, confidence, emotional and physical strength, and was a positive form of release. Participants also discussed physical and emotional challenges of the yoga program and how they contributed to self-judgment, vulnerability, and confrontation of uncomfortable feelings. The results of this pilot study are promising and warrant consideration of more rigorous study designs to explore the potential of a body image specific therapeutic yoga program to aid those in eating disorder treatment to improve body image disturbances.

Clinical Implication

- Yoga instructed with a body-positive theme has the potential to be an effective modality to improve negative body image in people diagnosed with an eating disorder
- A weekly body-positive yoga and process group lead by an eating disorder trained yoga teacher and licensed therapist could enhance the eating disorder treatment process by offering another option to explore negative body image
- Incorporating yoga with a body-positive theme and therapy lead process group demonstrates a promising option for those receiving eating disorder treatment at the outpatient level of care.

Introduction

A poor body image can lead to engagement in dieting, other forms of weight and food manipulation, disordered eating and, at times, can act as a catalyst in developing an eating disorder (Mehler & Andersen, 2017). Body image disturbances commonly coincide with an eating disorder diagnosis and a reduction in disturbances are one of the diagnostic criteria for partial and full remission of an eating disorder diagnosis according to the DSM-5 (American Psychiatric Association, 2013). Often, when someone is suffering from an eating disorder, there is an impaired ability to notice, describe, and/or properly care for sensations in the body (Cook-Cottone, 2015). During an active eating disorder, a distorted or negative relationship to one's body is common, and frequently there is a significant disconnect between self-perceptions of one's body versus the reality of it or how others view it (Herrin & Larkin, 2013; Mehler & Andersen, 2017). Having poor body image can be a pervasive struggle for people who have an eating disorder (Hrabosky et al., 2009).

Body dissatisfaction is multifaceted, persistent, and often considered a challenging aspect of eating disorder recovery, leaving clinicians pressed to discover what mode or modes of intervention can be most effective in managing or improving body dissatisfaction (Alleva et al., 2015). The well-known and respected intervention of Cognitive Behavioral Therapy (CBT) is one modality that can be used to address dysfunctional thoughts, feelings, and behaviors that contribute to negative body image. CBT is considered one of the primary interventions for body image disturbances (Cash, 2002; Jarry & Cash, 2011). Recently, some studies have explored techniques within body image interventions, such as CBT and others, to determine which techniques may be most helpful and why they are effective. A 2015 meta-analytic review of interventions to improve body image by Alleva and colleagues analyzed specific change techniques used in body image interventions to begin to explore why these specific interventions are, or are not, effective and how to use them in future interventions. Although physical activity, stress management, guided imagery, mindfulness, and mindful exercise were among some of the general techniques Alleva et al. listed as commonly used interventions for improving body image, yoga was not among the interventions named (Alleva et al., 2015). Yet, a large number of eating disorder treatment centers incorporate yoga as a therapeutic tool to support recovery; in fact, a 2006 study on services offered within 18 U.S. residential eating disorder programs found that 66.7% of programs offered yoga as part of regular programming (Frisch et al., 2006). There is a growing acknowledgment that a body-centered approach to eating disorder recovery is not only complementary but critical for creating an opportunity to flourish in the recovery process (Cook-Cottone, 2015).

Yoga, by nature, calls for a curious, reflective, and caring connection to one's body (Desikachar et al., 2005). When instructed with a body positive/ body acceptance, eating disorder informed, trauma sensitive, and therapeutic approach, yoga may be a useful tool in the healing and recovery process. Yoga is an encompassing practice of health and well-being. Indeed, according to the Yoga Sutras of Patanjali (Desikachar et al., 2005), widely considered a major authority on yoga, the practice of yoga addresses all dimensions of the human system: body, breath, mind, personality, and emotions. There are four overlying fundamentals to the teachings and practices of the system of yoga: 1) the human system is a holistic entity; 2) each individual is unique; 3) yoga is self-empowering; and 4) the quality and state of a person's mind is crucial to healing (Desikachar et al., 2005). When practiced wholly and attending to individual needs, yoga may help practitioners trust the healing process. Yoga can serve as a multidimensional tool used to approach the multi-faceted nature of an eating disorder. These tools may have the potential to impact the recovery process, including body image, awareness, and acceptance (Diers, 2016).

Yoga is becoming more regularly integrated into mental health treatment and increasingly being used as an adjunct therapeutic modality in eating disorder treatment. As a result, there is greater opportunity to evaluate yoga's role and effectiveness in body image recovery (Douglass, 2011; Klein & Cook-Cottone, 2013; Neumark-Sztainer, 2014). Recently, professional reports have described the potential benefits of yoga. These reports measure and explore clinical efficacy, participant satisfaction, the potential effectiveness of yoga's role in the treatment of eating disorders, anxiety, body image, traumatic disorders, and eating disorder prevention (Boudette, 2006; Diers, 2016; Diers & Neumark-Sztainer, 2019; Douglass, 2011; Neumark-Sztainer, 2014, 2016). Yoga therapy may be a particularly promising modality to promote embodiment, which is impaired to varying degrees in an active eating disorder. The yoga therapist can guide the student through a practice in a way that is attentive to his or her specific needs which could ultimately lead to a greater sense of embodiment (Cook-Cottone, 2016).

A randomized controlled trial of 38 individuals receiving treatment in a residential eating disorder treatment center, associated with the treatment center where the current study was implemented, found that participants exhibited significantly lower negative affects before consuming a meal when participating in yoga designed to target eating disorder symptoms as compared to treatment as usual (Pacanowski et al., 2017). However, the focus of this intervention was not on improving body image per se but rather was aimed at decreasing pre-meal eating anxiety. A 2019 systemic review of 12 trials (eight of which were randomized controlled trials) validated the need for more research to better understand the potential yoga may have in eating disorder treatment (Ostermann et al., 2019). Overall, there appears to be a promising place for yoga interventions in eating disorder treatment and prevention, particularly yoga's role in impacting self-perception, negative body image, and attending to the needs of the body (Boudette, 2006; Diers, 2016; Diers & Neumark-Sztainer, 2019; Douglass, 2011; Neumark-Sztainer, 2016).

In light of the promising results of previous studies, further research exploring innovative ways to incorporate yoga into residential and out-patient eating disorder treatment is warranted. Given the heterogeneity in both yoga interventions and eating disorder treatment programs, it is important to provide detailed descriptions of the yoga intervention and how it is incorporated into treatment. These descriptions can help health professionals accurately evaluate the intervention's quality, effectiveness, and transferability to their own programs. Currently, there is very little in the literature to help guide these developing programs.

The present feasibility study aims to describe and evaluate the integration of an innovative therapeutic yoga approach into an existing treatment program. The program described in this paper focuses primarily on the improvement of body image among individuals with eating disorders through a combined approach of yoga instruction followed by group therapy. We are unaware of any published programs that have utilized, provided an in-depth intervention description, and evaluated such an approach. Thus, our primary goal is to provide details on the intervention and its evaluation in order to inform other treatment programs interested in exploring such approaches and conducting evaluations under real-life constraints (e.g., billing, resistance to randomization, accepted norms of practice). The yoga program as well as the use of a mixed-methods approach in this pilot study to gather information on the potential for this type of intervention to impact body image is described. The study examines the program's acceptability and perceived impact on body image as reported by participants before and after the program.

Methods

Study overview

This pilot study describes an innovative yoga program aimed at improving body image among individuals receiving outpatient treatment for eating disorders. Both quantitative and qualitative data were collected from participants prior to, and following, program participation in order to learn more about the potential for the intervention to impact body image. First, survey data were used to quantitatively examine changes in body image concern scores before and after the program. Second, data from open-ended survey questions were used to help understand observed changes in body image scores and as a phenomenological exploration of the mechanisms through which the yoga program might influence body image concerns.

Participants included individuals who took part in the therapeutic yoga groups focused on body image (Yoga and Body Image: YBI), that were offered as part of an outpatient eating disorder treatment program in the Minneapolis–St. Paul metropolitan area. Overall, 91 individuals expressed interest in the group study. However, of the 91 participants who were taking the YBI classes for the first time, 67 participants completed both pre-and post-questionnaires and therefore were included in this study. The study was approved by both The Emily Program, an entity that offers psychological, nutritional, medical, and psychiatric care for those suffering from eating disorders and the Internal Review Board at the University of Minnesota. Data for this study were gathered from classes held between late 2011 and early 2014. Only one male patient expressed an interest in participating in this study, the rest were female with various eating disorder diagnoses.

Description of intervention

The YBI program was developed to address body image concerns common among individuals with varying eating disorder diagnoses. Sessions consisted of weekly, 90-minute sessions, over an 8-week period. Each yoga class was led by a registered yoga instructor, who received the minimum of a 200 h registered yoga certification approved by a registered yoga school. A mental health therapist performed yoga with the participants to aid in relatability and following the class, proceeded to co-facilitate the process portion of the group with the yoga instructor.

The yoga instructors and therapists who facilitated groups over the course of the study were trained by the first author (LD) regarding specific techniques for the YBI program. The yoga teachers were trained to incorporate language and physical instruction sensitive to eating disorders, varying levels of mobility, trauma, and negative body image. Additionally, the yoga teachers received training in facilitating client experiences from the yoga practice to aid in the verbal process portion of the group experience. The therapists were trained in the nuances of facilitating a process group focused on body-centered experiences evoked in yoga (e.g., encouraging exploration of sensations, emotions, yogic philosophy and strategies for managing and supporting participants in the event of a trauma response, avoidant behaviors, and more).

Weekly meetings between the yoga teachers and group therapists were held to ensure clinical communication, quality, and consistency between the therapeutic delivery of the groups. Although treatment adherence across the groups was not assessed, there was a general structure to the sessions, while allowing the facilitators the ability to modify in accordance with issues emerging in the group on any specific day. Additionally, random classes were observed by team leaders and monthly Yoga and Body Image team meetings were held with all facilitators of the multi-location groups. These observations and meetings provided professional consultation, direction, and ensured consistency of approach within the program.

Each yoga class had approximately seven participants who were referred to the group by a therapist or registered dietitian who used clinical judgment to determine whether the program would be effective and not bring about negative consequences. In addition to the professional referral, participants attended an informational group intake where they had the opportunity to meet the group facilitators, communicate any injuries or concerns to the yoga teacher, familiarize themselves with the space, and better understand the group focus. This process helped to ensure participant readiness as well as reinforce the expectations of the group. Like the co-facilitators, participants were also educated on effective group processing, specifically as it related to body image and yoga, in an effort to try to reduce the tendency of avoiding discussions of struggles with negative body image or sensations (Shafran et al., 2004; Wildes et al., 2010). The education on effective group processing continued throughout the 8-week series with both participants and facilitators, though separately. The primary goal was to aid in group facilitation as well as provide participants with tools to connect to, describe, and verbalize uncomfortable sensations and emotions that often arose as a result of the group experience.

The weekly sessions began with approximately 45 minutes of therapeutic yoga that incorporated aspects of hatha, vinyasa, and viniyoga and ended with a 45-minute group discussion. Each session focused on a theme related to body image and awareness. Specific yoga postures (asanas), breath technique (pranayama), and guided imagery were selected to support the overall themes (see Table 1).

The yoga instructed was adapted to support participants' needs such that each yoga session was individualized and unique. For example, a posture such as "downward facing dog" would be adapted for accessibility in the chair, against the wall, or on the floor depending on a participants' particular needs. Another example of how teaching was adapted for each individual was

Table 1. Description of yoga and body image (YBI) class content areas related to body image and awareness. *.

Content area	Description
Poses of Stability or Neutrality	Participants encouraged to familiarize themselves with poses which provided a sense of stability and safety. They were frequently reminded of their choice to return to these postures as needed during the class (e.g., mountain pose, child's pose, comfortable seated posture).
Breathing	Education in basic breath awareness, including instruction on ujjayi pranayama.
Body-Mind Capabilities/ Resiliency	Participants encouraged to experiment with poses and variations of accessibility (in Body, Mind and Emotion) that worked for them (e.g., modifications, adaptations or use of props); Encouraged to find stability/ window of tolerance and therapeutic expansion of this window; Used journaling intermittently throughout asana practice to collect thoughts, feelings and sensations.
Body Awareness	Education and experientials incorporated regarding Interoceptive Awareness; Spatial Awareness; Techniques used to aid in the mind-body connection (e.g.: anxiety in mind, restless in body; worry in mind) Provided words to help describe sensations (eg.: tight; constricted; open; warm; cool; tingly; tense; vibrating; smooth; pulsing; tender; stuck; numb; heavy; light; hot; spacey).
Body Appreciation	A "Function vs. Form" approach to yoga instruction to aid in connection to the felt experience and effects of the practice. Practices invited appreciation for the body's functions and capabilities; Body Gratitude Affirmations (e.g.: Inhale: "I am" Exhale "Enough") and other body gratitude meditations.
Free Movement	Guided to move body in free and creative ways in silence and to live music performed by a trained music therapist; Practiced moving the body based on what felt good vs. a "right or wrong" way to move.
Non-judgement	Regular reminders given to practice a "curious, but not furious" approach to judgmental thoughts and actions that may be present. Radical Acceptance. Non-reactive Stance encouraged.
Emotional Connection	Participants encouraged to describe the emotions that accompanied sensations in the body during class.

* Individual YBI classes focused on one or multiple content areas throughout the 8-week course.

by providing instruction for the most accessible version of a pose first, encouraging participants to stay in that version, if needed, or move to the next level of the pose. Participants were encouraged to explore their intentions with the choices they made to see if they matched what they needed in the moment. Additionally, participants were regularly prompted to consider the class theme and to notice any thoughts or feelings that arose related to body image. The discussion portion was co-led by the yoga instructor and therapist and aimed to aid in the participant's verbal processing of their experience in relation to sensation, emotion, and overall experience.

To help increase body awareness, participants were encouraged to notice and describe the sensations felt in their bodies (e.g., tingly, warm, empty; see Table 1). These types of group interactions appeared to aid in bridging the gap between the mind-body experience and enhancing the experience of embodiment (Piran & Neumark-Sztainer, 2020). Other benefits of the group discussion included increased awareness to judgmental or negative body descriptors (e.g., bad arm, lousy knee, fat stomach), which created a unique opportunity to highlight negative self-talk and offer suggestions for alternative ways to think about and describe one's body.

Additionally, a peer-based perspective was encouraged by the facilitators. For example, group members would respectfully comment or question other members shared experience, make a gentle observation about discrepancy between a participants' topic of discussion and physical expression (e.g., smiling while sharing an emotionally painful experience), or offer words of encouragement to one another.

Goal setting was regularly used to encourage positive change. Participants created goals related to various topics such as initiating a self-care routine, attending a public yoga class, wearing more comfortable clothing in yoga, practicing a yoga pose when food anxiety arose (Alleva et al., 2015). For example, one participant regularly wore baggy clothes to yoga as an attempt to hide her figure. She noticed that the baggy clothes hindered her ability to participate fully in class and described feeling distracted by them, especially during inverted postures. This participant set a goal to wear more fitting yoga clothes during the next class. She was able to accomplish this goal and discussed the triumphs and challenges of the experience and its relation to other body image concerns she held.

Measures

To better understand changes to participants' body image concerns before and after the yoga program, as well as to explore participants' perceived experiences participating in the yoga program, the authors developed a self-administered questionnaire for participants to complete at baseline and after completion of the YBI program. The questionnaire was informed both by constructs present in the Body Shape Questionnaire (Cooper & Taylor, 1987) and the clinical experience of both the first author (LD) and the primary therapist of the YBI groups. The questionnaire consisted of 10 quantitative items assessing body image preoccupations and concerns typical amongst those with diagnosed eating disorders (presented in Table 2), along with five open-ended questions. These qualitative questions were developed so that participants could reflect on the therapeutic process and share their experiences from the yoga classes, their feelings on the potential applicability of the yoga program to body image recovery, and the perceived impact of yoga on their relationship to self and others. The five open-ended questions were as follows: 1) I would describe my relationship to my body as_____; 2) How are your body image issues affecting your relationships with yourself and others?; 3) How are you hoping yoga will change your relationship with yourself and others?; 4) What yoga poses do you find the most challenging and why?; and 5) What yoga poses do you find the most empowering and why?

Table 2. Mean scores on body image concerns at baseline and after completion of the yoga and body image (YBI) group process program (n = 67).

Questionnaire item*	Baseline	Completion	Mean change (95% CI)	p-value
I tend to avoid looking at my body in full-length mirrors. † mean (SD)	1.6 (1.4)	1.9 (1.3)	0.24 (−0.02–0.51)	0.07
I am able to think about or experience my body without getting emotionally reactive. mean (SD)	1.3 (1.2)	1.7 (1.0)	0.43 (0.17–0.69)	<0.01
I have avoided social situations because I felt uncomfortable with my body.† mean (SD)	1.8 (1.1)	2.3 (1.0)	0.53 (0.25–0.81)	<0.001
I feel confident about my body shape and appearance. mean (SD)	0.5 (0.7)	1.1 (1.1)	0.60 (0.39–0.81)	<0.001
I have avoided romantic relationships, dating, or physical intimacy based on how I feel about my body.† mean (SD)	1.3 (1.2)	1.9 (1.3)	0.54 (0.25–0.83)	<0.001
I feel connected to my body (physically connected to its sensations, aware of how it feels). mean (SD)	1.7 (1.2)	2.2 (1.1)	0.49 (0.24–0.74)	<0.001
I am kind to my body by my thoughts and behaviors (speaking of it positively, keeping it comfortable, meeting its needs, giving it pleasure). mean (SD)	1.1 (0.7)	1.8 (1.1)	0.72 (0.50–0.94)	<0.001
My mood and self-esteem are connected to my body. † mean (SD)	1.0 (1.0)	1.3 (1.1)	0.27 (0.01–0.53)	0.04
Percent of day spent thinking about body. % (n)	50% (29)	43% (28)	−7.7 (−12.7—2.7)	<0.01
Level of body shame or embarrassment‡ mean (SD)	7.7 (1.8)	6.5 (2.2)	−1.1 (−1.6—0.71)	<0.001

*Scores based on scale with the following response options: 0 = Never, 1 = Sometimes, 2 = Moderately Often, 3 = Often, 4 = Always/Almost Always.
†Reverse-coded scores are displayed.
‡Assessed on a scale of 1–10 where 1 = least amount and 10 = most.

Analyses

To assess changes in scores on quantitative survey items before and after the yoga program, the mean and standard deviation of each question was descriptively examined and mean changes in item scores were examined by paired t-test with a p-value<0.05 indicating a statistically significant change. Data were analyzed using SAS 9.3. Since this pilot study was intended as a feasibility study, no a priori power calculations were conducted.

To understand how participants experienced the yoga program, if yoga had a perceived impact on body image, and identify potential mechanisms through which yoga might impact body image, open-ended survey data were analyzed using principles of content analysis (Hsieh & Shannon, 2005). Qualitative data were coded in two phases. First, the responses to each open-ended question were read carefully for overall content to develop an initial coding scheme. Next, an iterative process was undertaken whereby three raters independently coded each response, discussed any discrepancies until consensus was reached, and updated the coding scheme. Lastly, codes were grouped into broader themes and changes from baseline to follow-up were examined to determine the direction of change within a participant from pre-class to post-class, where applicable. This process of review, iteration, and consensus building amongst our experienced research team members were important steps to enhance the trustworthiness of the data, ensure analysis accurately reflected the participants intended meanings, and reduce potential bias. A detailed description of the study site, participants, and intervention context are also provided so that the transferability of the results can be assessed by the reader (Hsieh & Shannon, 2005).

Results

Quantitative findings

Participation in the YBI class yielded statistically significant improvements in body image concerns (Table 2). The majority of survey items were asked on a 0–4 point rating scale, and the mean change in scores before and after the YBI class ranged from 0.2 to 0.7 points. Scores for tending to avoid looking at one's body in full-length mirrors decreased by a mean change of −0.24 (95% CI: 0.02—−0.51, $p = .07$). The mean score for the ability to think about or experience one's body without getting emotionally reactive increased by 0.43 (95% CI: 0.17–0.69, $p < .01$). Scores for avoiding social situation because one felt uncomfortable with one's body decreased by a mean of 0.53 (95% CI: −0.25—−0.81, $p < .001$); similarly, mean participant scores decreased by 0.54 (95% CI: −0.25—−0.83, $p < .001$) when reporting on the avoidance of romantic relationships, dating, or physical intimacy based on how one felt about one's body. The mean score for reporting that one's mood and self-esteem were connected to one's body decreased by 0.27 (95% CI: 0.01–0.53, $p = .04$). Scores for feeling confident about one's body shape and appearance increased by a mean of 0.60 (95% CI: 0.39–0.81, $p < .001$). After participating in the YBI classes participants reported a mean change score of 0.49 (95% CI: 0.24–0.74, $p < .001$) when reflecting on feeling [physically] connected to one's body. Scores for being kind to one's body by one's thoughts and behaviors increased by a mean change score of 0.72 (95% CI: 0.50–0.94, $p < .001$).

Participants also reported a 7% decrease in the percentage of the day spent thinking about their body ($p < .01$) and a 1.2 point reduction in shame or embarrassment about their body after taking the YBI course (on a scale of 1–10 where 10 is considered the most shame/embarrassment; $p < .001$). Responses to the item, I tend to avoid looking at my body in full-length mirrors, did not change ($p = .7$).

Qualitative findings

Baseline body image concerns

Prior to commencing the YBI program, all but one participant reported that their body image concern was negatively affecting their relationships, with participants discussing four reasons why. The primary reason, which was endorsed by the majority of participants, was that body image concerns caused discord with friends, family, and partners. Other reasons included body image concerns were making participants less social; body image concerns promoted feelings of isolation; and body image concerns prevented intimacy. For example, one participant indicated that her body image concern *"annoys her friends and family."* Another said, *"I am isolated. I am often grumpy or down due to body image, which strains my relationships,"* while another stated *"I am self-conscious and have low confidence, I don't believe and deserve I am worthy of a relationship."*

Expected benefits of the YBI program

Prior to the program, participants indicated that they hoped that yoga would change their relationship with themselves and others. Many participants indicated that they hoped for improved self-acceptance (e.g., *"I am hoping that I might be able to enjoy, like, and appreciate my body"*), and a third of the participants expressed a hope for improved self-awareness (e.g., *"I want to practice slowing down and become more aware of what my body is saying"*). To a lesser extent, participants indicated that they hoped for emotional benefits (e.g., *"I hope it will give me a sense of peace as well as an appreciation for how my body works"*), physical benefits (e.g., *"I hope it will connect me more to my body's sensations and increase strength and flexibility"*), and improved self-confidence and connection with others (e.g., *"I want to feel strong and confident of my physical body … then I can be more confident in loving others"*).

Perceived changes experienced by participants after the YBI program

Upon completion of the YBI program, the directional change in how participants felt about their bodies was assessed. Many participants described positive changes in their body image. For example, one participant described her relationship toward her body as follows: *"Getting better, more peaceful, caring, loving and accepting every day,"* while another stated, *"I am learning to be kind to myself, head-to-toe, and this is helping reduce my resistance to exercise, to stop 'should' thinking about exercise and to move to feel good."* Positive changes were also acknowledged as part of an ongoing journey: *"a very challenging work in progress."* Despite the positive changes reported by many participants, about one-third of the women reported a continued negative relationship that was described using terms such as *"abusive," "negative and hateful," "uncomfortable," "unforgiving,"* and *"non-loving."*

A handful of others who began the class described their relationship to their body as one with either ups and downs or one where improvements were slowly being made, reported that they were on the same trajectory as when they started. A few individuals reported feelings that seemed to indicate more negativity or disappointment in not having achieved a more positive body image through the program. For example, participants described their relationship with their bodies as "*conflicted*" and "*trying to reconnect*" prior to the YBI and as "*disappointing*" and "*fraught with tension*" after the YBI. These comments may reflect, at least in part, greater self-awareness.

Following the YBI program with respect to relationships with others, several participants reported positive changes following the program. For example, one participant indicated, "*it's a work [in] progress, practicing patience, forgiveness, and love is new and hard but seeing positive changes b/c of it.*" Another said, "*As I love myself more, others seem to enjoy being around me.*"

More broadly, benefits of the program described most frequently by participants were emotional benefits and improved self-acceptance and awareness: "*Yoga has increased my compassion for myself and others. It has increased overall awareness and has cultivated a positive outlook on life.*" Nearly half of the participants found that yoga left them feeling empowered because they experienced increased confidence, and emotional and physical strength: "*I feel so strong and confident in myself when balancing. I feel beautiful,*" and "*I feel strong, grounded and connected to the earth.*" To a lesser extent, participants also found that yoga provided a form of release: "*[heart openers] are a wonderful relief and letting go.*"

Challenging aspects of yoga

Many aspects of yoga require flexibility, balance, and strength and several participants reported difficulty in these areas (e.g., difficulty balancing, low flexibility, and back pain). For other women, these physical challenges brought about self-judgment (e.g., "*[the positions] make me feel like I'm not good enough*") and perpetuated feelings of negative body image (e.g."*[In triangle] I feel my midsection most and it makes me most aware of my size*"). For other women, the yoga classes exposed emotional challenges because they caused women to feel vulnerable or to confront feelings that they were uncomfortable with: "*Any poses where I'm embracing myself because it's hard for me to be nurturing/loving to myself,*" and "*Heart openers always pull out emotion when I may not want to experience it,*" and "*Child's pose [makes me feel] submissive, vulnerable, and I can't see (imaginary) potential threats.*"

Discussion

The goal of this study was to describe a unique yoga therapy program that was designed to address body image concerns among individuals with eating disorders and to conduct a pilot study to evaluate the program's perceived impact on body image. Results revealed that participants' body image concerns improved modestly after the 8-week YBI program, and that participants described many positive impacts of the YBI program on their body image perceptions. Overall, findings from this pilot evaluation study, although preliminary, suggest that yoga may impact body image when offered within an eating disorder treatment program, while also suggesting the difficulties inherent in improving body image. Given the real-world nature of this study, we had limited information on sources of potential bias related to participants' personal characteristics, specific treatment, and referral method; therefore, we present our findings as preliminary. Further research is needed to confirm these findings using a larger, more robust study design, and to explore more fully the mechanisms through which yoga impacts body image within the eating disorder treatment context.

All but one survey measure of participants' body image concerns improved from baseline to completion of the YBI program. Although modest, observed improvements in body image concern after only 8 weeks of participation in the YBI program are encouraging and may reflect the value of delivering specifically focused yoga classes by trained instructors, supplemented by therapist-led discussions, within eating disorder treatment programs to help improve participants' ability to access aspects of body image, awareness, and emotions during a group session. Other observational studies have also reported that individuals participating in yoga have a more positive body image than those who do not participate in a yoga practice (Mahlo & Tiggemann, 2016; Neumark-Sztainer, MacLehose et al., 2018; Neumark-Sztainer, Watts et al., 2018). Interestingly, in a longitudinal study of young adults, Neumark-Sztainer et al. found that individuals with lower levels of body satisfaction saw greater improvements in body image over time with a regular practice of yoga as compared to those who had higher body satisfaction prior to practicing yoga. Moreover, in a related qualitative study, young adults practicing yoga described primarily a positive impact on body image, although some participants described a negative impact along with a positive impact. For the present study, a longer program may yield greater improvements in measures of body image concern. Therapeutic yoga needs to be complementary to other approaches to repairing body image issues and eating disorder treatment, as individuals may respond differently to yoga therapy. In order to better understand how yoga can help to improve body image and eating disorder outcomes, and for whom it is most effective, more research with rigorous study designs is needed (Neumark-Sztainer, 2014; Cook-Cottone, 2015).

Perhaps of more interest were the comments made by participants in response to open-ended survey questions. In general, their comments indicated that yoga had a positive impact on their body image, in addition to their self-esteem, self-compassion, and relationships with others. That said, some expressed a sense of disappointment that they still had not reached the point of having a positive body image. Responses also suggested participants' ability to recognize poses that have a positive effect, thus creating potential to use these poses to reinforce positive change, as well as the participant's ability to recognize poses that evoke negative or challenging emotions and internal dialogue. Including the psychotherapy component created a potential opportunity for participants to further explore these areas and how they may parallel similar emotional responses in the treatment process, potentially strengthening internal and external awareness and the effect internal dialogue has on choices in recovery, self-care, and relationships to others. These findings suggesting that yoga is generally perceived as having a positive impact on body image among participants with eating disorders are in alignment with an in-depth qualitative study examining perceptions of yoga's impact on body image in a general population-based sample of young adults (Neumark-Sztainer, MacLehose et al., 2018).

Despite many positive descriptions and stories about their experiences in the YBI program, participants also described many challenging aspects of yoga such as poses that bring about physical pain, or negative attention to a particular aspect of their bodies. Although these responses may appear discouraging, they may be reflective of a connection to uncomfortable emotions and experiences in the body that may typically be avoided. This potential connection could possibly have therapeutic benefits over time. It is common for unpleasant experiences to arise when trauma is present, for example, or feelings often avoided become uncovered while practicing yoga. A safe environment for the participant to explore these challenges, with trauma-informed and therapeutically minded instructors, is key to the success of a participant connecting to and possibly transforming unhelpful patterns and experiences.

Strengths of this study include the collection of both quantitative and qualitative data to assess the feasibility, acceptability, and effectiveness of the yoga-based program. It is crucial to provide models for designing preliminary evaluations of novel intervention approaches being introduced into real-life treatment settings, while being upfront about limitations of such evaluation designs and cautious in the interpretation of findings. A particular strength of the yoga-based program evaluated in this study is the high quality of program facilitators. The yoga instructors and mental health therapists who delivered the program were specifically trained in yoga approaches for those with all types of eating disorders, mental health diagnosis, trauma, all levels of yoga experience, mobility, body size, gender, gender identity, and other individualized needs. In our experience, programs such as this one work best when people have both similarities (e.g., body concerns) and differences (e.g., eating patterns, body shape, and size) since everyone can learn from, and help, each other.

Despite these strengths, several limitations need to be taken into account when interpreting the study findings. This study did not include a control group, therefore, observed changes in body image may have been the result of other aspects of eating disorder treatment and not specific to the YBI program. Our study design did not allow for the isolation of the effects of the YBI program above and beyond other aspects of treatment. Nevertheless, findings were supported by qualitative descriptions of participant experiences that revealed information about how the yoga program may have positively influenced their body image. The next step is to conduct a larger, more rigorous study using a randomized-controlled design evaluating the approach utilized here. Furthermore, in-depth qualitative interviews or focus groups may have elicited more nuanced and detailed description of participants experiences than our open-ended survey questions. The survey measures of body image concern adapted from the BSQ were not validated and survey responses were based on self-report. Participants were aware they were participating in a yoga program to improve their body image; therefore, social desirability bias may have led participants to over report positive changes in their body image. A portion of the participants did not complete surveys at baseline and/or at follow-up, and information about people who did not complete the surveys was not collected. It is possible that the experiences of those who did not complete the surveys were quite different than those who participated and this may have biased our results. Because this was a small feasibility pilot study, we did not conduct power calculations. We also collected very limited personal information on participants such that specific eating disorder diagnosis, medications use, type or frequency of outpatient treatment, prior yoga experience, or the ethnicity of participants were not assessed. We also have limited information about how participants were referred to the yoga program, which may have biased the results. Overall, the lack of data on participants' personal characteristics, specific treatment, and referral method remain important sources of bias in our study and mean that results need to be interpreted with caution. It will be important for future studies to understand how the type of disorder, gender, ethnicity, and other contextual/personal factors may impact the effectiveness of such programs.

Moving forward, a critical next step will be to examine the effect of the YBI program within eating disorder treatment centers using a randomized study design. Another line of inquiry could focus on whether a therapeutically designed yoga course with a multidisciplinary support team that includes a psychotherapist leads to a greater improvement in body satisfaction than one taught by instructors using body-positive language alone. Future studies could also examine differential intensities or durations of yoga therapy and its impact on body image based on eating disorder diagnosis and severity and/or longevity of negative body image. These studies should be complimented with qualitative approaches in order to fully understand the impact of yoga on individuals suffering with eating disorders.

Conclusions

Findings from this pilot study suggest that yoga, paired with a therapist-led group discussion, may help impact body image in an outpatient sample of eating disordered individuals. The results of the present study warrant consideration of more research in this area, with future studies being designed to address the limitations of the current study. Future research in this area will aid in the development of specific yogic techniques and therapeutic approaches that are most effective at promoting a positive body image among those suffering from eating disorders. When instructed intentionally and in a clinically informed way, yoga may serve as a powerful tool in finding peace with one's body. As negative body image can be a catalyst to dieting and disordered eating (Mehler & Andersen, 2017), therapeutic yoga programs targeting a positive body image may have a role to play in the prevention of disordered eating.

ORCID

Sarah A. Rydell ⓘ http://orcid.org/0000-0001-9712-2116

References

Alleva, J. M., Sheeran, P., Webb, T. L., Martijn, C., & Miles, E. (2015). A meta-analytic review of stand-alone interventions to improve body image. *PloS One, 10*(9), e0139177. https://doi.org/10.1371/journal.pone.0139177

American Psychiatric Association. (2013). *Eating Disorders*. American Psychiatric Press.

Boudette, R. (2006). Question & answer: Yoga in the treatment of disordered eating and body image disturbance: How can the practice of yoga be helpful in recovery from an eating disorder? *Eating Disorders, 14*(2), 167–170. https://doi.org/10.1080/10640260500536334

Cash, T. F. (2002). Cognitive-behavioral perspectives on body image. In T. F. Cash & T. Pruzinsky (Eds.), *Body image: A handbook of theory, research, and clinical practice* (pp. 38–46). Guilford Press.

Cook-Cottone, C. (2016). Yoga for the re-embodied self: The therapeutic journey home. *Yoga Therapy Today, Winter, 40-42*(1), 48 http://www.sytar.org/YTTwinter2016/index.html.

Cook-Cottone, C. P. (2015). Incorporating positive body image into the treatment of eating disorders: A model for attunement and mindful self-care. *Body Image, 14*, 158–167. https://doi.org/10.1016/j.bodyim.2015.03.004

Cooper, P., & Taylor, M. (1987). The development and validation of the body shape questionnaire. *International Journal of Eating Disorders, 6*(4), 485–494. https://doi.org/10.1002/()1098-108X

Desikachar, K., Bragdon, L., & Bossart, C. (2005). The yoga of healing: Exploring yoga's holistic model for health and well-being. *International Journal of Yoga Therapy, 15*(1), 17–39. https://doi.org/10.17761/ijyt.15.1.p501l33535230737

Diers, L. (2016). Discovering the role of yoga in eating disorder treatment. *Scan's pulse: Official Publication of Sports, Cardiovascular, and Wellness Nutrition (SCAN)*, *35*(1), 10–13.

Diers, L., & Neumark-Sztainer, D. (2019). *The principles of yoga and how they apply to eating disorders recovery.* Gurze-Salucore Eating Disorders Resource Catalogue, https://www.edcatalogue.com/principles-yoga-apply-eating-disorders-recovery/

Douglass, L. (2011). Thinking through the body: The conceptualization of yoga as therapy for individuals with eating disorders. *Eating Disorders*, *19*(1), 83–96. https://doi.org/10.1080/10640266.2011.533607

Frisch, M. J., Herzog, D. B., & Franko, D. L. (2006). Residential treatment for eating disorders. *International Journal of Eating Disorders*, *39*(5), 434–442. https://doi.org/10.1002/()1098-108X

Herrin, M., & Larkin, M. (2013). *Nutrition counseling in the treatment of eating disorders.* Routledge.

Hrabosky, J. I., Cash, T. F., Veale, D., Neziroglu, F., Soll, E. A., Garner, D. M., Strachan-Kinser, M., Bakke, B., Clauss, L. J., & Phillips, K. A. (2009). Multidimensional body image comparisons among patients with eating disorders, body dysmorphic disorder, and clinical controls: A multisite study. *Body Image*, *6*(3), 155–163. https://doi.org/10.1016/j.bodyim.2009.03.001

Hsieh, H. F., & Shannon, S. E. (2005). Three approaches to qualitative content analysis. [peer reviewed]. *Qualitative Health Research*, *15*(9), 1277–1288. https://doi.org/10.1177/1049732305276687

Jarry, J. L., & Cash, T. F. (2011). Cognitive-behavioral approaches to body image change. In T. F. Cash & L. Smolak (Eds.), *Body image: A handbook of science, practice, and prevention* (2nd ed., pp. 415–423). Guilford Press.

Klein, J., & Cook-Cottone, ca. 2013. The effects of yoga on eating disorder symptoms and correlates: A review. *International Journal of Yoga Therapy*, *23*(2), 41–50. [Review]

Mahlo, L., & Tiggemann, M. (2016). Yoga and positive body image: A test of the embodiment model. *Body Image*, *18*, 135–142. https://doi.org/10.1016/j.bodyim.2016.06.008

Mehler, P. S., & Andersen, A. E. (2017). *Eating disorders: A guide to medical care and complications.* JHU Press.

Neumark-Sztainer, D. (2014). Yoga and eating disorders: Is there a place for yoga in the prevention and treatment of eating disorders and disordered eating behaviours? *Advances in Eating Disorders*, *2*(2), 136–145. https://doi.org/10.1080/21662630.2013.862369

Neumark-Sztainer, D. (2016). Eating disorders prevention: Looking backward, moving forward; looking inward, moving outward. *Eating Disorders*, *24*(1), 29–38. https://doi.org/10.1080/10640266.2015.1113825

Neumark-Sztainer, D., MacLehose, R. F., Watts, A. W., Pacanowski, C. R., & Eisenberg, M. E. (2018). Yoga and body image: Findings from a large population-based study of young adults. *Body Image*, *24*, 69–75. https://doi.org/10.1016/j.bodyim.2017.12.003

Neumark-Sztainer, D., Watts, A. W., & Rydell, S. (2018). Yoga and body image: How do young adults practicing yoga describe its impact on their body image? *Body Image*, *27*, 156–168. https://doi.org/10.1016/j.bodyim.2018.09.001

Ostermann, T., Vogel, H., Boehm, K., & Cramer, H. (2019). Effects of yoga on eating disorders–a systematic review. *Complementary Therapies in Medicine*, *46*, 73–80. https://doi.org/10.1016/j.ctim.2019.07.021

Pacanowski, C. R., Diers, L., Crosby, R. D., & Neumark-Sztainer, D. (2017). Yoga in the treatment of eating disorders within a residential program: A randomized controlled trial. *Eating Disorders*, *25*(1), 37–51. https://doi.org/10.1080/10640266.2016.1237810

Piran, N., & Neumark-Sztainer, D. (2020). Yoga and the experience of embodiment: A discussion of possible links. Eating Disorders, January 10. [Online ahead of print]

Shafran, R., Fairburn, C. G., Robinson, P., & Lask, B. (2004). Body checking and its avoidance in eating disorders. *International Journal of Eating Disorders*, *35*(1), 93–101. https://doi.org/10.1002/()1098-108X

Wildes, J. E., Ringham, R. M., & Marcus, M. D. (2010). Emotion avoidance in patients with anorexia nervosa: Initial test of a functional model. *International Journal of Eating Disorders*, *43*(5), 398–404. https://doi.org/10.1002/eat.20730

Yoga practice in a college sample: associated changes in eating disorder, b ody image, and related f actors over time

Rachel Kramer ⓘD and Kelly Cuccolo ⓘD

ABSTRACT

Yoga practice is associated with improvements in eating disorder (ED) symptoms and body dissatisfaction. This study continued to evaluate this relationship while also assessing changes in variables negatively associated with ED symptoms (self-compassion, mindfulness, body appreciation, self-efficacy) that are emphasized throughout yoga. Men were also included in this study given studies have predominantly focused on women. Participants (N = 99, 77.8% women) were recruited from a university-implemented yoga course and completed assessments at the beginning (Time 1 (T1)) and end (Time 2 (T2)) of an eight-week yoga course meeting three times a week for fifty minutes. Body dissatisfaction (ps <.05) and ED pathology (p = .02) were lower at T2. Body appreciation (p < .001), self-compassion (p = .01), yoga self-efficacy (p = .004) were higher at T2. Some gender differences emerged. Men reported greater reductions in concern with being overweight, (Overweight Preoccupation) from T1 (M = 2.46, SD = 0.61) to T2 (M = 2.13, SD = 0.61) compared to women, T1 (M = 2.75, SD = 0.98) to T2 (M = 2.69, SD = 0.97) associated with yoga practice. Men also reported greater improvements in body satisfaction (Appearance Evaluation) from T1 (M = 3.60, SD = 0.49) to T2 (M = 3.90, SD = 0.34) compared with women, T1 (M = 3.48, SD = 0.58) to T2 (M = 3.39, SD = 0.52) associated with yoga practice. Results suggest yoga may be associated with concurrent changes in protective and risk factors for ED in a college population.

Clinical Implications

- Frequent yoga practice may be associated with reductions in eating disorder symptoms.
- Yoga practice may be associated with reductions in body dissatisfaction.
- Men reported greater improvements in body dissatisfaction associated with yoga practice.
- Yoga practice may be associated with improvements in self-compassion, body appreciation, and self-efficacy.

Introduction

Yoga has been incorporated as an adjunct to treatment for many psychological (Büssing, Michalsen, Khalsa, Telles, & Sherman, 2012) and physiological concerns (Banerjee et al., 2007; Field, 2011; Park, Braun, & Siegel, 2015), and is one of the most popular complementary medicine practices in the United States. Notably, yoga has also been incorporated as part of eating disorder (ED) treatment (Frisch, Herzog, & Franko, 2006) and empirical support for the use of yoga during ED treatment is amassing (see Carei, Fyfe-Johnson, Breuner, & Marshall, 2010; Hall, Ofei-TEnkorang, Machan, & Gordon, 2016; McIver, O'Halloran, & McGartland, 2009; Pacanowski, Diers, Crosby, & Neumark-Sztainer, 2017).

Studies assessing yoga as a preventative method against ED symptomology and body dissatisfaction (a key risk factor for ED) also yield promising results (Cook-Cottone, Talebkhah, Guyker, & Keddie, 2017; Scime & Cook-Cottone, 2008). For instance, incorporating yoga with an ED prevention curriculum resulted in reductions in ED symptoms among youth (Cook-Cottone et al., 2017; Scime & Cook-Cottone, 2008). Youth also reported decreases in body surveillance and greater body appreciation after participation in physical education courses incorporating yoga (Cox, Ullrich-French, Howe, & Cole, 2017). In college samples, yoga practice was associated with improvements in ED risk factors such as self-objectification and appearance evaluation (Ariel-Donges, Gordon, Bauman, & Perri, 2018; Cox et al., 2017), and protective factors (e.g. body appreciation and mindfulness; Ariel-Donges et al., 2018; Cox & McMahon, 2019; Cox et al., 2017).

While researchers demonstrate yoga incorporated during ED treatment and prevention is effective, understanding skills emphasized during yoga practice, which negatively or positively relate to ED symptoms will enable researchers to examine mediating and moderating factors of how yoga is beneficial. Therefore, in addition to assessing changes in ED symptoms and body dissatisfaction associated with frequent yoga practice (to support extant literature), the current study assessed changes in skills including mindfulness, self-compassion (SC), body appreciation, and yoga self-efficacy.

Mindfulness may be one way yoga positively impacts ED symptoms and body dissatisfaction. Yoga improves mindfulness by encouraging practitioners to non-judgmentally identify their thoughts and work to coordinate breath with body movement (Ariel-Donges et al., 2018; Cox & McMahon, 2019; Eastman-Mueller, Wilson, Jung, Kimura, & Tarrant, 2013; Freeman, 2004). Such skills learned throughout yoga may enable practitioners to become less critical of themselves in the moment which may facilitate reductions in body dissatisfaction, ED symptoms, and enhance body appreciation.

Indeed, mindfulness is negatively associated with ED symptoms (Butryn et al., 2013; Lavender et al., 2009), body dissatisfaction (Butryn et al., 2013; Pidgeon & Appleby, 2014; Lavender, Gratz, & Anderson, 2012), and body surveillance (Dijkstra & Barelds, 2011) and positively associated with body satisfaction (Dijkstra & Barelds, 2011; Lavender et al., 2012). Mindfulness interventions have yielded positive outcomes in ED samples (Baer, Fischer, & Huss, 2005; Butryn et al., 2013; Kristeller, Baer, & Quillian Wolever, 2006). In studies assessing changes in mindfulness related to yoga, state mindfulness improved (Cox et al., 2017) and predicted lower self-objectification, a risk factor for ED development. Cox and McMahon (2019) also found improvements in mindfulness related to yoga practice predicted improvements in body appreciation.

Additionally, yoga's focus is akin to self-compassion (SC), which involves kindness towards oneself (self-kindness), non-judgmental awareness of individual flaws and strengths (mindfulness), and the belief that one's experience is universal (common humanity; Neff, 2003a, 2003b). Yoga may enable participants to perceive their body more kindly and respond more compassionately to self-criticism instead of pushing their body's limit, often an unfortunate feature of ED pathology (e.g. over-exercise). Yoga may also encourage participants to appreciate how others may feel similarly about their body appearance and abilities; everyone works hard to master, without perfection, poses.

Preliminary research indicates a link between SC and yoga practice, with yoga practitioners experiencing improvements in SC, which predicted improvements in perceived quality of life (Gard et al., 2012). To date, no other studies have examined changes in SC associated with yoga practice, which would be beneficial given SC is negatively associated with body dissatisfaction and ED symptoms (Breines, Toole, Tu, & Chen, 2014; Kelly, Vimalakanthan, & Miller, 2014; Wasylkiw, MacKinnon, & MacLellan, 2012) and unrealistic expectations of one's body positively associated with body appreciation (Tylka & Wood-Barcalow, 2015b). Further, including SC during ED treatment is associated with earlier improvements in ED symptoms (Kelly, Carter, & Borairi, 2014). Additional support that yoga practice is associated with improvements in SC may provide further rationale to assess SC as an additional mechanism of action predicting symptom change.

Body appreciation, another protective factor against ED and body dissatisfaction (Andrew, Tiggemann, & Clark, 2015; Cotter, Kelly, Mitchell, & Mazzeo, 2015), is also encouraged during yoga. Body appreciation is defined as an individual's ability to perceive positive qualities of their body beyond appearance (e.g. body functionality) while accepting perceived flaws, showing one's body respect, and rejecting unrealistic expectations of their body (Avalos, Tylka, & Wood-Barcalow, 2005; Foroughi, Zhu, Smith, & Hay, 2019). Body appreciation is also closely associated with embodiment which increases as individuals engage in tasks focusing on body functionality, competence, and mind-body connection (Mahlo & Tiggemann, 2016; Menzel & Levine, 2011). Yoga may enhance body appreciation, as yoga philosophy often emphasizes gratitude for one's abilities on the mat while focusing on form and function over appearance and perfection. Indeed, Ariel-Donges et al. (2018) and Cox and McMahon (2019) experimentally demonstrated frequent yoga practice predicted increases in body appreciation.

One additional and minimally explored mechanism of yoga is associated with prevention or reduction of ED symptoms and body dissatisfaction is an individual's perception of their competence and growth during yoga practice, i.e. yoga self-efficacy. While an individual's perception of their yoga abilities may not in and of itself predict or prevent lower ED symptoms or body dissatisfaction, perceptions of competence or growth related to yoga practice may be associated with a greater self-efficacy, which may lead to greater body appreciation, SC, and increased willingness to engage in physical activity such as yoga. Research demonstrates self-efficacy predicts engagement in physical activity and positive body image (Kołoło, Guszkowska, Mazur, & Dzielska, 2012) as well as embodiment (Cook-Cottone, 2015, 2016; Piran, 2015) often associated with positive body image, and reduced ED sympto-mology (Kinsaul, Curtin, Bazzini, & Martz, 2014). In a recent study, Cox, Ullrich-French, Cole, and D'Hondt-Taylor (2016) found yoga practice was associated with greater confidence in their body's abilities as well as increased motivation to engage in physical activity for health-related versus appearance reasons.

However, researchers have studied the impact of yoga on ED symptoms and body image among women (Carei et al., 2010; Pacanowski et al., 2017) more so than men (see Cox et al., 2017; Flaherty, 2014). In the few studies focusing on men, similar positive effects observed in women are identified. Flaherty (2014) notes yoga practice is associated with lower body dissatisfac-tion in men. In an experimental study, yoga practice was associated with increases in state mindfulness which predicted decreased self-objectification among men and women (Cox et al., 2016). Further, Conboy and colleagues (2013) reported perceived increases in body awareness related to yoga prac-tice among men. Therefore, findings suggest yoga may also be beneficial in reducing body dissatisfaction and risk factors among men.

In sum, there were several aims of the current study. Aim one was to further assess changes in body dissatisfaction and ED symptomology asso-ciated with yoga practice in a college sample, who are often considered at higher risk for ED pathology (Eisenberg, Nicklett, Roeder, & Kirz, 2011). Aim two was to assess changes in body appreciation, SC, and mindfulness associated with yoga practice. Such factors are emphasized considerably during yoga practice and predict lower ED symptomology and body dissatisfaction (Ariel-Donges et al., 2018; Cox et al., 2017; Field, 2011). While the current study design limits our ability to make firm assertions about mechanisms of action or claim the yoga course was the sole influence of change in the variables of interest, findings will help us understand which factors could be assessed as mediators or moderators in future studies. Lastly, the novelty and ecological validity of this study was increased by the inclusion of men who also experience negative body image and struggle with ED (Grogan & Richards, 2002; McCabe & Ricciardelli, 2004; Tiggerman, Martins, & Kirkbride, 2007). Since yoga courses are not limited by gender, it is imperative to include men in studies especially since the majority of studies have examined benefits of yoga among women.

Hypotheses

Hypothesis one

Participants would report a change (increase) in yoga self-efficacy and knowledge, SC, body appreciation, and mindfulness from Time 1 (T1) to Time 2 (T2).

Hypothesis two

Participants would report a change (decrease) in ED pathology and body dissatisfaction from T1 to T2.

Exploratory hypotheses. Men will report lower ED symptoms than women as per previous findings using the EDE-Q (Lavender, De Young, & Anderson, 2010). Women and men will report similar changes in ED symptoms, body image, and other factors at T1 and T2.

Method

Participants

Participants were recruited from a one-credit yoga course offered by a public Midwestern university. A total of 99 participants completed at least one part of the study with the majority identifying as female (n = 76, 76.7%) and Caucasian (n = 88, 89.8%). Full demographics are in Table 1.

Procedure

Participants were recruited at two time points during the spring semester of 2017. Time 1 (T1) was the first day of the eight-week yoga course. Time 2 (T2) occurred on the second to last or last day of the course. The yoga classes, which met three times a week for 50 minutes, included discussions on

Table 1. Demographics.

	N	%	
	83	100	
Gender			
Cisgender Women	63	77.8	
Cisgender Men	18	22.2	
Ethnicity			
Caucasian	73	90.1	
African American	2	2.5	
Hispanic	4	4.9	
American Indian	2	2.5	
Sexual Orientation			
Heterosexual	75	98.7	
Bisexual	1	1.3	
Grade			
Freshman	18	22.2	
Sophomore	20	24.7	
Junior	15	18.5	
Senior	28	34.6	
Practiced Yoga Before			
Yes	37	46.3	
No	43	53.8	
	Female M(SD)	Male M(SD)	t-test of Gender Differences
Age	20.00 (1.46)	20.78 (1.67)	$t(79) = -2.08, p = .04$
BMI	23.59 (3.55)	25.84 (2.88)	$t(79) = 0.52, p = .61$
Years of Yoga	2.18 (1.75)	1.50 (1.61)	$t(36) = 0.88, p = .38^{a,b}$
Hours of Yoga Per Week	0.83 (1.08)	0.50 (0.55)	$t(37) = 0.73, p = .47^a$
Hourly Exercise/Week	6.74(6.26)	9.00 (13.04)	$t(75) = -1.01, p = .32^b$

[a]only included participants who have tried yoga before at T1
[b]assessed prior to T1

yoga philosophy (first 10 minutes), with instruction on breathing, mindfulness, and yoga poses occurring simultaneously during the following 40 minutes. At T1 and T2, participants responded to a packet of questionnaires assessing ED symptoms, body dissatisfaction, body appreciation, self-compassion, mindfulness, and yoga self-efficacy. The T1 packet included a demographics questionnaire. The T2 packet inquired about participants' participation, enjoyment, and knowledge gained during the yoga course. Participants were entered into a raffle for a $25 Target gift card for completing T1 and given $5 for completing T2.

Measures

Demographic questionnaire
Participants reported age, ethnicity, sexual orientation, gender identity, grade, exercise frequency, and height (inches) and weight (pounds) to obtain BMI. Previous yoga practice was assessed (e.g. which forms, frequency of participation, knowledge, etc.). See Table 1.

Eating disorder pathology

ED symptoms were assessed using the *Eating Disorder Examination-Questionnaire* (EDE-Q; Fairburn & Beglin, 2008). The EDE-Q is a self-report measure widely used in research with norms for women (Luce, Crowther, & Pole, 2008) and men (Lavender et al., 2010) in clinical and non-clinical settings (Aardoom, Dingemans, Op't Landt, & Van Furth, 2012; Welch, Birgegård, Parling, & Ghaderi, 2011). The EDE-Q demonstrates acceptable test-retest reliability (Luce et al., 2008) and internal consistency. The EDE-Q can be averaged to provide an overall score (Global EDE-Q) and also has four subscales. Only the Global EDE-Q was utilized given recent research suggesting a single factor loading (Allen, Bryne, Lampard, Watson, & Fursland, 2011). Internal consistency was acceptable at both time points; T1 (α = .92) and T2 (α = .93).

Body dissatisfaction

Three subscales from the *Multidimensional Body-Self Relations Questionnaire-Appearance Subscales* (MBSRQ-AS; Cash, 2000) were utilized to assess body image. The MBSRQ-AS utilizes a 5-point Likert scale; each subscale consists of averages of items in the scale. The first subscale, *Appearance Evaluation (AE)* assesses individuals' perception of physical attractiveness. Higher scores indicate greater body satisfaction. The *Appearance Orientation (AO)* scale assessed the amount of investment an individual has in their appearance with higher scores suggesting more per-severation. The last scale, *Overweight Preoccupation (OP)* assesses distress about being overweight; higher scores suggest greater concern. The MBSRQ demonstrates promising internal consistency and test-retest reliability (Cash, 2000; Vossbeck-Elsebusch et al., 2014). Internal consistency for most AE, T1 (α = .87) and T2 (α = .91) and AO T1 (α = .84) and T2 (α = .81) were acceptable, with OP being T1 (α = .75) and T2 (α = .78) marginally acceptable.

Body appreciation

Body appreciation was assessed using the *Body Appreciation Scale-2* (BAS-2; Tylka & Wood-Barcalow, 2015a). The BAS-2 is a 10-item self-report scale using a 5-point Likert score and demonstrates adequate internal consistency and retest reliability. Internal consistency at T1 (α = .86) and T2 (α = .96) were good.

Self-compassion

Self-compassion was assessed using the *Self-Compassion Scale* (SCS; Neff, 2003b) which demonstrates adequate validity and reliability over time (Neff, Rude, & Kirkpatrick, 2007) in addition to good discriminant and convergent validity. The SCS is a 26-item, 5-point Likert, self-report questionnaire consisting of an overall score (average of all items) and six subscales. Only the overall SCS score was used for this study. Internal consistency was acceptable at T1 (α = .86) and T2 (α = .90).

Mindfulness

Mindfulness was assessed using an average of all items of the *Five Facet Mindfulness Questionnaire* (FFMQ; Baer, Smith, Hopkins, Krietemeye, & Toney, 2006). The 39-item self-report scale assesses participants' ability to observe, describe, respond non-judgmentally and without becoming reactive, and also stay present in the moment. Internal consistency for the FFMQ at T1 (α = .84) and T2 (α = .91) were adequate.

Yoga self-efficacy

Yoga Self-Efficacy Scale assessed participant's yoga skills and knowledge (YSES; Birdee, Sohl, & Wallston, 2015). The YSES is a 12-item, 10-point Likert scale. Higher scores indicated greater knowledge and confidence in practicing yoga. While total YSES scores were used, subscales examined mindfulness, breath-work, and abilities in postures. Internal consistency for T1 (α = .94) and T2 (α = .95) were excellent.

Yoga knowledge and experience

At T1, participants responded to a 7-point Likert scale where higher scores implied greater knowledge of yoga. At T2, enjoyment was assessed using a 10-point Likert scale; higher scores indicated greater enjoyment. Participants also reported how many classes they missed.

Statistical analyses

Prior to running main analyses, demographic data were assessed and T-tests and Chi-Square tests were conducted to assess for differences between T1 and T2 completers and non-completers for validity purposes. T-tests were also run to assess differences between participants who have never tried yoga compared to individuals who have practiced yoga prior to participating in the study. T-tests were also conducted to look at gender differences on demographic factors (See Table 1). Assumptions for later analyses were assessed by examining histograms, skew, and kurtosis. Global EDE-Q was positively skewed and AE was negatively skewed. Square root and reflected square root transformations were conducted respectively to meet assumptions for analyses. Correlations (Pearson and Spearman's Rho, when variables were not normally distributed) were run to evaluate the relationship between dependent variables of the study. To assess changes over time, repeated measures ANOVAs were conducted using only participants who had completed T1 and T2. Bootstrapping was used to protect against Type II error. If BMI correlated with a dependent variable it was included as a covariate. While there were gender differences in age ($p = .04$), age was not included as a covariate as it was not correlated with any dependent variable ($p > .05$).

Results

To address validity concerns given some drop out in participation from T1 to T2 (predominantly due to absences on one of the days participants completed assessments), differences between participants who completed both time points (completers, n = 83, 73.5%) versus participants who did not complete both time points (non-completers, n = 30, 26.5%) were assessed. Comparisons between completers and non-completers are limited; demographics questionnaires were only included at T1 to decrease participant burden. As a result, comparisons between individuals who completed both time points and non-completers can only be based on individuals who responded at T1 but not T2 (n = 18, 15.9%). There were no significant differences in completers and non-completers on the dependent variables or average exercise weekly (all $ps > .05$).

Around half of the participants, n = 43, (53.8%) reported never trying yoga prior to the yoga course. A greater portion of women (54.1%) reported practicing yoga before compared to men (22.2%), Fisher's exact test, $p= .03$. Of the 37 participants who have tried yoga before, four participants (10.3%) reported trying Bikram, 13 (33.3%) Flow, one (2.6%) Iyengar, one (2.6%) Sivananda, 15 (38.5%) Vinyasa, one (2.6%) Yin, and eight (20.5%) reported doing Pilates. Most participants who have practiced yoga before reported minimal knowledge of yoga ($M = 2.47$, $SD = 2.04$). Interestingly, there were no differences between participants who have practiced yoga before or who have never tried yoga (all $ps > .05$) on dependent variables at T1. At T2, class attendance was reported to be high; students missed on average 1.72 classes ($SD = 1.32$). Class enjoyment, rated on a 0 to 10 scale (10 is most enjoyment), was also high. Gender differences were also assessed; the only significant difference between men and women was age (See Table 1). Men ($M = 1.71$, $SD = 1.31$) and women ($M = 1.70$, $SD = 1.34$) missed a similar amount of courses $t(73) = -0.21$, $p = .94$. ($M = 9.05$, $SD = 1.46$) and men ($M = 9.44$, $SD = 0.71$) and women ($M = 8.92$, $SD = 1.62$) reported no statistically significant differences in enjoyment of yoga, $t(75) = -1.34$, $p = .18$. Men ($M = 5.36$, $SD = 5.05$) and women ($M = 5.97$, $SD = 7.42$) reported similar overall exercise (including yoga), $t(74) = 0.32$, $p = .75$.

Correlations were run assessing relationships between dependent variables. See Table 2.

Repeated measures ANOVAs assessed differences in variables over time (within-subjects), gender differences (between subjects), and whether change

Table 2. Correlations between dependent variables at T1.

	BMI[#]	BAS-2	FFMQ	SCS	YSES	AE	AO	OP
BAS-2	−.19							
FFMQ	−.13	.36***						
SCS	−.12	.57***	.64***					
YSES	−.09	.35*	.22	.32**				
AE	−.28*	.75***	.24*	.404***	.24*			
AO	−.18	−.22	−.11	−.26*	.04	−.11		
OP	.12	−.33**	−.20	−.32**	.06	.37***	.40***	
EDE-Q[#]	.11	−.61***	−.20	−.45***	−.20	−.57***	.30**	.77***

BMI = Body Mass Index, BAS-2 = Body Appreciation Scale −2, FFMQ = Five Facet Mindfulness Questionnaire, SCS = Self-Compassion Scale, YSES = Yoga Self-Efficacy Scale, AE = Appearance Evaluation, AO = Appearance Orientation, OP = Overweight Preoccupation, EDE-Q = Eating Disorder Examination-Questionnaire, * $p < .05$, ** $p < .01$, ** $p < .001$, [#] = Spearman's Rho statistic

varied by gender. Hypothesis 1, suggesting YSES, SC, BAS-2, and FFMQ would be higher at T2 than T1 was partially supported. YSES, SC, and BAS-2 were higher at T2 compared to T1 (all $ps < .05$). FFMQ did not significantly change ($p = .37$). Interaction and between subject factor effects were not significant (all $ps > .05$).

Hypothesis two, that yoga practice would be associated with lower ED symptoms, AO, and OP and higher AE[1] was also partially supported. Gender differences were noted in overall EDE-Q scores ($p = .02$). Interactions effects of AE and gender ($p = .001$) and OP and gender ($p = .04$) demonstrated steeper improvements in AE and reductions in OP among men than women. Global EDE-Q, AO, and OP (all $ps < .05$) were lower and AE ($p < .001$) was higher at T2 compared to T1. See Table 3 for M, SD, ANOVA results, effect size (ω^2) and power.[2]

Discussion

It was hypothesized eight weeks of regular yoga practice would be associated with increases in perceived yoga skills and knowledge, self-compassion (SC), body appreciation, and mindfulness, as well as decreases in ED symptoms and negative body image. In addition to assessing associated changes over time, this study assessed overall differences between women and men and whether change over time differed due to gender (interaction effects).

Results indicated a probable association between frequent yoga practice and ED symptoms such that participants reported lower ED symptoms at the end of the eight weeks compared with the first week. In line with previous research, men generally reported lower ED symptoms than women (Lavender et al., 2010; Smith et al., 2017). This finding is promising, as Neumark-Sztainer, MacLehose, Watts, Pacanowski, and Eisenberg (2018) suggest yoga may be an efficient and accessible way to decrease ED risk given the popularity of yoga.

Table 3. Repeated measures ANOVA assessing within and between subject differences and interaction effects.

Variable	Time 1 M (SD)	Time 2 M (SD)	Analysis	F	ω^2	Power
YSES						
Total	72.54 (14.41)	78.26 (14.66)	Within (Time)	9.17**	.11	.85
Women	71.86 (13.96)	77.16 (15.29)	Between (Gender)	1.02	<.01	.17
Men	74.59 (16.97)	81.59 (12.41)	Gender x Time	0.18	<.01	.07
SCS						
Total	2.99 (0.56)	3.08 (0.62)	Within (Time)	6.73**	.07	.73
Women	2.98 (0.61)	3.04 (0.36)	Between (Gender)	0.47	<.01	.10
Men	3.04 (0.69)	3.20 (0.26)	Gender x Time	0.99	<.01	.17
BAS-2						
Total	36.18 (6.74)	37.87 (7.40)	Within (Time)	15.21***	.16	.97
Women	35.64 (7.23)	36.86 (7.57)	Between (Gender)	3.33	.03	.40
Men	37.94 (4.56)	41.11 (5.95)	Gender x Time	2.98	.03	.40
FFMQ						
Total	3.25 (0.42)	3.26 (0.48)	Within (Time)	0.82	<.01	.15
Women	3.24 (0.47)	3.22 (0.52)	Between (Gender)	0.85	<.01	.15
Men	3.30 (0.23)	3.38 (0.26)	Gender x Time	1.69	<.01	.20
AE[a]						
Total	3.43 (0.68)	3.49 (0.75)	Within (Time)	2.62	<.01	.36
Women	3.37 (0.83)	3.36 (0.80)	Between (Gender)	10.91***	.12	.90
Men	3.60 (0.49)	3.90 (0.34)	Gender x Time	12.37***	.13	.94
AO						
Total	3.43 (0.56)	3.33 (0.53)	Within (Time)	7.87**	.08	.79
Women	3.48 (0.58)	3.39 (0.52)	Between (Gender)	2.49	.02	.34
Men	3.27 (0.46)	3.13 (0.55)	Gender x Time	0.25	<.01	.08
OP						
Total	2.68 (0.97)	2.55 (0.93)	Within (Time)	9.99**	.11	.88
Women	2.75 (0.98)	2.69 (0.97)	Between (Gender)	3.30	.03	.43
Men	2.46 (0.61)	2.13 (0.61)	Gender x Time	4.31*	.04	.54
EDEQ						
Total	1.49 (1.16)	1.34 (1.26)	Within (Time)	6.34**	.07	.70
Women	1.67 (1.24)	1.56 (1.34)	Between (Gender)	7.32**	.08	.76
Men	0.87 (0.50)	0.62 (0.47)	Gender x Time	0.88	<.01	.15

YSES = Yoga Self-Efficacy Scale, SCS = Self-Compassion Scale, BAS-2 = Body Appreciation Scale-2, FFMQ = Five Facet Mindfulness Questionnaire, AE = Appearance Evaluation, AO = Appearance Orientation, OP = Overweight Preoccupation, EDEQ = Eating Disorder Examination-Questionnaire.
Time = Within-Subjects analysis (T1 versus T2), Gender = Between-Subjects Analyses (Women vs. Men), Gender x Time = Interaction of Gender by Time.
*$p < .05$, **$p < .01$, ***$p < .001$.
[a]BMI was included as a covariate as it was correlated with AE but was noted to not be significant, $F(1, 72) = 1.32$, $p= .25$.

One of the most studied ED risk factors, body dissatisfaction, was assessed by examining changes associated with yoga practice in concern of being overweight, perception of attractiveness, and degree of focus on their appearance. Specifically, participants reported reduced concern with their physical appearance, likely associated with frequent yoga practice, at T2. While men and women reported lower fear of becoming overweight (OP) and more favourable body image perceptions (AE) at T2, men appeared to report greater improvements over time compared to women. The difference noted between men and women may relate to social experiences; males are raised to focus on their body's abilities and strengths (Daniel & Bridges, 2010;

Tatangelo & Ricciardelli, 2013). A practice emphasizing body functionality may elicit greater benefits in men as a result.

Further, body dissatisfaction among males typically results from concerns of being muscular versus thin or lower weighted like women (Grogan, 2006). It may be men perceived greater improvements in muscularity while women did not note the physical changes in line with gender specific body image goals (Grogan, 2006). Hausenblas and Fallon (2006) also note greater improvements in body image factors among men compared to women related to exercise supporting our findings. An alternative explanation may be that more men reported never practicing yoga prior to taking the yoga course which may have been associated with larger improvements in variables due to the novelty of the experience.

This study was one of the first to demonstrate changes in perceived yoga skills associated with eight weeks of regular yoga practice. This is notable since perceptions of body competency may relate to greater body appreciation. Researchers hypothesize practices which increase body awareness, body capabilities, and demonstrable improvements in body functionality may predict greater body appreciation, embodiment, and motivation to engage in physical activity for intrinsic purposes (e.g. Cook-Cottone, 2015, 2016; Piran, 2015) which may be protective against ED and body dissatisfaction.

While previous research has indicated positive relationships between mindfulness and yoga practice (Butryn et al., 2013; Cox & McMahon, 2019; Eastman-Mueller et al., 2013), we failed to observe such a relationship. The style of yoga practiced may have influenced mindfulness scores (Birdee et al., 2015). The nature of the course, which was offered for course credit, may have also impacted results; individuals who seek yoga at yoga studios or gyms may have had different objectives than individuals seeking course credit as in our sample (Douglass, 2009; Delaney and Anthis, 2010; Mahlo & Tiggemann, 2016). Further the FFMQ assesses trait mindfulness while researchers reporting improvements in mindfulness related to yoga assessed state mindfulness. (Cox & McMahon, 2019; Cox et al., 2016) which could have also explained the differing results of this study compared with previous research.

SC is another ability emphasized through the practice of yoga. Practitioners are instructed to accept their body's performance with minimal judgment and with kindness. We observed SC was higher at Time 2 compared to T1 which may have been associated with yoga practice, supporting previous research (e.g. Gard et al., 2012). This is encouraging since SC is negatively related to ED risk (Kelly, Vimalakanthan, & Carter, 2014), disordered eating (Breines et al., 2014), and body dissatisfaction (Wasylkiw et al., 2012). It is possible teachings of yoga, which emphasize greater acceptance and reductions in critical evaluation of one's abilities lead to increases in SC. Research demonstrates early improvements in SC are associated with improvement during ED treatment (Kelly et al., 2014). As such, yoga may be one viable method of improving SC thus reducing ED risk and body dissatisfaction.

Body appreciation was also higher at T2 compared to T1; women and men in this study reported higher gratitude for their body's functionality, potentially associated with eight weeks of yoga practice. It has been hypothesized the more an individual perceives their body as functional and a vessel to achieve values versus as an object, the less likely they are to experience body dissatisfaction and thus, disordered eating (Cook-Cottone, 2015; Piran, 2015). Similar to SC, as participants learn to appreciate their body's ability to move, they may be at lower risk for ED pathology and body dissatisfaction. Our study provides further evidence for previous research noting improvements in body appreciation related to yoga practice (Ariel-Donges et al., 2018; Cox et al., 2017).

As with any research study, there are important limitations which should be addressed. First, this study was quasi-experimental and did not recruit controls or a comparison group which reduces our ability to claim yoga itself was responsible for changes demonstrated over time. We can only surmise associations in change over time related to yoga. However, repeated measures ANOVA were used given that within subject designs account for variance between and within factors, are associated with less "noise" in assessing change, and may better control against random uncontrolled differences in conditions seen in independent designs (Field, 2013).

While this is one of the first studies to include men while assessing yoga and ED related factors, the sample size was small. Due to a smaller sample size, repeated measures ANOVA yielded suboptimal power in assessing gender differences and interaction effects. Therefore, differences between genders, which support some research findings (Lavender et al., 2010), should be considered with caution. Regardless, assessment of the impact of yoga on body image, disordered eating, and related factors among men is essential as men are also at risk for ED development (McCabe & Ricciardelli, 2004; Graham et al., 2005) and also present in ED treatment settings that offer yoga.

Another limitation of the study was that participants chose to enroll in the yoga courses. This may limit the generalizability of the findings especially as some participants did not complete all time points. However, this study possesses ecological validity since it is examining a sample participating in yoga volitionally, which is the usual motivator for practice. Reasons why an individual is practicing yoga may be important (Douglass, 2009; Mahlo & Tiggemann, 2016). Given this sample was seeking course credit, participants' goals may have been different than individuals who are going to yoga studios or even practicing yoga as an adjunct to ED treatment. Participants completing questionnaires at both time points could have also been more interested in yoga, however most missed data occurred due to absence on recruitment days.

The majority of the sample identified as White/Caucasian. While the sample reflects the regional demographics of the area, this may limit the generalizability of our results. Previous research suggests ethnic minorities use complementary alternative medicine practices less than Caucasian individuals (Graham et al., 2005). Understanding the effect of yoga in such populations and the disparity of use represents an important avenue for future research. Future studies could also assess impact of yoga on other populations (e.g. body functionalities, ages).

In all, regular yoga practice appears to be associated with decreases in ED pathology and negative body image as well as concurrent increases in self-compassion, body appreciation, and perceived yoga skills and abilities in a college sample. The concurrent decreases in ED symptoms and improvements in protective factors associated with yoga practice is promising; both independently predict ED pathology (Tylka & Wood-Barcalow, 2015b). Incorporating yoga into physical education, as health requirements, or offering courses in college or similar settings could yield numerous benefits. Such findings are also supported by existing prevention and intervention studies on yoga (Ariel-Donges et al., 2018; Cox & McMahon, 2019; Halliwell, Dawson, & Burkey, 2019). In sum, yoga appears to be associated with improvements in many protective factors (i.e., self-compassion and body appreciation), risk factors (i.e., body dissatisfaction), and ED symptoms among young adults. Future research should continue to assess mechanisms of action by which yoga practice is associated with reductions in ED symptoms and risk to incorporate the most effective elements in the practice for ED prevention and treatment.

Notes

1. AE is scored such that high scores suggest lower body dissatisfaction while higher scores on all other subscales of the MBSRQ-AS indicate greater body dissatisfaction.
2. Between-subjects and some interaction analyses yielded results that were low-powered and should be considered cautiously.

Acknowledgments

Authors would like to thank Julian Paul Keenan, Ph.D., Abigail Matthews, Ph.D., and Andrea Meisman, M.A. for their helpful comments and feedback on earlier versions of this manuscript.

Funding

Funding to compensate participants was provided by first author's department [a] through a departmental research grant.

Conflicts of interest

In accordance with Taylor & Francis policy and our ethical obligation as researchers, the authors report that no conflicts of interest.

ORCID

Rachel Kramer ⓘ http://orcid.org/0000-0001-5698-0712
Kelly Cuccolo ⓘ http://orcid.org/0000-0002-0358-7113

References

Aardoom, J. J., Dingemans, A. E., Op't Landt, M. C. S., & Van Furth, E. F. (2012). Norms and discriminative validity of the Eating Disorder Examination Questionnaire (EDE-Q). *Eating Behaviors, 13*(4), 305–309. doi:10.1016/j.eatbeh.2012.09.002

Allen, K. L., Bryne, S. M., Lampard, A., Watson, H., & Fursland, A. (2011). Confirmatory factor analysis of the Eating Disorder Examination-Questionnaire (EDE-Q). *Eating Behaviors, 12*(2), 143–151. doi:10.1016/j.eatbeh.2011.01.005

Andrew, R., Tiggemann, M., & Clark, L. (2015). The protective role of body appreciation against media-induced body dissatisfaction. *Body Image, 15*, 98–104. doi:10.1016/j.bodyim.2015.07.005

Ariel-Donges, A. H., Gordon, E. L., Bauman, V., & Perri, M. G. (2018). Does yoga help college-aged women with body-image dissatisfaction feel better about their bodies? *Sex Roles, 80*(1–2), 1–11.

Avalos, L., Tylka, T. L., & Wood-Barcalow, N. (2005). The body appreciation scale: Development and psychometric evaluation. *Body Image, 2*(3), 285–297. doi:10.1016/j.bodyim.2005.06.002

Baer, R. A., Fischer, S., & Huss, D. B. (2005). Mindfulness and acceptance in the treatment of disordered eating. *Journal of Rational-Emotive and Cognitive-Behavior Therapy, 23*(4), 281–300. doi:10.1007/s10942-005-0015-9

Baer, R. A, Smith, G. T, Hopkins, J, Krietemeyer, J, & Toney, L. (2006). Using self-report assessment methods to explore facets of mindfulness. *Assessment, 13*(1), 27-45. doi:10.1177/1073191105283504

Banerjee, B., Vadiraj, H. S., Ram, A., Rao, R., Jayapal, M., & Gopinath, K. S., ... & Hegde, S. (2007). Effects of an integrated yoga program in modulating psychological stress and radiation-induced genotoxic stress in breast cancer patients undergoing radiotherapy. Integrative cancer therapies, 6(3), 242–250. doi: 10.1177/1534735407306214

Birdee, G. S., Sohl, S. J., & Wallston, K. (2015). Development and psychometric properties of the Yoga Self-Efficacy Scale (YSES). *Complementary and Alternative Medicine, 16*(1), 1–9. doi:10.1186/s12906-015-0981-0

Breines, J., Toole, A., Tu, C., & Chen, S. (2014). Self-compassion, body image, and self reported disordered eating. *Self and Identity, 13*(4), 432–448. doi:10.1080/15298868.2013.838992

Büssing, A., Michalsen, A., Khalsa, S. B. S., Telles, S., & Sherman, K. J. (2012). Effects of yoga on mental and physical health: A short summary of reviews. *Evidence-Based Complementary and Alternative Medicine, 2012*. doi:10.1155/2012/165410

Butryn, M. L., Juarascio, A., Shaw, J., Kerrigan, S. G., Clark, V., O'Planick, A., & Forman, E. M. (2013). Mindfulness and its relationship with eating disorders symptomatology in women receiving residential treatment. *Eating Behaviors, 14*(1), 13–16. doi:10.1016/j.eatbeh.2012.10.005

Carei, T. R., Fyfe-Johnson, A. L., Breuner, C. C., & Marshall, M. A. (2010). Randomized controlled clinical trial of yoga in the treatment of eating disorders. *Journal of Adolescent Health, 46*(4), 346–351. doi:10.1016/j.jadohealth.2009.08.007

Cash, T. F. (2000). *Multidimensional body-self relations questionnaire (MBSRQ)*. Norfolk, VA: Author.

Conboy, L. A, Noggle, J. J, Frey, J. L, Kudesia, R. S, & Khalsa, Sat Bir S. (2013). Qualitative evaluation of a high school yoga program: feasibility and perceived benefits. *Explore: The Journal Of Science and Healing, 9*(3), 171-180. doi: 10.1016/j.explore.2013.02.001

Cook-Cottone, C., Talebkhah, K., Guyker, W., & Keddie, E. (2017). A controlled trial of a yoga-based prevention program targeting eating disorder risk factors among middle school females. *Eating Disorders, 25*(5), 392–405. doi:10.1080/10640266.2017.1365562

Cook-Cottone, C. P. (2015). Incorporating positive body image into the treatment of eating disorders: A model for attunement and mindful self-care. *Body Image, 14*, 158–167. doi:10.1016/j.bodyim.2015.03.004

Cook-Cottone, C. P. (2016). Embodied self-regulation and mindful self-care in the prevention of eating disorders. *Eating Disorders, 24*(1), 98–105. doi:10.1080/10640266.2015.1118954

Cotter, E. W., Kelly, N. R., Mitchell, K. S., & Mazzeo, S. E. (2015). An investigation of body appreciation, ethnic identity, and eating disorder symptoms in Black women. *Journal of Black Psychology, 41*(1), 3–25. doi:10.1177/0095798413502671

Cox, A. E., & McMahon, A. K. (2019). Exploring changes in mindfulness and body appreciation during yoga participation. *Body Image, 29*, 118–121. doi:10.1016/j.bodyim.2019.03.003

Cox, A. E., Ullrich-French, S., Cole, A. M., & D'Hondt-Taylor, M. (2016). The role of state mindfulness during yoga in predicting self-objectification and reasons for exercise. *Psychology of Sport and Exercise, 22*, 321–327. doi:10.1016/j.psychsport.2015.10.001

Cox, A. E., Ullrich-French, S., Howe, H. S., & Cole, A. N. (2017). A pilot yoga physical education curriculum to promote positive body image. *Body Image, 23*, 1–8. doi:10.1016/j.bodyim.2017.07.007

Daniel, S., & Bridges, S. K. (2010). The drive for muscularity in men: Media influences and objectification theory. *Body Image, 7*, 32–38. doi:10.1016/j.bodyim.2009.08.003

Delaney, K., & Anthis, K. (2010). Is women's participation in different types of yoga classes associated with different levels of body awareness and body satisfaction? *International Journal of Yoga Therapy, 20*, 62–71.

Dijkstra, P, & Barelds, Dick P.H. (2011). Examining a model of dispositional mindfulness, body comparison, and body satisfaction. *Body Image, 8*(4), 419-422. doi: 10.1016/j.bodyim.2011.05.007

Douglass, L. (2009). Yoga as an intervention in the treatment of eating disorders. *Does It Help, Eating Disorders, 17*, 126–130. doi:10.1080/10640260802714555

Eastman-Mueller, H., Wilson, T., Jung, A. K., Kimura, A., & Tarrant, J. (2013). iRest yoga-nidra on the college campus: Changes in stress, depression, worry, and mindfulness. *International Journal of Yoga Therapy, 23*(2), 15–24.

Eisenberg, D., Nicklett, E. J., Roeder, K., & Kirz, N. E. (2011). Eating disorder symptoms among college students: Prevalence, persistence, correlates, and treatment-seeking. *Journal of American College Health, 59*(8), 700–707. doi:10.1080/07448481.2010.546461

Fairburn, C. G., & Beglin, S. J. (2008). Eating Disorder Examination Questionnaire (EDE-Q6. 0). In C. G. Fairburn (Ed.), *Cognitive behavior therapy and eating disorders* (pp. 309–314). New York, NY: Guilford Press.

Field, A. (2013). Repeated measures designs: GLM-4. In *Discovering statistics using IBM statistics – Fourth Edition* (pp. 543–590). London, England: Sage.

Field, T. (2011). Yoga clinical research review. *Complementary Therapies in Clinical Practice*, *17*, 1–8. doi:10.1016/j.ctcp.2010.09.007

Flaherty, M. (2014). Influence of yoga on body image satisfaction in men. *Perceptual and Motor Skills*, *119*(1), 203–214. doi:10.2466/27.50.PMS.119c17z1

Foroughi, N., Zhu, K. C. Y., Smith, C., & Hay, P. (2019). The perceived therapeutic benefits of complementary medicine in eating disorders. *Complementary Therapies in Medicine*, *43*, 176–180. doi:10.1016/j.ctim.2019.01.025

Freeman, R. (2004). Richard Freeman on yoga as a path to physical and spiritual health. Interview by Bonnie Horrigan. *Alternative Therapies in Health and Medicine*, *10*(2), 64–72.

Frisch, M. J., Herzog, D. B., & Franko, D. L. (2006). Residential treatment for eating disorders. *International Journal of Eating Disorders*, *39*(5), 434–442. doi:10.1002/(ISSN) 1098-108X

Gard, T., Brach, N., Hölzel, B. K., Noggle, J. J., Conboy, L. A., & Lazar, S. W. (2012). Effects of a yoga-based intervention for young adults on quality of life and perceived stress: The potential mediating roles of mindfulness and self-compassion. *The Journal of Positive Psychology*, *7*(3), 165–175. doi:10.1080/17439760.2012.667144

Graham, R. E., Ahn, A. C., Davis, R. B., O'Connor, B. B., Eisenberg, D. M., & Phillips, R. S. (2005). Use of complementary and alternative medical therapies among racial and ethnic minority adults: Results from the 2002 national health interview survey. *Journal of the National Medical Association*, *97*(4), 535–545.

Grogan, S. (2006). Body image and health: Contemporary perspectives. *Journal of Health Psychology*, *11*(4), 523–530. doi:10.1177/1359105306065013

Grogan, S, & Richards, H. (2002). Body image: focus groups with boys and men. *Men and Masculinities*, *4*(3), 219-232. doi: 10.1177/1097184X02004003001

Hall, A., Ofei-TEnkorang, N. A., Machan, J. T., & Gordon, C. M. (2016). Use of yoga in outpatient eating disorder treatment: A pilot study. *Journal of Eating Disorders*, *4*, 38. doi:10.1186/s40337-016-0130-2

Halliwell, E., Dawson, K., & Burkey, S. (2019). A randomized experimental evaluation of yoga-based body image intervention. *Body Image*, *28*, 119–127. doi:10.1016/j.bodyim.2018.12.005

Hausenblas, H. A., & Fallon, E. A. (2006). Exercise and body image: A meta-analysis. *Psychology and Health*, *21*(1), 33–47. doi:10.1080/14768320500105270

Kelly, A. C., Carter, J. C., & Borairi, S. (2014). Are improvements in shame and self-compassion early in eating disorders treatment associated with better patient outcomes? *International Journal of Eating Disorders*, *47*(1), 54–64. doi:10.1002/eat.v47.1

Kelly, A. C., Vimalakanthan, K., & Carter, J. C. (2014). Understanding the roles of self-esteem, self-compassion, and fear of self-compassion in eating disorder pathology: An examination of female students and eating disorder patients. *Eating Behaviors*, *15*(3), 388–391. doi:10.1016/j.eatbeh.2014.04.008

Kelly, A. C., Vimalakanthan, K., & Miller, K. E. (2014). Self-compassion moderates the relationship between body mass index and both eating disorder pathology and body image flexibility. *Body Image*, *11*(4), 446–453. doi:10.1016/j.bodyim.2014.07.005

Kinsaul, Jessica A.E, Curtin, L, Bazzini, D, & Martz, D. (2014). Empowerment, feminism, and self-efficacy: relationships to body image and disordered eating. *Body Image*, *11*(1), 63-67. doi: 10.1016/j.bodyim.2013.08.001

Kołoło, H, Guszkowska, M, Mazur, J, & Dzielska, A. (2012). Self-efficacy, self-esteem and body image as psychological determinants of 15-year-old adolescents' physical activity levels. *Human Movement*, *13*(3), 264-270. doi: 10.2478/v10038-012-0031-4

Kristeller, J. L., Baer, R. A., & Quillian Wolever, R. (2006). Mindfulness-based approaches to eating disorders. In R. A. Baer (Ed.), *Mindfulness-based treatment approaches: Clinician's guide to evidence base and applications* (pp. 75–91). San Diego, CA: Elsevier Academic Press.

Lavender, J. M., De Young, K. P., & Anderson, D. A. (2010). Eating Disorder Examination Questionnaire (EDE-Q): Norms for undergraduate men. *Eating Behaviors, 11*(2), 119–121. doi:10.1016/j.eatbeh.2009.09.005

Lavender, J. M., Gratz, K. L., & Anderson, D. A. (2012). Mindfulness, body image, and drive for muscularity in men. *Body Image, 9*(2), 289–292. doi:10.1016/j.bodyim.2011.12.002

Lavender, J. M., Jardin, B. F., & Anderson, D. A. (2009). Bulimic symptoms in undergraduate men and women: Contributions of mindfulness and thought suppression. *Eating Behaviors, 10*(4), 228–231. doi:10.1016/j.eatbeh.2009.07.002

Luce, K. H., Crowther, J. H., & Pole, M. (2008). Eating Disorder Examination Questionnaire; Norms for undergrad women. *International Journal of Eating Disorders, 41*(3), 273–276. doi:10.1002/eat.20504

Mahlo, L., & Tiggemann, M. (2016). Yoga and positive body image: A test of the embodiment model. *Body Image, 18*, 135–142. doi:10.1016/j.bodyim.2016.06.008

McCabe, M. P, & Ricciardelli, L. A. (2004). Body image dissatisfaction among males across the lifespan: a review of past literature. *Journal Of Psychosomatic Research, 56*(6), 675-685. doi: 10.1016/S0022-3999(03)00129-6

McIver, S., O'Halloran, P., & McGartland, M. (2009). Yoga as a treatment for binge eating disorder: A preliminary study. *Complementary Therapies in Medicine, 17*(4), 196–202. doi:10.1016/j.ctim.2009.05.002

Menzel, J. E., & Levine, M. P. (2011). Embodying experiences and the promotion of positive body image: The example of competitive athletics. In R. M. Calagero, S. Tantleff-Dunn, & J. K. Thompson (Eds.), *Self-objectification in women: Causes, consequences, and counter-actions* (pp. 163–186). Washington, DC: American Psychological Association.

Neff, K. D. (2003a). Self-compassion: An alternative conceptualization of a healthy attitude toward oneself. *Self & Identity, 2*(2), 85–101. doi:10.1080/15298860309032

Neff, K. D. (2003b). The development and validation of a scale to measure self-compassion. *Self and Identity, 2*(3), 223–250. doi:10.1080/15298860309027

Neff, K. D., Rude, S. S., & Kirkpatrick, K. L. (2007). An examination of self-compassion in relation to positive psychological functioning and personality traits. *Journal of Research in Personality, 41*(4), 908–916. doi:10.1016/j.jrp.2006.08.002

Neumark-Sztainer, D., MacLehose, R. F., Watts, A. W., Pacanowski, C. R., & Eisenberg, M. E. (2018). Yoga and body image: Findings from a large population-based study of young adults. *Body Image, 24*, 69–75. doi:10.1016/j.bodyim.2017.12.003

Pacanowski, C. R., Diers, L., Crosby, R. D., & Neumark-Sztainer, D. (2017). Yoga in the treatment of eating disorders within a residential eating disorders program: A randomized controlled trial. *Eating Disorders, 25*(1), 37–51. doi:10.1080/10640266.2016.1237810

Park, C. L., Braun, T., & Siegel, T. (2015). Who practices yoga? A systematic review of demographic health-related, and psychosocial factors associated with yoga practice. *Journal of Behavioral Medicine, 38*, 460–471. doi:10.1007/s10865-015-9618-5

Pidgeon, A. M, & Appleby, L. (2014). Investigating the role of dispositional mindfulness as a protective factor for body image dissatisfaction among women. *Current Research in Psychology, 5*(2), 96-103. doi: 10.3844/crpsp.2014.96.103

Piran, N. (2015). New possibilities in the prevention of eating disorders: The introduction of positive body image measures. *Body Image, 14*, 146–157. doi:10.1016/j.bodyim.2015.03.008

Scime, M., & Cook-Cottone, C. (2008). Primary prevention of eating disorders: A constructivist integration of mind and body strategies. *International Journal of Eating Disorders, 41*(2), 134–142. doi:10.1002/eat.20480

Smith, K. E, Mason, T. B, Murray, S. B, Griffiths, S, Leonard, R. C, Wetterneck, C. T, & Lavender, J. M. (2017). Male clinical norms and sex differences on the eating disorder inventory (edi) and eating disorder examination questionnaire (ede-q). *International Journal Of Eating Disorders, 50*(7), 769–775. doi: 10.1002/eat.22716

Tatangelo, G. L., & Ricciardelli, L. (2013). A qualitative study of preadolescent boys' and girls' body image: Gendered ideals and sociocultural influences. *Body Image, 10*, 591–598. doi:10.1016/j.bodyim.2013.07.006

Tiggemann, M, Martins, Y, & Kirkbride, A. (2007). Oh to be lean and muscular: body image ideals in gay and heterosexual men. *Psychology Of Men & Masculinity, 8*(1), 15. doi: 10.1037/1524-9220.8.1.15

Tylka, T. L., & Wood-Barcalow, N. L. (2015a). The body appreciation scale-2: Item refinement and psychometric evaluation. *Body Image, 12*, 53–67. doi:10.1016/j.bodyim.2014.09.006

Tylka, T. L., & Wood-Barcalow, N. L. (2015b). What is and what is not positive body image? Conceptual foundations and construct definition. *Body Image, 14*, 118–129. doi:10.1016/j.bodyim.2015.04.001

Vossbeck-Elsebusch, A. N., Waldorf, M., Legenbauer, T., Bauer, A., Cordes, M., & Vocks, S. (2014). German version of the Multidimensional Body-Self Relations Questionnaire–Appearance Scales (MBSRQ-AS): Confirmatory factor analysis validation. *Body Image, 11* (3), 191–200. doi:10.1016/j.bodyim.2014.02.002

Wasylkiw, L., MacKinnon, A. L., & MacLellan, A. M. (2012). Exploring the link between self-compassion and body image in university women. *Body Image, 9*(2), 236–245. doi:10.1016/j.bodyim.2012.01.007

Welch, E., Birgegård, A., Parling, T., & Ghaderi, A. (2011). Eating Disorder Examination-Questionnaire and clinical impairment assessment questionnaire: General population and clinical norms for young adult women in Sweden. *Behaviour Research and Therapy, 49*(2), 85–91. doi:10.1016/j.brat.2010.10.010

Yoga's impact on risk and protective factors for disordered eating: a pilot prevention trial

CR Pacanowski, L Diers, RD Crosby, M Mackenzie ⓘ, and D. Neumark-Sztainer

ABSTRACT

Yoga has been proposed as a strategy for improving risk and protective factors for eating disorders, but few prevention trials have been conducted. The purpose of this pilot study was to assess the feasibility and acceptability of a yoga series in female college students (n = 52). Participants were randomized to a yoga intervention (three 50-minute yoga classes/week for 10 weeks conducted by certified yoga teachers who received a 3-day intensive training) or a control group. Risk and protective factors, assessed at baseline, 5 and 10 weeks, included body dissatisfaction, negative affect, loneliness, self-compassion, positive affect, and mindfulness. Mixed models controlling for baseline levels of outcome variables were run. On average, participants attended 20 out of 30 yoga classes, and the majority of participants reported high levels of satisfaction with the yoga series. Appearance orientation decreased and positive affect increased in the yoga group relative to the control group. After controlling for baseline levels, the yoga group had a significantly higher positive affect than the control group. Changes in other outcomes were not statistically significant, as compared to the control condition. Future yoga research directions are discussed including education about body image, measure and sample selection, and use of an implementation science framework.

Clinical Implications

- Yoga may increase positive affect in nonclinical groups.

Introduction

Yoga, which involves the practice of joining breath and movement, can be used as a tool to inhabit the body from the inside out; and for this reason, among others, has been suggested as a tool for prevention of eating disorders and disordered eating (Cook-Cottone, 2015; Hall et al., 2016; Klein & Cook-Cottone, 2013; Neumark-Sztainer, 2016). A mindful focus on nonjudgmental awareness of the present moment, in conjunction with an appreciation for what one's body can do, rather than how it looks, has been found to improve body dissatisfaction (e.g., Alleva et al., 2015), a key risk factor for disordered eating. In addition to theoretical reasons to expect yoga to offer healing properties to those with eating disorders, empirical data show reduced levels of risk factors and enhanced levels of protective factors in individuals practicing yoga. Considering the interest in and availability of yoga on college campuses, this practice is a natural fit for the prevention of disordered eating in college women.

Risk factors: body dissatisfaction, negative affect, and loneliness

Body dissatisfaction remains a concerning risk factor for disordered eating among college-aged women (Dakanalis et al., 2016; Karazsia et al., 2017). Because yoga promotes embodiment, much research has focused on body dissatisfaction as a risk factor. Cross-sectional data shows that yoga practitioners report lower body dissatisfaction and lower negative affect as compared to non-practitioners (e.g., Neumark-Sztainer et al., 2018). A large, observational, population-based study, young adults who practiced yoga had significantly higher body satisfaction than those who did not practice, controlling for prior body satisfaction and Body Mass Index (BMI) (Neumark-Sztainer et al., 2018). Daubenmier (2005) found that yoga practitioners not taking aerobic exercise classes self-reported significantly higher body satisfaction, after adjusting for BMI, as compared to aerobic exercisers who did not take yoga or participants who engaged in neither activity (Daubenmier, 2005). Gammage et al. (2016) assessed state-level body satisfaction in college women before and after either a yoga class or a resistance training class. They found that body satisfaction significantly improved after yoga, but not after resistance training (Gammage et al., 2016). Finally, two studies investigating the effects of yoga on college women that employed randomized designs: one found no significant difference between yoga and control conditions, though the yoga group's scores on body image distress did decrease minimally (Mitchell et al., 2007), and the other found significant improvements in both the yoga and control groups; however, the yoga group improved to a greater degree (Ariel-Donges et al., 2019).

In addition to body dissatisfaction, negative affect has been linked to disordered eating (e.g., Dakanalis et al., 2016). In an experimental study of individuals with eating disorders, negative affect was significantly reduced after participating in a yoga program (Pacanowski et al., 2017). A systematic review reported several studies indicate that yoga decreases negative mood states, such as anxiety and depressive symptoms (Pascoe & Bauer, 2015). A study of college women found a significant decrease in negative affect after one yoga session (Sullivan et al., 2019). Thus, there is evidence that suggests that yoga may reduce negative affect, a known risk factor for disordered eating.

While studied less than body dissatisfaction or negative affect in the context of eating disorders, loneliness, or perceived social isolation, is common among college students and implicated in many mental health problems (Diehl et al., 2018). Loneliness has been indicated in binge eating and other eating disorders (Levine, 2012; Mason et al., 2016). Yoga is often practiced in a community setting, which has the potential to create a sense of community, ameliorating feelings of loneliness (Wang, 2010), and in this way serves to reduce a risk factor for disordered eating.

Protective factors: self-compassion, positive affect, and mindfulness

Factors protecting against the onset of disordered eating have been identified and are important to address within prevention interventions. Self-compassion may mitigate body dissatisfaction and also is associated with less disordered eating behavior (Albertson et al., 2015; Braun et al., 2016; Duarte et al., 2015). Pilot evidence suggests that even a 5-day yoga intervention can increase self-compassion (Braun et al., 2012). A systematic review cited self-compassion as one of the potential mediators between yoga and stress (Riley & Park, 2015).

The role of positive affect has been understudied with regards to disordered eating, but positive affect represents an important and conceptually different targets from negative affect. Positive affect has been found to increase with body satisfaction (Stern & Engeln, 2018). Within a yoga context, specifically, the language used by yoga instructors that focuses on functionality rather than appearance can improve body image and increase positive affect (Engeln et al., 2018). A week-long yoga class significantly improved positive affect in a sample of adults (Narasimhan et al., 2011)

Finally, mindfulness is inversely related to disordered eating and body dissatisfaction (Barrington & Jarry, 2019; Wilson & O'Connor, 2017). One study found that participants with greater mindfulness surveyed their bodies less, which is a known symptom associated with disordered eating (Cox et al., 2017). Mindfulness may also be associated with internal reasons to exercise as opposed to appearance-based reasons (Cox et al., 2015). Cox and McMahon (2019) fond that university students electing to take a 16-week yoga class experienced a linear increase in mindfulness (Cox & McMahon, 2019).

The purpose of the current pilot study is twofold: (a) to report the development, feasibility and acceptability of conducting a yoga intervention for prevention of eating disorders among college females and (b) to report findings on risk (body dissatisfaction, negative affect, loneliness) and protective (self-compassion, positive affect, mindfulness) factors for eating disorders. Weight and height were measured for the inclusion of Body Mass Index as a covariate.

Methods

Participants and assessment

Participants were recruited from a state university on the east coast of the United States. Recruitment flyers were displayed on campus and distributed electronically to students via academic advisors. Handing out flyers at tables in student hubs, emailing student groups and clubs (e.g., sororities), and Facebook were also used to recruit. Inclusion criteria were being a female of freshman, sophomore, or junior standing, preferably having little to no yoga experience, being free during the time of the yoga class on Mondays, Wednesdays, and Fridays, physically able to participate in yoga, and between the ages of 18 and 26. Individuals who did not practice yoga regularly were targeted to assess the feasibility and acceptability of the program for the general population of female college students. The flyer informed participants that they would be either part of a group offered three yoga classes per week or a control group that only participated in assessments. Seniors were excluded from the study because compensation provided to the control group consisted of a group fitness pass, allowing for students to take yoga classes the following Fall semester, as the trial was conducted in the Spring. Thus, seniors would not be able to use this group fitness pass because they would have graduated. In addition, the recruitment flyer noted that participants would be compensated for the 10-week study.

Participants were screened for eligibility via email, and once they committed to participating in the study, were scheduled for a baseline assessment visit (in groups of six to seven, every 15 minutes, within a 2-hour period). Participants were randomized (using Google's random number generator) to either the yoga group or control group. Upon arrival, participants checked in with a Research Assistant (RA) and proceeded through "assessment stations." The first station consisted of a RA going through the consent form with potential participants. The study was described to participants in the consent form as follows: "*The purpose of this study is to assess the effects of a regular yoga practice on college women. The primary aim of this study is to evaluate change in body image resulting from a yoga intervention compared to a control group.*" After consenting, participants completed a questionnaire, then were individually invited to an area blocked-off by large screens, where weight and height were measured by a trained anthropometrist. Weight was measured in kilograms and not reported to the participants unless they requested this information. Finally, participants proceeded to the "check out" station, where they received a card with their group assignment, mat if they were in the yoga group, and compensation. Each assessment (baseline, 5-week, and 10-week) was done this way, at the same time of day, on a Saturday, in the same large room, with participants arriving in groups at scheduled 15-minute intervals based on their availability. Make-up assessments took place the following Monday, if needed. Only members of the research team were present for these visits; none of the yoga interventionists were present during assessments or collected data.

Participants were compensated 10 USD for the baseline assessment, 10 USD for the mid-point assessment, and 20 USD for the end-of-treatment assessment. Yoga group participants were provided with their own mat at baseline, and control participants were provided with a mat and the ability to take a comparable number of free yoga classes at the end-of-treatment assessment. All procedures were approved by the University's Institutional Review Board.

Implementation of intervention

Interventionists

Yoga instructors who taught for the University were interviewed as potential study instructors. Three selected instructors met the minimum requirements of a 200-hr Registered Yoga Teacher (RYT) and completed an in-person three-day intensive training conducted by an Experienced Registered Yoga Teacher (E-RYT) with over 10 years of eating disorder and body image yoga specialty instruction (LD). Each yoga teacher was educated about body image, the importance of language choice in instruction, and the relationship of triggering words to disordered eating. Instruction and peer-led instruction (practicum components) were included in this training. The three yoga interventionists were all female, between the ages of 40 and 65, and of thin-to-moderate body size. Each instructor taught one class, the same day of the week (Monday, Wednesday, or Friday) for 10 weeks, except for the few instances in which substitutions were necessary.

Environment

A large, spacious room was reserved and rented at the university. Due to recent work suggesting potential adverse effects of mirrors for some individuals when practicing yoga (Frayeh & Lewis, 2018), classes were instructed facing away from the mirrored wall, and care was taken to board windows into the hallway every time class was held to prevent self-consciousness or distraction from onlookers. Yoga group participants were advised to wear clothing that they felt comfortable moving in, with additional suggestions provided by yoga instructors (e.g., hoods could be distracting). The same room was used both for yoga intervention classes (Mondays, Wednesdays, and Fridays) and for assessment visits (Saturdays).

Intervention development

In a previous study, the yoga sequence was designed (by LD) for inpatient residential eating disorder clients (Pacanowski, Diers, Crosby, & Neumark-Sztainer, Cox et al., 2017) and led to a decrease in pre-meal negative affect. This sequence was modified to meet the needs of a general college-aged female sample, based on knowledge gained from the previous trial and over a decade of experience with yoga training and teaching to individuals with body weight and shape concerns. Techniques used included breath-centric asana (postures), breath-centric affirmations, and non-triggering language used in instruction (discussed more in depth in the following section: '*Language*').

Table 1 details the yoga intervention sequence and Figure 1 provides visuals of poses described. The first 5 minutes of class were devoted to centering, when participants lay on their backs and perform affirmation-focused breathing. The affirmation changed weekly, and specific affirmations used (e.g., inhale "*I am*"; exhale "*enough*") are listed in the table. For consistency and replication/dissemination of the intervention, an outline of asanas accessible to all levels of experience, mobility, and body size and specific breathing techniques using body neutral or body-positive language was designed. After the series of postures concluded, participants were instructed to rest and reflect, led through a guided imagery practice, and finally, invited to assimilate benefits of their practice in savasana, or corpse pose, a supine resting posture, while again repeating the affirmation to themselves while breathing. This general structure was intended to allow for individual modification by instructor, but also to allow for dissemination to other college campuses.

Language

Yoga teachers were trained to avoid language that could potentially trigger an external, objectified focus, such as "*you look beautiful*" or "*that's perfect*." Instead of using directives such as "*engage or hollow out your core/abs*" instructors were taught to use "*feel your inner strength*"; instead of "*feel your weight in your feet*", directives like "*notice where your feet connect to the floor*" were provided. Phrases promoting students' self-inquiry and connection to internal discovery were used. Examples included: "*Notice how you feel*", "*Consider making any adjustments that feel best to your body*"; "*There is no 'perfect' pose*", and "*Listening to your body is a sign of strength*" were used. The instructor training provided instructional language to guide the student to focus more on

Table 1. Yoga intervention sequence (for associated visuals see Figure 1).

Allotted Time (Minutes)	Category	Instruction	Affirmation (In = Inhale; Ex = Exhale)
5	Centering	Lie on back Take 3 In & 3 Ex Reflection on relationship to body in: Thought, Emotion, Sensation	Announce Affirmation Weeks 1 &6: In "I am" Ex "Enough" Weeks 2&7: In "I am" Ex "Whole" Weeks 3&8: In "I honor" Ex "My Body" Weeks 4&9: In "I inhale Courage" Ex "I exhale fear" Weeks 5&10: In "I am Free" Ex "To be myself"
5	Integration	Invite organic Movement (suggestions- gentle body stretch, wrists, ankles) Apanasana (knees-to-chest pose) Knees to Chest Movements with Affirmations Spinal Twists with feet on floor Apanasana (knees-to-chest pose)	Inhale & Exhale affirmation 3 times (internally repeat) 3 times each side, paired with breath Inhale & Exhale affirmation 3 times (internally repeat) with 3 sets
0.5 – 1 8	Rest & Reflect Flow	Cakravakasana (cat/puppy (cow) pose)Vajrasana (forward bend, Seated, Kneel-standing) adding cakravakasana (cat/puppy (cow) pose), Adho mukha svanasana (downward facing dog)	6 times, paired with breath 3 times; 3 times with additional two postures In Adho mukha svanasana In & Ex affirmation each time
0.5–1	Rest & Reflect	What do you notice? Invite awareness to thought, emotion, sensation	
12	Flow		

(Continued)

Table 1. (Continued).

Allotted Time (Minutes)	Category	Instruction	Affirmation (In = Inhale; Ex = Exhale)
		Samasthiti (Mountain pose)	Intermittently incorporate affirmations throughout
		Uttanasana (forward fold)	Complete on each side
		VirabhadrasanaII(Warrior II)	Goddess- 3 times each side
		Utkata Konasana (Goddess pose)	
		Samasthiti (Mountain pose)	
		Tree Pose	
		Tree Nyasa (Warrior I with dynamic movement and audible affirmation)	
		Breath of Joy	
0.5–1	Rest and Reflect	Invite awareness to thought, emotion, sensation	
6 mins	Floor Practice	Apanasana (knees-to-chest pose)	3 times
		Makarasana (Crocodile pose)	Inhale & Exhale affirmation 3 times (internally repeat) with 3 sets of
		Bhujangasana (Cobra pose)	
		Supta Kapotāsana (Supine Pigeon)	
		Spinal Twists with feet on floor	
		Apanasana (knees-to-chest pose)	
		Knees to Chest Movements with Affirmations	
0.5 – 1	Rest and Reflect	Invite awareness to thought, emotion, sensation	
5	Guided Imagery		
2	Savasana	Savasana (corpse pose)	Breathe in affirmation
3	Gentle wake up Seated; End of Practice		

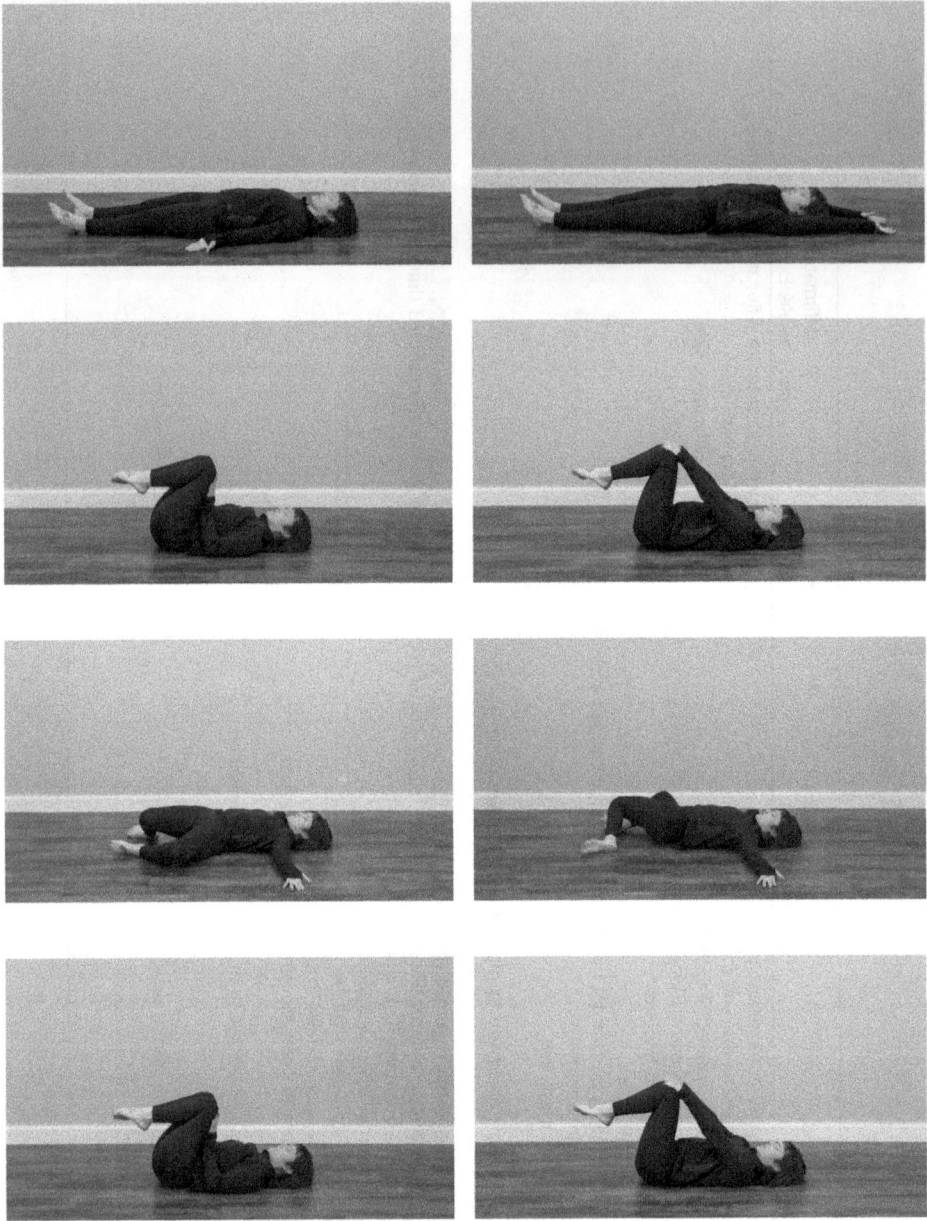

Figure 1. Yoga sequence poses.

the function of the yoga posture instead of the form (e.g., "*notice how the posture feels in your body today*" or "*it's not about how it looks, it is about how the pose is working for your body.*"). Instructors were provided with example phrases of language to promote inclusivity and curiosity, for example, "*Invite your arms toward the ground*" versus "*Bring the arms to the ground.*" Additionally, slight modifications in wording promoted connection to the body: "*your* arm to the ground" versus "*the* arm to the ground." To further

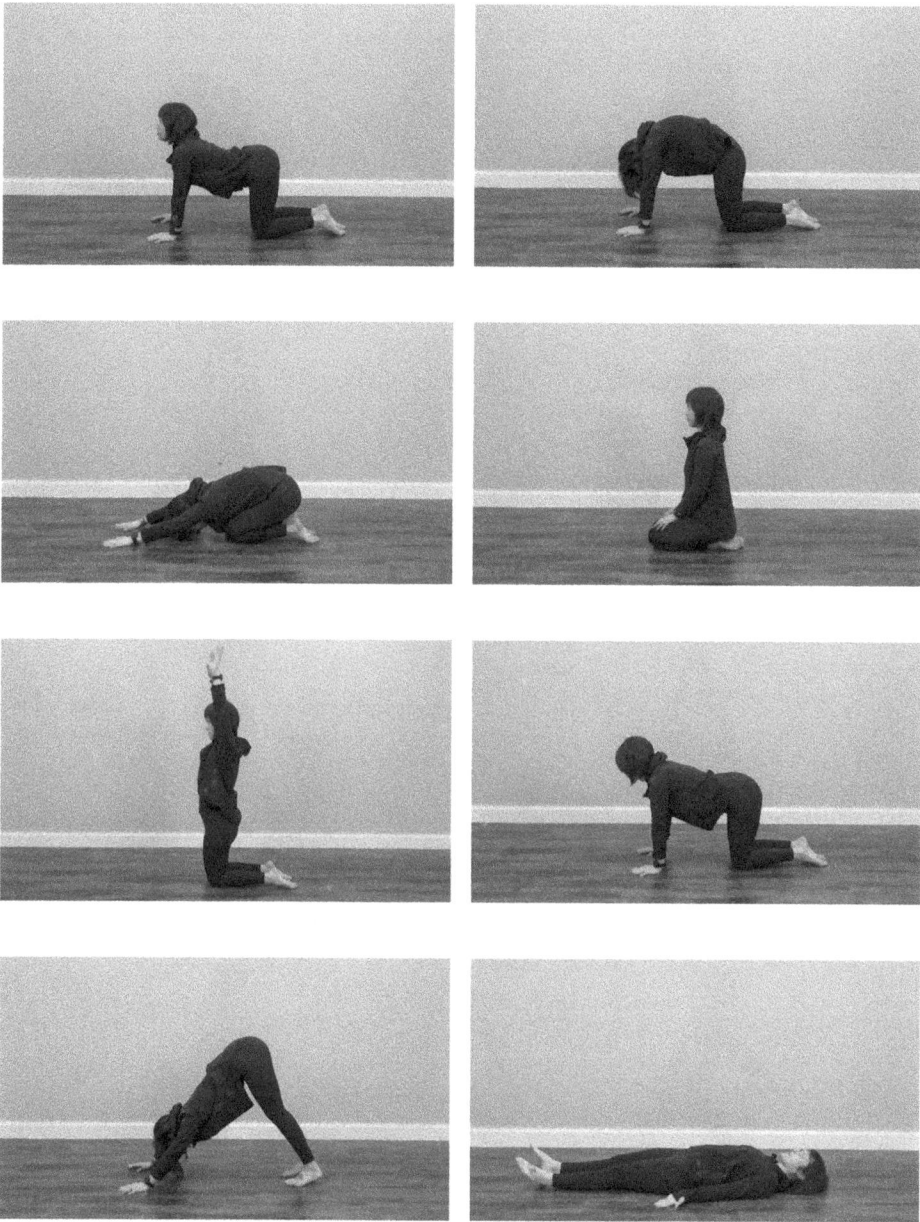

Figure 1. (Continued).

emphasize how yoga feels rather than what it looks like, the practice focused on verbal cues first, and demonstrations second/only if necessary. Instructors were advised to layer options for poses. Option 1 would be the most adaptable and presented before more demanding options, "*consider your needs, stay here, or if it feels right consider this next movement*" .... and so on.

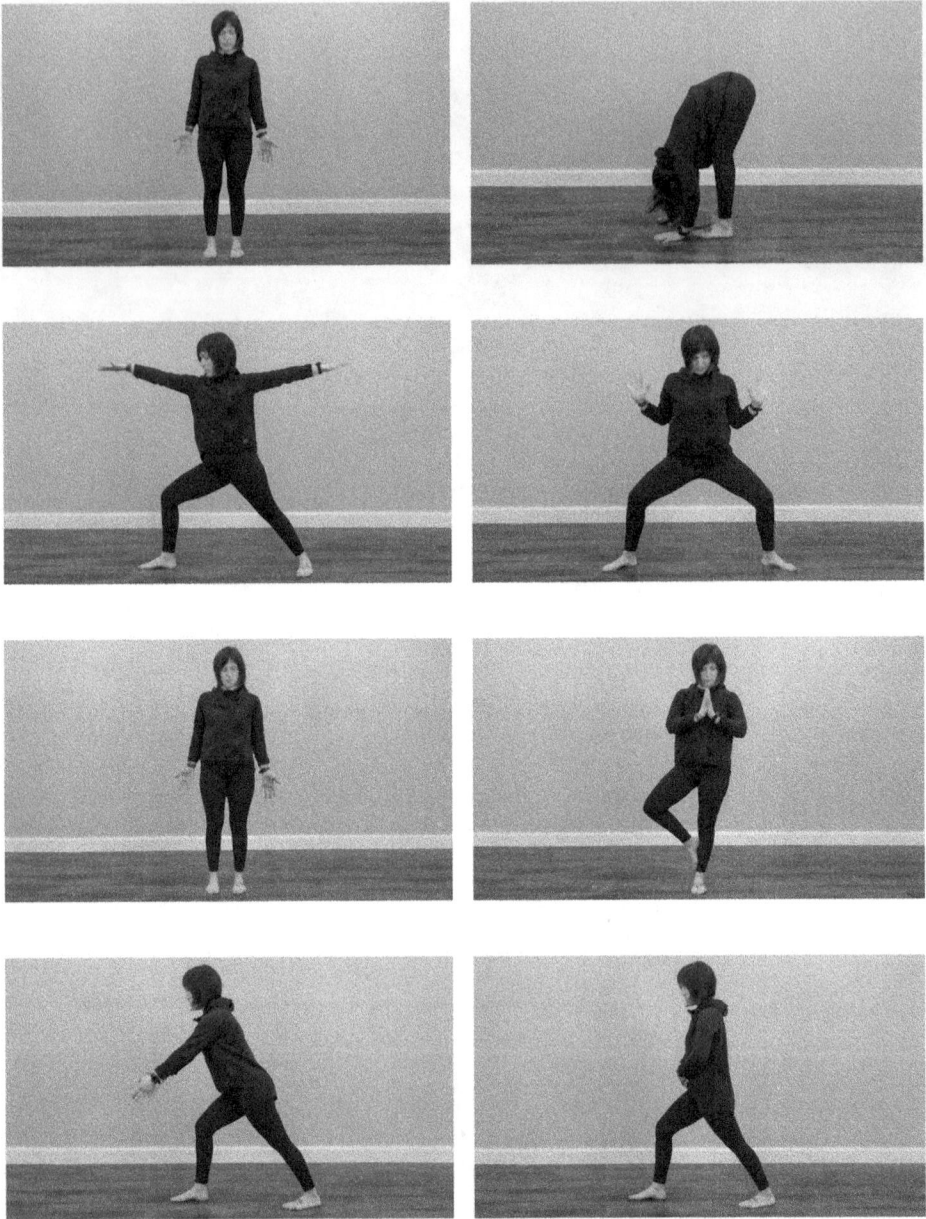

Figure 1. (Continued).

Process evaluation

Throughout the 10-week trial, weekly fidelity calls took place with the intervention developer (LD), yoga interventionists, and Principal Investigator (CP). These calls were scheduled for instructors to discuss anything notable that occurred during their class the previous week, any questions they had about affirmations or specific poses, and general comments regarding how the intervention was proceeding. LD was present to

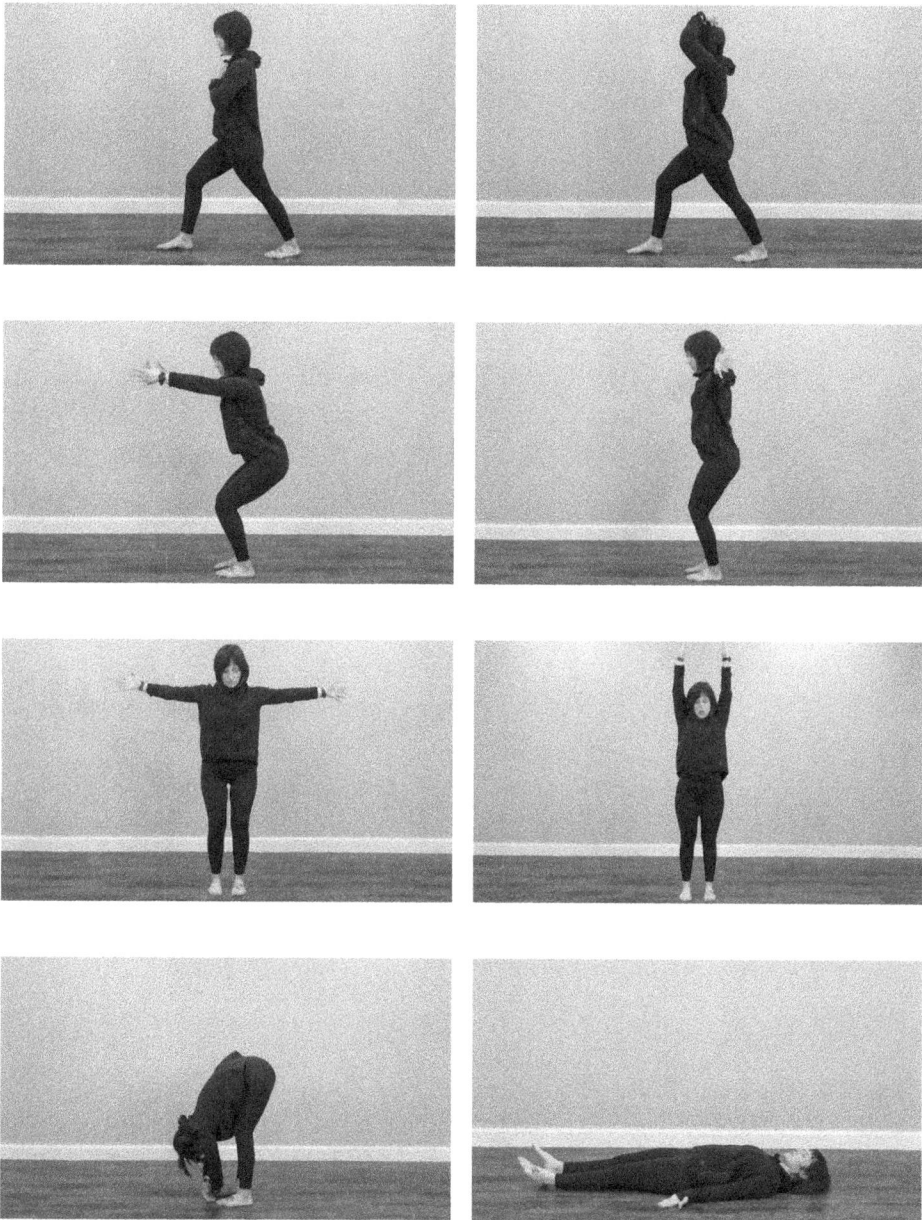

Figure 1. (Continued).

clarify any language or pose adjustments needed and CP was present to clarify whether the addition of elements (e.g., music, journaling) would impact the study design. It was decided that to isolate the effects of the yoga itself, additional components such as music and journaling would not be part of the intervention.

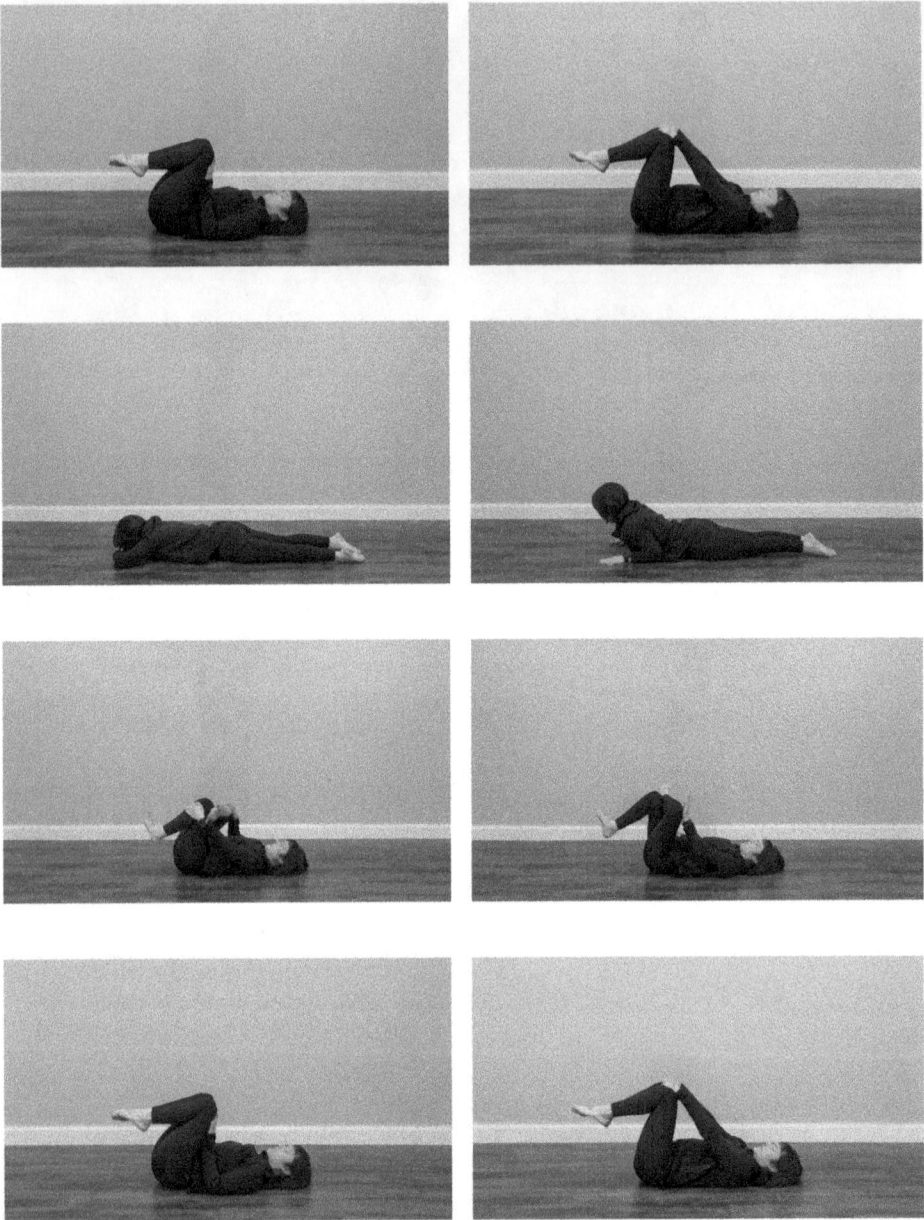

Figure 1. (Continued).

Acceptability

Acceptability was assessed via semi-structured survey offered to those who were randomized to the yoga group and participated in at least the first yoga class (n = 25). Participants responded to the following question: "*On a scale of 1 (very unsatisfied) to 5 (very satisfied), how satisfied were you with the yoga series?*" Other questions allowed for participants to provide anonymous written feedback in terms of how the practice related to their body and

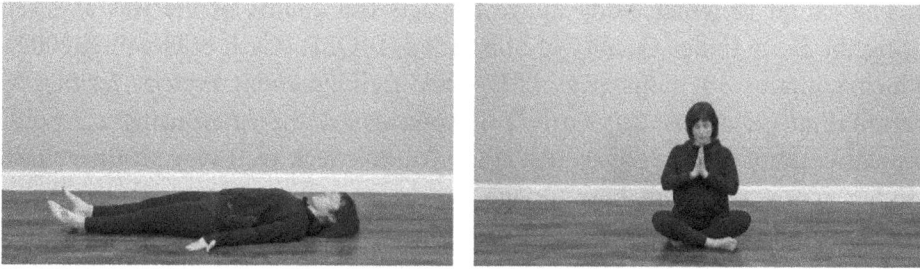

Figure 1. (Continued).

included: '*describe how participating in this yoga series impacted the way you feel about your body*', '*To what degree do you feel that participating in these yoga classes changed the way you feel about your body (i.e., your body image)?*' Response options included '*1 = I feel much worse about my body than I did before starting the yoga study; 2 = I feel worse about my body than I did before starting the yoga study; 3 = I don't feel any differently about my body than I did before starting the yoga study; 4 = I feel better about my body than I did before starting the yoga study; 5 = I feel much better about my body than I did before starting the yoga study)*', and response options for satisfaction with the yoga series included '*1 = very unsatisfied to 5 = very satisfied*'. Finally, we asked whether participants planned to continue practicing yoga.

Measures

Measures were collected at baseline, and after 5- and 10-weeks of intervention.

Body dissatisfaction

Body dissatisfaction was assessed using subscales of the Multidimensional Body-Self Relations Questionnaire (MBSRQ) (Cash, 2000). The MBSRQ contains 69 items (e.g., "*Before going out in public, I always notice how I look.*") with response options on a 5-point Likert response from (1) *definitely disagree* to (5) *definitely agree*. The following four subscales of the MBSRQ were selected to operationalize body image: Appearance Evaluation (AE, satisfaction, or dissatisfaction with physical self), Appearance Orientation (AO, how much investment one puts on how they look), Overweight Preoccupation (OWP, anxiety about fatness, weight control), and Body Area Satisfaction Subscale (BASS, satisfaction with separate parts of one's body, e.g.,, arms, chest, stomach). Higher scores represent greater attention placed on appearance/weight as determined by AE, AO, and OWP subscale. Higher scores on the BASS represent greater satisfaction with one's body. Baseline Cronbach's alphas for the current sample were 0.89 for MBSRQ-AE, 0.72 for MBSRQ-AO, 0.72 for MBSRQ-OWP, and 0.75 for MBSRQ-BASS.

The extent to which body image impacts the quality of life was assessed using the Body Image Quality of Life Index (BIQLI) (Cash & Fleming, 2002), which contains 19 items (e.g., *"My basic feelings about myself—feelings of personal adequacy and self-worth"*). Responses are indicated using a 7-point bipolar scale of (−3) *very negative effect*; (0) *no effect*; (+3) *very positive effect*. Higher scores represent body image having a positive impact on aspects of life; scores close to zero represent minimal impact; negative scores represent body image having a negative impact on aspects of life. Baseline Cronbach's alpha was 0.93 for the BIQLI in this sample.

Both the MBSRQ and BIQLI have shown evidence of internal consistency, convergent validity, and test-retest reliability without intervention in young adult samples (Brown et al., 1990; Cash et al., 2004).

Negative affect

Negative affect (PANAS-NA) was measured using the Positive and Negative Affect Schedule. Using a scale of (1) *very slightly or not at all* to (5) *extremely*, participants rated the degree to which they felt a list of 60 emotions within the past week, 10 of which comprise the PANAS-NA (e.g., *nervous; dissatisfied with self*). Higher scores reflect greater negative affect. Baseline Cronbach's alphas for the current sample was 0.86 for PANAS-NA.

Loneliness

Loneliness was measured by the NIH's social isolation construct short survey (Hahn et al., 2010). Participants responded to eight items (e.g., *"I feel left out …"*) by checking a box to indicate *Never—often—rarely—sometimes—usually—always*. Higher scores reflect greater loneliness. Cronbach's alpha was 0.95 for loneliness at baseline in this sample.

Self-compassion

Self-compassion was measured using a 26-item scale (e.g., *"I'm disapproving and judgmental about my own flaws and inadequacies."*) Response options ranged from (1) *almost never* to (5) *almost always* (Neff, 2003). Higher Scores reflect greater self-compassion. Cronbach's alpha was 0.95 for self-compassion at baseline in this sample.

Positive affect

Positive affect (PANAS-PA) was measured by the Positive and Negative Affect Schedule (Watson et al., 1988). Using a scale of (1) *very slightly or not at all* to (5) *extremely*, participants rated the degree to which they felt a list of 60 emotions over the past week, 10 of which comprise the PANAS-PA (e.g., *excited; inspired*). Higher scores reflect greater positive affect. Baseline Cronbach's alphas for the current sample was 0.73 for PANAS-PA.

Mindfulness

Mindfulness was assessed by the Five Facet Mindfulness Questionnaire (Baer et al., 2006). Participants responded to 39 items (e.g., *"When I'm walking, I deliberately notice the sensations of my body moving."*) using a scale of (1) *never or very rarely true* to (5) *very often or always true*. Higher scores reflect greater mindfulness. Cronbach's alpha was 0.91 for mindfulness at baseline in this sample.

Disordered eating

The Eating Attitudes Test (EAT-26) is a 26-item (e.g., *"Find myself preoccupied with food"*) questionnaire for assessing eating behaviors in the non-clinical college population (Garner et al., 1982). Participants rated each item on a 6-point Likert scale *(never to always)*. Responses were assigned a value of 3 *(always)*, 2 *(usually)*, 1 *(often)* and 0 *(sometimes, rarely,* or *never)*. The EAT-26 has three subscales: dieting, bulimia and food preoccupation, and oral control. Baseline Cronbach's alphas for the current sample were 0.93 for dieting, 0.71 for bulimia, and 0.74 for oral control.

The Binge Eating Scale (BES) is a 16-question survey that assesses the severity of binge eating (Gormally et al., 1982). Each item contains four options and the participant notes which option best describes them. (e.g., *"It is rare that I eat so much that I felt uncomfortably full; About once a month I eat so much that I felt uncomfortably full; There are regular periods during the month when I eat large amounts of foods at meals or between meals; I eat so much that usually, after eating, I feel pretty bad and I have nausea."*) Higher scores represent more binge eating symptoms. Baseline Cronbach's alpha for the current sample was 0.89.

Body Mass Index (BMI; kg/m^2) was calculated using measured height and weight using a SECA portable stadiometer and Tonita BWB-800 scale.

Analysis

Feasibility was presented via the use of a consort diagram and numbers and percentages of participants withdrawing or continuing the intervention and the study. Acceptability was assessed via collating individual responses and quantifying answers that appeared in multiple from the semi-structured survey. Responses were collated according to evaluation question, and mean scores were computed when appropriate. In addition, to behaviorally assess feasibility and acceptance, research assistants took attendance at each of the 30 offered yoga classes and ensured that the instructor was present and taught the class.

Outcome variables were assessed for normality. All variables approximated the normal distribution with the exception of subscales of the EAT-26 and BES. Accordingly, analyses using the EAT-26-dieting, EAT-26-bulimia, EAT-

26-oral control, and BES as dependent variables were repeated using a nonparametric test, which did not change results. Data were analyzed for missingness, and missing data were imputed in two ways: first, using maximum likelihood estimation, and second, using multiple imputation. This resulted in three sets of data: available data, maximum likelihood imputed dataset, and a multiple imputed dataset.

Mixed models were run using the outcome as the dependent variable, controlling for baseline level of the dependent variable, with interest in a main effect of group or a group by time interaction. First, a mixed model was run using the complete dataset where maximum likelihood imputation was used for missing values. Second, available data were used as a sensitivity analysis for any significant main effect of group or group by time interaction. Finally, if the significant main effect of group or a group by time interaction had a p-value less than 0.10, as appropriate for pilot studies (International Journal of Eating Disorders, 2008; Lee et al., 2014), the mixed model was run once more using the multiple imputation dataset. Effect size was calculated for significant effects.

Analyses followed an intention-to-treat approach, except for when available data were used. Due to the pilot nature of this trial, in an attempt to balance exploration with multiple comparison problems (International Journal of Eating Disorders, 2008) patterns of significance and directionality of results are emphasized. Data were analyzed using IBM SPSS v 24.0.

Results

Feasibility of recruitment, randomization, and retention

A consort flow diagram (Figure 2) shows the number of interested, eligible, randomized, and analyzed participants and reasons for exclusion. Descriptive characteristics of the analytic sample are displayed in Table 2. On average, participants were approximately 20 years old, about half (25 out of 51) were freshmen, 16 were sophomores, and 10 were juniors. Three of the 51 participants self-identified as Hispanic/Latino. Forty-three participants self-identified as white, five as Asian, two as Black/African American, and one as American Indian or Alaska Native. Participants' majors spanned a variety of fields; the most frequent being Dietetics, Human Services, Fashion Merchandising, and Psychology (for each major, n = 3). Regarding previous yoga experience, 40 participants had no experience or reported going to classes a couple of times per year, one reported going to class once a month, two reported going to class once a week, one participant reported going to class multiple times per week. Other responses (written in) ranged from practicing years ago to taking three classes in ones' lifetime. The average BMI of the sample was 23.7 ± 4.6 kg/m^2. Scores on body image assessments were slightly more favorable than published

Enrollment

Contacted research team with interest (n= 182)

Excluded (n=111)
- Did not respond (n=82)
- Did not meet inclusion criteria (n=29)
  - Class time (n=15)
  - Experience (n=2)
  - Senior (n=3)
  - Over 26 (n=1)
  - Male (n=1)
  - Time (n=4)
  - Contacted after study started (n=3)

Eligible (n=71)

Declined to participate (n=8)
- Surgery (n=1)
- Time (n=1)
- Other/no response (n=6)

Allocation

Randomized (n=63)

Allocated to yoga (n=32)
- Received yoga intervention (n=26)
- Did not receive yoga intervention (n=6)
  - Surgery, withdrew before baseline (n=1)
  - Waitlist (n=5)

Allocated to control (n=31)
- Participated in study (n=26)
- Did not participate in study (n=5)
  - Waitlist (n=5)

Baseline

Attended baseline (n=26)
- Lost to follow-up (n=0)
- Discontinued intervention (n=1)
  - Work; attended baseline did not start intervention

Attended baseline (n=26)
- Lost to follow-up (n=0)
- Discontinued study (n=0)

Follow-Up (Mid-Point)

Attended midpoint (n=25)
- Lost to follow-up (n=0)
- Discontinued intervention (n=5)
  - Joint pain (n=1)
  - Academics (n=3)
  - Injury unrelated to yoga(n=1)

Attended midpoint (n=25)
- Withdrew (n=1; due to academics)

End of Treatment (EOT)

Attended EOT (n=24)
- Lost to follow-up (n=1; no show)
- Discontinued intervention (n=2)
  - Schedule (n=1)
  - Academics (n=1)

Attended EOT (n=25)
- Lost to follow-up (n=0)

Analysis

Analysed (n= 25)
Excluded from analysis (n= 0)

Analysed (n= 26)
Excluded from analysis (n= 0)

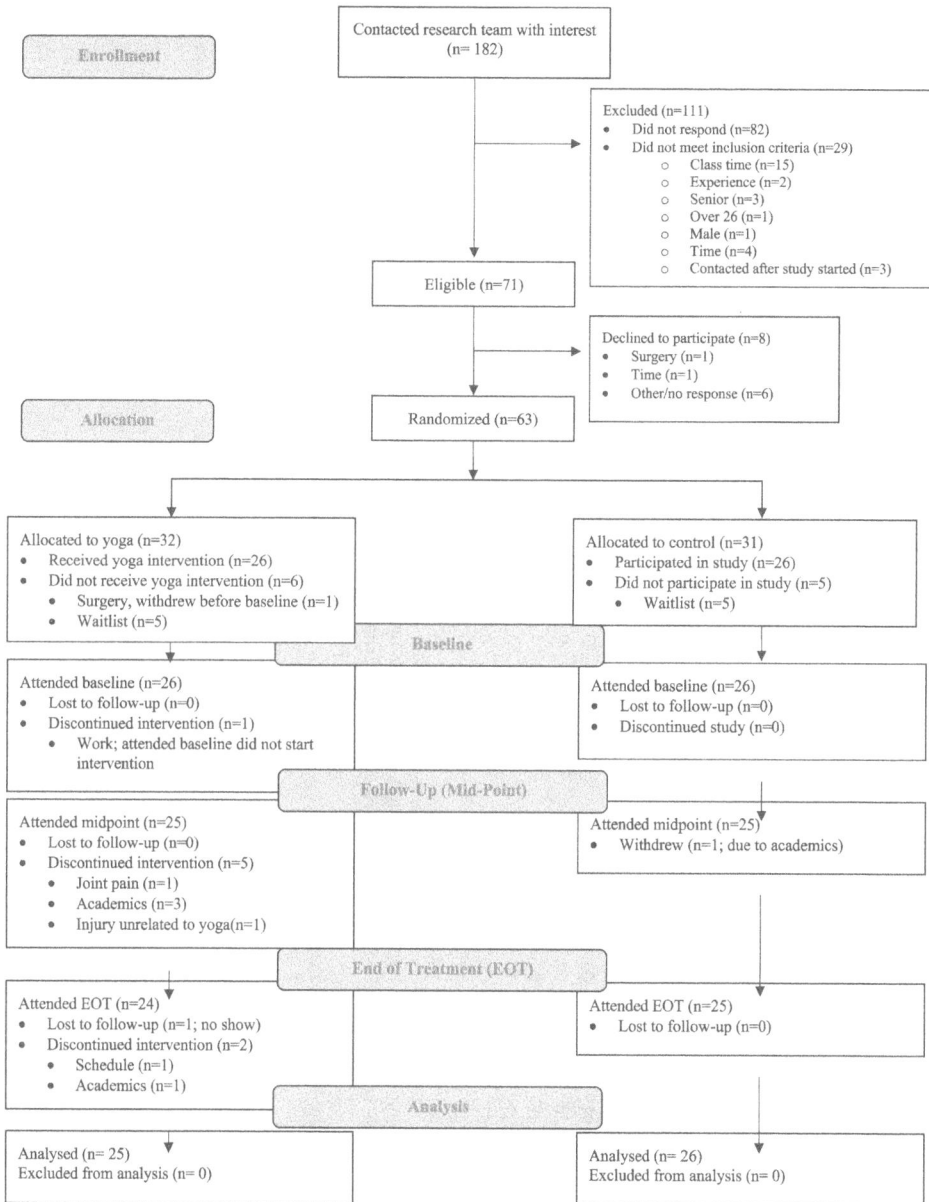

Figure 2. Consort flow diagram.

normative values for college women (see Table 2, rightmost column). The only difference between participants randomized to the yoga and control groups at baseline was on positive affect; however, all analyses presented controlled for baseline levels of dependent variables.

Out of 26 participants randomized to the yoga group, 25 participants attended the first class and comprised the analytic sample. The average number of classes attended was 19.8 ± 9.1, with a range of 3–30 classes

Table 2. Baseline comparisons between yoga and control group participants and published values for comparable samples.

Variable	Yoga n = 25 M	SD	Control n = 26 M	SD	t(df)	95% CI for difference lower	upper	p	Total sample n = 51 M	SD	Published values for comparable sample M	SD
Age	19.51	0.90	19.74	1.03	-0.84(48)	0.78	0.32	0.403	19.63	0.96		
Body Mass Index (kg/m²)	24.33	5.74	23.07	2.99	0.99(49)	-1.30	3.82	0.329	23.69	4.55		
MBSRQ-AE	3.15	0.80	2.90	0.84	1.10(49)	-0.21	0.71	0.276	3.02	0.82	3.36	0.87
MBSRQ-AO	3.61	0.65	3.76	0.53	-0.92(49)	-0.49	0.18	0.361	3.69	0.59	3.91	0.60
MBSRQ-OWP	2.63	0.82	2.90	0.92	-1.12(49)	-0.77	0.22	0.269	2.77	0.88	3.03	0.96
MBSRQ-BASS	3.21	0.56	2.99	0.55	1.43(49)	-0.09	0.53	0.160	3.10	0.56	3.23	0.74
BIQLI	0.90	1.01	0.50	0.93	1.46(49)	-0.15	0.53	0.151	0.70	0.98	1.02	1.17
PANAS Negative	20.44	6.55	19.65	8.03	0.38(49)	-3.35	-0.63	0.704	20.04	7.28	20.4	7.0
PANAS Positive	30.00	4.86	33.62	5.71	-2.43(49)	-6.60	-0.63	0.018	31.84	5.57	32.4	7.3
Self-Compassion	2.78	0.80	2.91	0.65	-0.64(49)	-0.54	0.28	0.525	3.01[a]	0.84	2.95	0.62
Loneliness	21.28	8.73	21.28	7.62	-0.12(49)	-4.63	4.58	0.990	21.29	8.10	Not available	
Mindfulness	121.32	20.21	118.38	18.94	0.54(49)	-8.08	13.95	0.595	119.82	19.43	112.7	16.9
EAT-D	7.16	8.42	10.31	10.84	-1.15(49)	-8.63	2.33	0.254	8.76	9.77	7.1	7.2
EAT-B	2.00	2.58	2.61	3.42	-0.72(49)	-2.33	1.09	0.473	2.31	3.02	1.0	2.1
EAT-OC	1.52	1.56	2.36	3.75	-1.03(48)	-2.47	0.79	0.306	1.94	2.87	1.9	2.1
BES	11.20	9.16	11.85	8.32	-2.64(49)	-5.56	4.27	0.793	11.53	8.66	11.9	6.9

MBSRQ = Multidimensional Body-Self Relations Questionnaire, AE = Appearance Evaluation, AO = Appearance Orientation, OWP = Overweight Preoccupation, BASS = Body Areas Satisfaction Scale, BIQLI = Body Image Quality of Life Inventory, PANAS = Positive and Negative Affect Schedule, EAT = Eating Attitudes Test, D = Dieting, B = Bulimia, OC = Oral Control, BES = Binge Eating Scale, [a]n = 49.

Published values for comparable samples are from the following sources:

MBSRQ_AE: Cash (2000).

MBSRQ_AO: Cash (2000).

MBSRQ_OWP: Cash (2000).

MBSRQ_BASS: Cash (2000).

BIQLI: Cash and Fleming (2002).

PANAS Negative & PANAS Positive

*PANAS values from PANAS-X manual—include both males and females, not just females.

Self-Compassion: Neff (2003).

*because overall self-compassion score was totaled, for comparison purposes we here divided by the number of subscales.

Mindfulness: Lattimore et al. (2011).

EAT-D, -B, and -OC: Garner et al. (1982).

BES: Sala and Levinson (2017).

attended out of 30 classes offered. Seven participants withdrew from the study during the intervention period and gave reasons unrelated to the yoga intervention (see Figure 2).

A comparison of baseline characteristics between those who completed the study ('completers' n = 43) versus those who withdrew ('withdrew' n = 8; 7/8 in the yoga group) revealed significant differences on several variables. Table 3 shows these comparisons along with comparisons between those who withdrew and those who continued the study within the yoga group. In general, at baseline, completers were higher on Appearance Orientation, Overweight Preoccupation, EAT-26-dieting, EAT-26-bulimia, and binge eating symptoms and lower on self-compassion.

Acceptability

Twenty-three out of 25 participants filled out the semi-structured survey after the 10-week trial was completed. Thus, some individuals who withdrew from the study after taking a few yoga classes also provided feedback. In terms of satisfaction with the yoga series (*1 = very unsatisfied to 5 = very satisfied*), 22 participants responded to this question, and the mean response was 4.09 ± 0.87. Responses ranged from 2 (reported only once) to 5 and more than 75% of participants reported that they were satisfied (4) or very satisfied (5). Responses to how the yoga series made them feel about their body ranged from "*It made me feel better that I can do the positions and gave me a sense that my body can accomplish things*" to "*Empowering class, definitely helped my confidence but also made me realize how unflexible I am*" and "*It did not impact the way I felt about my body.*" When asked to rate the degree to which the yoga classes changed how participants felt about their body (*1 = feel much worse about body to 5 = feel much better about body*), the mean response was 3.78 ± 0.80. Fifteen of the 23 respondents (65%) selected either a '4' or '5', indicating that the yoga series made them feel better about their bodies. Finally, of the 22 participants who responded to the question about whether they would continue yoga, approximately 73% said yes, 9% said maybe/they hoped to, 9% said probably not, and 9% said no, they would not continue practicing yoga.

Outcomes

The amount of missing data varied according to variable and assessment time point; overall the amount of missing data was very low. Only one variable at one time point had missing data exceeding 5% (5.9%, EAT-26 bulimia subscale). Many variables had no missing data, or were missing 1 or 2 participant responses (2.0% and 3.9% missing, respectively).

Table 3. Baseline comparisons between completers and withdrawals for all participants and those randomized to the yoga group.

| | All participants (n = 51) | | | | | Randomized to the yoga group (n = 25) | | | | |
| | Completers (n = 43) | | Withdrawals (n = 8) | | | Completers (n = 18) | | Withdrawals (n = 7) | | |
Variable	M	SD	M	SD	p-value	M	SD	M	SD	p-value
MBSRQ-AE	2.97	0.84	3.30	0.69	0.291	3.06	0.83	3.37	0.72	0.404
MBSRQ-AO	3.80	0.55	3.11	0.50	0.002	3.84	0.57	3.01	0.44	0.002
MBSRQ-OWP	2.89	0.86	2.13	0.73	0.022	2.82	0.78	2.14	0.79	0.063
MBSRQ-BASS	3.03	0.54	3.47	0.55	0.040	3.10	0.53	3.51	0.58	0.103
BIQLI	0.69	0.93	0.73	1.32	0.922	0.94	0.86	0.80	1.41	0.820
PANAS NA	20.72	7.44	16.38	5.34	0.122	22.06	6.24	16.29	5.77	0.045
PANAS PA	31.98	5.79	31.13	4.39	0.695	29.72	5.07	30.71	4.57	0.657
Self-Compassion	2.73	0.68	3.46	0.68	0.007	2.53	0.69	3.41	0.72	0.009
Loneliness	21.84	8.04	18.38	8.33	0.271	22.56	8.56	18.00	8.93	0.250
Mindfulness	118.81	18.86	125.25	22.86	0.395	119.39	18.7	126.29	24.49	0.455
EAT-D	10.16	10.00	1.25	2.05	0.000	9.39	8.93	1.43	2.15	0.002
EAT-B	2.63	3.16	0.63	1.19	0.004	2.50	2.81	0.71	1.25	0.039
EAT-OC	2.10	3.09	1.13	0.99	0.110	1.78	1.73	0.86	0.69	0.070
BES	12.67	8.67	5.38	5.71	0.027	13.33	9.39	5.71	6.07	0.060
Body Mass Index (kg/m^2)	23.98	4.78	22.12	2.74	0.294	25.05	6.48	22.47	2.76	0.324

MBSRQ = Multidimensional Body-Self Relations Questionnaire, AE = Appearance Evaluation, AO = Appearance Orientation, OWP = Overweight Preoccupation, BASS = Body Areas Satisfaction Scale, BIQLI = Body Image Quality of Life Inventory, PANAS = Positive and Negative Affect Schedule, NA = Negative Affect, PA = Positive Affect, EAT = Eating Attitudes Test, D = Dieting, B = Bulimia, OC = Oral Control, BES = Binge Eating Scale.

Table 4 displays the means and standard deviations by group at baseline, 5 weeks, and 10 weeks. In the first set of analyses using the maximum likelihood imputed dataset, significant effects were found for both group and time on the MBSRQ-Appearance Orientation (AO) subscale, favoring the yoga group (Beta estimate for group = − 0.136, SE = 0.074, t = − 1.823, p = .072; beta estimate for time = 0.094, SE = 0.054, t = 1.756, p = .085). On average, controlling for baseline levels of MBSRQ-AO, scores improved for the whole sample between weeks 5 and 10 of the trial, but significantly more in the yoga group (at 10-weeks: M ± SD: yoga = 3.57 ± 2.65; control = 3.44 ± 0.27; Cohen's d = 0.07). Positive affect also increased significantly between weeks 5 and 10 in the yoga group, controlling for baseline positive affect (beta estimate for group = − 3.537, SE = 1.768, t = − 2.000, p = .049; at 10-weeks: M ± SD: yoga = 32.89 ± 6.24; control = 26.36 ± 6.24; Cohen's d = 0.57).

Using the available data for sensitivity analysis, MBSRQ-AO subscale favored the yoga group (beta estimate for group = − 0.136, SE = 0.076, t = − 1.783, p = .079; at 10-weeks: M ± SD: yoga = 3.48 ± 0.57; control = 3.50 ± 0.82; Cohen's d = 0.03). Positive affect increased in the yoga group compared to the control group (beta estimate for group = − 3.090, SE = 1.814, t = − 1.704, p = .093; at 10-weeks: M ± SD: yoga = 31.54 ± 6.30;

Table 4. Means and standard deviations for outcome variables by group at baseline, 5- and 10-weeks.

| | Yoga | | | | | | Control | | | | | |
| | Baseline (n = 25) | | 5 weeks (n = 25) | | 10 weeks (n = 24) | | Baseline (n = 26) | | 5 weeks (n = 25) | | 10 weeks (n = 25) | |
Variable	M	SD	M	SD	M	SD	M	SD	M	SD	M	SD
MBSRQ-AE	3.15	0.80	3.28	0.79	3.32	0.75	2.90	0.84	3.03	0.76	3.10	0.82
MBSRQ-AO	3.61	0.65	3.61	0.58	3.48	0.57	3.76	0.53	3.57	0.51	3.50	0.43
MBSRQ-OWP	2.63	0.82	2.58	1.00	2.39	0.85	2.90	0.92	2.90	0.97	2.92	0.92
MBSRQ-BASS	3.21	0.61	3.46	0.61	3.44	0.62	2.99	0.55	3.12	0.57	3.21	0.61
BIQLI	0.90	1.01	1.03	1.00	1.05	0.99	0.50	0.93	0.77[b]	1.17	0.99	1.24
PANAS NA	20.44	6.55	18.44	6.39	19.71	7.20	19.65	8.03	19.96	8.70	19.76	7.13
PANAS PA	30.00	4.86	31.60	6.56	31.54	6.30	33.62	5.71	29.12	7.49	30.12	6.69
Self-Compassion	2.78	0.80	2.90	0.76	2.99	0.92	2.91	0.65	2.94	0.69	3.03	0.78
Loneliness	21.28	8.73	18.28	7.69	17.33	8.20	21.31	7.62	20.56	7.88	18.28	6.99
Mindfulness	121.32	20.21	125.00	20.95	128.00	24.85	118.38	18.94	121.40	18.71	124.4	19.73
EAT-D	7.16	8.42	5.76	6.78	4.61[c]	6.32	10.31	10.84	10.08[b]	10.12	9.48	9.29
EAT-B	2.00	2.58	1.36	2.43	1.50	3.16	2.62	3.42	2.36	2.94	1.96	3.08
EAT-OC	1.52	1.56	1.48	1.85	1.21	1.32	2.36[a]	3.75	2.68	4.60	2.44	3.71
BES	11.20	9.16	10.28	8.63	8.58	8.83	11.85	8.32	11.12	6.78	10.80	7.76
Body Mass Index (kg/m²)	24.33	5.74	24.75	5.88	24.68	5.86	23.07	2.99	23.33	2.86	23.25	2.77

MBSRQ = Multidimensional Body-Self Relations Questionnaire, AE = Appearance Evaluation, AO = Appearance Orientation, OWP = Overweight Preoccupation, BASS = Body Areas Satisfaction Scale, BIQLI = Body Image Quality of Life Inventory, PANAS = Positive and Negative Affect Schedule, NA = Negative Affect, PA = Positive Affect, EAT = Eating Attitudes Test, D = Dieting, B = Bulimia, OC = Oral Control, BES = Binge Eating Scale.
[a]n = 25; [b]n = 24; [c]n = 23.

control = 30.12 ± 6.69; Cohen's d = 0.16). Neither BMI nor attendance was significant covariates in these analyses.

Using the multiple imputation dataset, MBSRQ-AO's group effect was no longer significant (beta estimate = − 0.147, SE = 0.108, t = − 1.362, p = .198; at 10-weeks: M ± SD: yoga = 3.55 ± 0.43; control = 3.42 ± 0.33; Cohen's d = 0.35). There was a main effect of group, favoring an increase in positive affect in the yoga group between weeks 5 and 10 as compared to the control group (beta estimate = − 4.103, SE = 1.423, t = − 2.883, p = .004; at 10-weeks: M ± SD: yoga = 32.62 ± 6.16; control = 29.13 ± 6.15; Cohen's d = 0.57).

Since the increase in positive affect in the yoga group as compared to control group between weeks 5 and 10, controlling for baseline was a consistently significant finding, estimates and effect sizes were computed. Controlling for baseline, averaging over visits 2 and 3, participants in the yoga group reported significantly higher positive affect than the control group (M ± SD: yoga = 32.5 ± 1.1; control = 28.6 ± 1.1; Cohen's d = 0.77) indicating a medium effect for the difference in positive affect between groups (Cohen, 1988).

Discussion

The aim of this study was to assess the feasibility and acceptability of a preventative yoga intervention on a college campus. Generally, the intervention was found to be acceptable; participants attended about two-thirds of the yoga classes on average and reported high satisfaction with the yoga series. The majority of participants had little to no prior yoga experience, signifying that this type of intervention may be palatable for college women who did not previously try yoga. Missing data were low, suggesting that our assessment and retention plan was acceptable for participants. On average, participants reported that the yoga sequence helped them to feel better about their bodies.

An increase in positive affect was observed in the yoga group as compared to the control group; lower positive affect has been theorized to make individuals more susceptible to disordered eating (Eggert et al., 2007). No significant intent-to-treat intervention effects were observed for validated measures of body dissatisfaction or other outcomes. It is possible that the present sample's relatively 'healthy' baseline body image contributed to lack of significant findings. A similar study (Ariel-Donges et al., 2019) found that yoga significantly improved body image. However, in contrast to the present study, Ariel-Donges and colleagues selected participants with poor body image—inclusion criteria required an MBSRQ-AE less than or equal to 3.0 (Appearance Evaluation, higher scores indicate a positive perception of one's looks—e.g., finding self sexually attractive, others think you are attractive, etc.). At baseline, their sample self-reported an MBSRQ-AE score of 2.4 ± 0.5, whereas in the present study's yoga group, baseline MBSRQ-AE score was 3.1 ± 0.8. This difference in baseline body dissatisfaction, combined with sample size (n = 37 as compared to n = 25) may partially explain why the present study did not observe statistically significant differences. In line with the idea that improvement may be visible for those with poorer body image, in an observational, population-based study Neumark-Sztainer et al. (2018) observed improvements in body image among yoga practitioners with prior low body satisfaction but not among those with high prior body satisfaction (Neumark-Sztainer et al., 2018).

Study strengths and limitations are important to consider in interpreting the findings. Strengths of this study included low amounts of missing data, use of a general sample, as compared to an at-risk group, training of yoga instructors, and retention of participants: we collected data from those who withdrew from the intervention. With regard to study limitations, it is important to note that the study was not powered to test the impact of the intervention on outcome measures, but rather was designed to assess the feasibility and acceptability of running such a trial. Though pilot studies are not intended for hypothesis testing (Leon et al., 2011), patterns of preliminary results displayed that the majority of findings aligned to support yoga having benefit, though most were not statistically significant. The sample was not diverse in terms of ethnicity, race, age, or gender; thus, we cannot generalize these results to other unstudied groups with different demographic characteristics. Lastly, one of the walls of the room in which yoga was practiced had mirrors; despite having participants face away from the wall, for some, this may have attenuated effects related to body image. However, a study examining the impact of mirrors on yoga practice found improvements in body image in both the mirrored and non-mirrored conditions (Frayeh & Lewis, 2018).

Extant literature encourages publication of pilot studies due to the information they provide for future trials (e.g., Feeley et al., 2009; Leon et al., 2011; Thabane et al., 2010). We have several recommendations moving forward. The present intervention did not include an educational component of body image's importance, and yoga's role in fostering positive body image. It is possible that the students did not make the connection without it being explicitly stated and reinforced. Participants stated improvement in how they felt about their bodies post yoga session on the questions we added, but this was not evidenced on validated body dissatisfaction questionnaires. Thus, we recommend evaluating the impact of adding an educational component about the importance of body image versus a more generalized yoga approach as done in the present study. Supplemental activities, for example, home practice, journaling, and processing prior to and after yoga can reinforce the messages of the yoga practice were not included here. In the present study, the majority of participants indicated that they did not practice outside of the scheduled yoga sessions. Offering additional resources for home practice may represent an acceptable way to increase the dosage. Additionally, screening for those with poor body image, who may experience the most benefit from a yoga intervention is one avenue in which to proceed; however, prevention remains an important strategy. In terms of measurement, assessing positive body image, as a protective factors and separate construct from body image concerns (Tylka & Wood-Barcalow, 2015) will be key, especially in prevention. To this effect, a recently published four-session yoga intervention found improvements in positive body image along with increased positive mood, like our study found (Halliwell et al., 2019). Another important avenue for future yoga intervention research will be examining trials from an implementation science framework—measuring details beyond individual-level participant factors, in this case, for example, the degree to which instructors were able to successfully implement the intervention. Future research should incorporate measures of how the implementation of a yoga intervention impacts the facility, organization, broader community, and policy environment (Bauer et al., 2015; Proctor et al., 2011).

In conclusion, this pilot study demonstrated the feasibility of a yoga series for women on a college campus and suggested that yoga may reduce appearance orientation and improve positive affect; however, in general, statistically significant differences were not found between the yoga and control group. Women qualitatively reported feeling more satisfied with their bodies after completing the yoga series. We welcome future research considering the aforementioned recommendations, and also investigating state-level in addition to trait-level body image, as done by Frayeh and Lewis (2018). Using Ecological Momentary Assessment to assess how risk and protective factors change throughout the day for those practicing yoga is an exciting and novel direction for future investigation.

Acknowledgments

The authors would like to express their gratitude to the yoga interventionists who worked on this trial: Gwen Hayes, Andrea Boulden, and Susan Smith. Additionally, research assistants, whose dedication, follow-through, and positivity were imperative to the success of conducting this trial, and deserve recognition: Brielle Evangelista, Alexa Nichols, Adrienne Fraczkowski, Haillie Tandon, and Hannah Lightcap.

Declaration of interest statement

The authors have no conflicts of interest to declare. Funding from the School of Public Health at the University of Minnesota was used to conduct this study.

ORCID

M Mackenzie ⓘ http://orcid.org/0000-0001-7792-2511

References

Albertson, E. R., Neff, K. D., & Dill-Shackleford, K. E. (2015). Self-compassion and body dissatisfaction in women: a randomized controlled trial of a brief meditation intervention. *Mindfulness*, 6(3), 444–454. https://doi.org/10.1007/s12671-014-0277-3

Alleva, J. M., Martijn, C., Van Breukelen, G. J. P., Jansen, A., & Karos, K. (2015). Expand your horizon: A programme that improves body image and reduces self-objectification by training women to focus on body functionality. *Body Image*, 15, 81–89. https://doi.org/10.1016/j.bodyim.2015.07.001

Ariel-Donges, A. H., Gordon, E. L., Bauman, V., & Perri, M. G. (2019). Does yoga help college-aged women with body-image dissatisfaction feel better about their bodies? *Sex Roles*, 80, 41–51. https://doi.org/10.1007/s11199-018-0917-5

Baer, R. A., Smith, G. T., Hopkins, J., Krietemeyer, J., & Toney, L. (2006). Using self-report assessment methods to explore facets of mindfulness. *Assessment*, 13(1), 27–45. https://doi.org/10.1177/1073191105283504

Barrington, J., & Jarry, J. L. (2019). Does thought suppression mediate the association between mindfulness and body satisfaction? *Mindfulness*, 10(4), 679–688. https://doi.org/10.1007/s12671-018-1012-2

Bauer, M. S., Damschroder, L., Hagedorn, H., Smith, J., & Kilbourne, A. M. (2015). An introduction to implementation science for the non-specialist. *BMC Psychology*, 3(1), 32. https://doi.org/10.1186/s40359-015-0089-9

Braun, T. D., Park, C. L., & Conboy, L. A. (2012). Psychological well-being, health behaviors, and weight loss among participants in a residential, Kripalu yoga-based weight loss program. *International Journal of Yoga Therapy*, 22, 9–22.

Braun, T. D., Park, C. L., & Gorin, A. (2016). Self-compassion, body image, and disordered eating: A review of the literature. *Body Image*, 17, 117–131. https://doi.org/10.1016/j.bodyim.2016.03.003

Brown, T. A., Cash, T. F., & Mikulka, P. J. (1990). Attitudinal body-image assessment: Factor analysis of the body-self relations questionnaire. *Journal of Personality Assessment*, 55(1–2), 135–144. https://doi.org/10.1080/00223891.1990.9674053

Cash, T. F. (2000). *User's manual for the multidimensional body-self relations questionnaire.* Old Dominion University.

Cash, T. F., & Fleming, E. C. (2002). The impact of body image experiences: Development of the body image quality of life inventory. *The International Journal of Eating Disorders*, 31 (4), 455–460. https://doi.org/10.1002/eat.10033

Cash, T. F., Jakatdar, T. A., & Williams, E. F. (2004). The body image quality of life inventory: Further validation with college men and women. *Body Image*, 1(3), 279–287. https://doi.org/10.1016/S1740-1445(03)00023-8

Cohen, J. (1988). *Statistical power analysis for the behavioral sciences* (2 ed.). Routledge.

Cook-Cottone, C. P. (2015). Incorporating positive body image into the treatment of eating disorders: A model for attunement and mindful self-care. *Body Image*, 14, 158–167. https://doi.org/10.1016/j.bodyim.2015.03.004

Cox, A. E., & McMahon, A. K. (2019). Exploring changes in mindfulness and body appreciation during yoga participation. *Body Image*, 29, 118–121. https://doi.org/10.1016/j.bodyim.2019.03.003

Cox, A. E., Ullrich-French, S., Cole, A. N., & D'Hondt-Taylor, M. (2015). The role of state mindfulness during yoga in predicting self-objectification and reasons for exercise. *Psychology of Sport and Exercise.* https://doi.org/10.1016/j.psychsport.2015.10.001

Cox, A. E., Ullrich-French, S., Howe, H. S., & Cole, A. N. (2017). A pilot yoga physical education curriculum to promote positive body image. *Body Image, 23,* 1–8. https://doi.org/10.1016/j.bodyim.2017.07.007

Dakanalis, A., Timko, A., Serino, S., Riva, G., Clerici, M., & Carrà, G. (2016). Prospective psychosocial predictors of onset and cessation of eating pathology amongst college women. *European Eating Disorders Review, 24*(3), 251–256. https://doi.org/10.1002/erv.2433

Daubenmier, J. J. (2005). The relationship of yoga, body awareness, and body responsiveness to self-objectification and disordered eating. *Psychology of Women Quarterly, 29*(2), 207–219. https://doi.org/10.1111/j.1471-6402.2005.00183.x

Diehl, K., Jansen, C., Ishchanova, K., & Hilger-Kolb, J. (2018). Loneliness at Universities: Determinants of emotional and social loneliness among students. *International Journal of Environmental Research and Public Health, 15*(9), 9. https://doi.org/10.3390/ijerph15091865

Duarte, C., Ferreira, C., Trindade, I. A., & Pinto-Gouveia, J. (2015). Body image and college women's quality of life: The importance of being self-compassionate. *Journal of Health Psychology, 20*(6), 754–764. https://doi.org/10.1177/1359105315573438

Eggert, J., Levendosky, A., & Klump, K. (2007). Relationships among attachment styles, personality characteristics, and disordered eating. *EAT International Journal of Eating Disorders, 40*(2), 149–155. https://doi.org/10.1002/eat.20351

Engeln, R., Shavlik, M., & Daly, C. (2018). Tone it down: How fitness instructors' motivational comments shape women's body satisfaction. *Journal of Clinical Sport Psychology, 12* (4), 508–524. https://doi.org/10.1123/jcsp.2017-0047

Feeley, N., Cossette, S., Côté, J., Héon, M., Stremler, R., Martorella, G., & Purden, M. (2009). The importance of piloting an RCT intervention. *The Canadian Journal of Nursing Research = Revue Canadienne De Recherche En Sciences Infirmieres, 41*(2), 85–99.

Frayeh, A. L., & Lewis, B. A. (2018). The effect of mirrors on women's state body image responses to yoga. *Psychology of Sport and Exercise, 35,* 47–54. https://doi.org/10.1016/j.psychsport.2017.11.002

Gammage, K. L., Drouin, B., & Lamarche, L. (2016). Comparing a yoga class with a resistance exercise class: effects on body satisfaction and social physique anxiety in University Women. *Journal of Physical Activity & Health, 13*(11), 1202–1209. https://doi.org/10.1123/jpah.2015-0642

Garner, D. M., Olmsted, M. P., Bohr, Y., & Garfinkel, P. E. (1982). The eating attitudes test: Psychometric features and clinical correlates. *Psychological Medicine, 12*(4), 871–878. https://doi.org/10.1017/S0033291700049163

Gormally, J., Black, S., Daston, S., & Rardin, D. (1982). The assessment of binge eating severity among obese persons. *Addictive Behaviors, 7*(1), 47–55. https://doi.org/10.1016/0306-4603(82)90024-7

Hahn, E. A., DeVellis, R. F., Bode, R. K., Garcia, S. F., Castel, L. D., Eisen, S. V., Bosworth, H. B., Heinemann, A. W., Rothrock, N., & Cella, D. (2010). Measuring social health in the patient-reported outcomes measurement information system (PROMIS): Item bank development and testing. *Quality of Life Research : An International Journal of Quality of Life Aspects of Treatment, Care and Rehabilitation, 19*(7), 1035–1044. https://doi.org/10.1007/s11136-010-9654-0

Hall, A., Ofei-Tenkorang, N. A., Machan, J. T., & Gordon, C. M. (2016). Use of yoga in outpatient eating disorder treatment: A pilot study. *Journal of Eating Disorders, 4*(1), 38. https://doi.org/10.1186/s40337-016-0130-2

Halliwell, E., Dawson, K., & Burkey, S. (2019). A randomized experimental evaluation of a yoga-based body image intervention. *Body Image, 28*, 119–127. https://doi.org/10.1016/j.bodyim.2018.12.005

International Journal of Eating Disorders. (2008). *IJED statistical reporting guidelines.* https://onlinelibrary-wiley-com.udel.idm.oclc.org/pb-assets/assets/1098108x/IJED_Statistical_Reporting_Guidelines_revisedFINAL.pdf

Karazsia, B. T., Murnen, S. K., & Tylka, T. L. (2017). Is body dissatisfaction changing across time? A cross-temporal meta-analysis. *Psychological Bulletin, 143*(3), 293–320. https://doi.org/10.1037/bul0000081

Klein, J., & Cook-Cottone, C. (2013). The effects of yoga on eating disorder symptoms and correlates: A review. *International Journal of Yoga Therapy, 2*(2), 41–50.

Lattimore, P., Fisher, N., & Malinowski, P. (2011). A cross-sectional investigation of trait disinhibition and its association with mindfulness and impulsivity. *Appetite, 56*(2), 241–248. https://doi.org/10.1016/j.appet.2010.12.007

Lee, E. C., Whitehead, A. L., Jacques, R. M., & Julious, S. A. (2014). The statistical interpretation of pilot trials: Should significance thresholds be reconsidered? *BMC Medical Research Methodology, 14*(1), 41. https://doi.org/10.1186/1471-2288-14-41

Leon, A. C., Davis, L. L., & Kraemer, H. C. (2011). The role and interpretation of pilot studies in clinical research. *Journal of Psychiatric Research, 45*(5), 626–629. https://doi.org/10.1016/j.jpsychires.2010.10.008

Levine, M. P. (2012). Loneliness and Eating Disorders. *The Journal of Psychology, 146*(1–2), 243–257. https://doi.org/10.1080/00223980.2011.606435

Mason, T. B., Heron, K. E., Braitman, A. L., & Lewis, R. J. (2016). A daily diary study of perceived social isolation, dietary restraint, and negative affect in binge eating. *Appetite, 97*, 94–100. https://doi.org/10.1016/j.appet.2015.11.027

Mitchell, K. S., Mazzeo, S. E., Rausch, S. M., & Cooke, K. L. (2007). Innovative interventions for disordered eating: Evaluating dissonance-based and yoga interventions. *International Journal of Eating Disorders, 40*(2), 120–128. https://doi.org/10.1002/eat.20282

Narasimhan, L., Nagarathna, R., & Nagendra, H. (2011). Effect of integrated yogic practices on positive and negative emotions in healthy adults. *International Journal of Yoga, 4*(1), 13–19. https://doi.org/10.4103/0973-6131.78174

Neff, K. D. (2003). Development and validation of a scale to measure self-compassion. *Self and Identity, 2*(3), 223–250. https://doi.org/10.1080/15298860309027

Neumark-Sztainer, D. (2016). Eating disorders prevention: Looking backward, moving forward; looking inward, moving outward. *Eating Disorders, 24*(1), 29–38.

Neumark-Sztainer, D., MacLehose, R. F., Watts, A. W., Pacanowski, C. R., & Eisenberg, M. E. (2018). Yoga and body image: Findings from a large population-based study of young adults. *Body Image, 24*, 69–75. https://doi.org/10.1016/j.bodyim.2017.12.003

Pacanowski, C. R., Diers, L., & Crosby, R. D., & Neumark-Sztainer, D. (2017). Yoga in the treatment of eating disorders within a residential program: A randomized controlled trial. *Eating Disorders, 25*(1), 37–51. https://doi.org/10.1080/10640266.2016.1237810

Pascoe, M. C., & Bauer, I. E. (2015). A systematic review of randomised control trials on the effects of yoga on stress measures and mood. *Journal of Psychiatric Research, 68*, 270–282. https://doi.org/10.1016/j.jpsychires.2015.07.013

Proctor, E., Silmere, H., Raghavan, R., Hovmand, P., Aarons, G., Bunger, A., Griffey, R., & Hensley, M. (2011). Outcomes for implementation research: Conceptual distinctions, measurement challenges, and research agenda. *Administration and Policy in Mental Health, 38*(2), 65–76. https://doi.org/10.1007/s10488-010-0319-7

Riley, K. E., & Park, C. L. (2015). How does yoga reduce stress? A systematic review of mechanisms of change and guide to future inquiry. *Health Psychology Review*, 9(3), 379–396. https://doi.org/10.1080/17437199.2014.981778

Sala, M., & Levinson, C. A. (2017). A longitudinal study on the association between facets of mindfulness and disinhibited eating. *Mindfulness*, 8(4), 893–902. https://link.springer.com/article/10.1007/s12671-016-0663-0

Stern, N. G., & Engeln, R. (2018). Self-compassionate writing exercises increase college women's body satisfaction. *Psychology of Women Quarterly*, 42(3), 326–341. https://doi.org/10.1177/0361684318773356

Sullivan, M., Carberry, A., Evans, E. S., Hall, E. E., & Nepocatych, S. (2019). The effects of power and stretch yoga on affect and salivary cortisol in women. *Journal of Health Psychology*, 24(12), 1658–1667. https://doi.org/10.1177/1359105317694487

Thabane, L., Ma, J., Chu, R., Cheng, J., Ismaila, A., Rios, L. P., Robson, R., Thabane, M., Giangregorio, L., & Goldsmith, C. H. (2010). A tutorial on pilot studies: The what, why and how. *BMC Medical Research Methodology*, 10(1), 1. https://doi.org/10.1186/1471-2288-10-1

Tylka, T. L., & Wood-Barcalow, N. L. (2015). What is and what is not positive body image? Conceptual foundations and construct definition. *Body Image*, 14, 118–129. https://doi.org/10.1016/j.bodyim.2015.04.001

Wang, D. S. (2010). Feasibility of a yoga intervention for enhancing the mental well-being and physical functioning of older adults living in the community. *Activities, Adaptation & Aging*, 34(2), 85–97. https://doi.org/10.1080/01924781003773559

Watson, D., Clark, L. A., & Tellegen, A. (1988). Development and validation of brief measures of positive and negative affect: The PANAS scales. *Journal of Personality and Social Psychology*, 54(6), 1063. https://doi.org/10.1037/0022-3514.54.6.1063

Wilson, D., & O'Connor, E. L. (2017). Mindfulness, personality and disordered eating. *Personality and Individual Differences*, 119, 7–12. https://doi.org/10.1016/j.paid.2017.06.033

Future directions

Future directions for research on yoga and positive embodiment

Catherine Cook-Cottone, Anne Elizabeth Cox, Dianne Neumark-Sztainer, and Tracy L. Tylka

ABSTRACT
This article provides the concluding thoughts on the special issue, *Yoga for Positive Embodiment in Eating Disorder Prevention and Treatment*, which illustrate the progress being made on the relationship between yoga practice and the different indicators of positive embodiment that is relevant for the prevention and treatment of eating disorders. Based on the current body or work, we offer recommendations for the next steps for researchers for population-based, qualitative, and prevention and intervention research.

The articles in this special issue, *Yoga for Positive Embodiment in Eating Disorder Prevention and Treatment*, illustrate the progress being made on the relationship between yoga practice and the different indicators of positive embodiment that is relevant for the prevention and treatment of eating disorders. There is a growing understanding of positive embodiment and associated constructs, as well as an increasingly sophisticated conceptualization of the potential mechanisms at work in the enhancement of embodied experience that appears to be associated with yoga practice (Borden & Cook-Cottone, 2020; Cox & Tylka, 2020; Cook-Cottone, 2020; Perry & Cook-Cottone, 2020; Piran & Neumark-Sztainer, 2020). There is also a body of empirical evidence including cross-sectional, longitudinal, intervention-based, and experimental studies offering preliminary support for the positive relationship between yoga practice and outcomes such as body appreciation and reduced eating disorder risk and symptomatology (Borden & Cook-Cottone, 2020).

The articles in this special issue have offered multiple theoretical frameworks that can be applied to examine and test this relationship (Cox & Tylka, 2020; Perry & Cook-Cottone, 2020; Piran & Neumark-Sztainer, 2020). Yet, in some ways, it feels like we are just getting started. The diversity of yoga practices and approaches, as well as the complex interactions among the components that make up a yoga practice, open the door for much more nuanced and rigorous research to take place as we move into the next decade of this work. Here we offer some suggestions on how to move this work forward in a systematic manner that will play a meaningful role in eating disorder treatment and prevention.

First, have we done enough population-based research to understand how yoga may be associated with body image, disordered eating, and embodiment among individuals representing diverse social identities (e.g., ethnicity, race, gender identity, sexual orientation, age, body size, socioeconomic status, and their interactions), as well as higher risk groups? Is the body of qualitative work sufficient enough to detail the connections between yoga and embodiment, particularly mechanisms of action (e.g., mediators and moderators) and ways to improve outcomes? It is clear that we need more research in these areas (Cox & Tylka, 2020; Neumark-Sztainer et al., 2018; Webb et al., 2020). Moreover, do we have enough well-designed, sufficiently powered research conducted in both eating disorder prevention and treatment contexts to conclude that yoga effectively contributes to a positive embodiment, prevents disordered eating, and supports treatment? At this point, the most recent comprehensive review and meta-analysis (Borden & Cook-Cottone, 2020) identified 43 articles, only 13 of those are randomized controlled trials representing a broad spectrum in terms of quality of evidence. Going forward, we need to increase the employment of rigorous experimental designs in population-based research. Empirical studies need to include appropriate comparison groups (i.e., other types of body image interventions, other movement modalities), use random assignment, control for key confounding variables (e.g., age, body image, gender), and describe the content of the yoga practice or intervention in detail. Studies with control groups that consist of participants that are adequately matched to those who are in the yoga intervention groups (e.g., those with the same level and type of risk or disordered eating) are needed. When these design elements are missing, we are precluded from drawing more confident conclusions about the effects of yoga on positive embodiment and disordered eating variables.

Second, we need to pay more careful attention to individual factors that potentially moderate the impact of yoga on positive embodiment. Future research needs to better account for characteristics such as participants' age, race, gender, gender identity, exercise behavior, disordered eating history, and extent of pathology, traumatic experiences, body size, and protective characteristics like body appreciation and self-compassion. Designing studies that incorporate larger sample sizes will allow us to test for any number of individual factors that potentially moderate the effect of yoga. Further, how can research address social justice, inclusivity, and access issues (Webb et al.,

2020). These findings will then inform the way that we customize recommendations for yoga practices for specific segments of the population.

Third, we need to take a much closer look at the mechanisms that are responsible for the relationship between yoga practice and positive embodiment and ground our investigations in strong theoretical or conceptual frameworks. How can we better isolate and test the potential mechanisms responsible such as the climate of the class, the characteristics of the instructor/other participants, the intensity of the practice, the content and tone of the instruction, the types of asanas practiced, and the state experiences of the participants throughout the class (Cook-Cottone & Douglass, 2017; Cox & Tylka, 2020)? For example, the Cox et al. (2020) RCT found that mindfulness-based yoga instruction showed better outcomes than appearance-based instruction. What is the role of yoga philosophy? What are the most potent ingredients in a yoga practice for cultivating positive embodiment (e.g., sensation focus, mindfulness, breathwork, postures; Cook-Cottone & Douglass, 2017)? Is there a prescriptive approach in which certain types of classes are recommended for particular levels of risk, symptomatic presentation, or stage of recovery? What are the contraindications across level of risk, symptom presentation, and stage of recovery? Research is needed to better understand how yoga affects embodiment, risk, and treatment outcomes associated with the various eating disorder diagnostic categories throughout the etiological and treatment trajectories of each disorder.

Fourth, is there a unique approach to teaching yoga for those at-risk for and manifesting disordered eating that can more specifically and intentionally increase embodiment for this population? For example, is it important for yoga instructors to teach to experiences such as acceptance of the body, sensations, and emotions; distress tolerance; riding the wave of emotion; self-worth, self-determination and agency, and coping during yoga classes (Cook-Cottone & Douglass, 2017). For example, a critical aspect to risk reduction and recovery associated with embodiment is getting comfortable with the uncomfortable whether it be body sensations, emotions, life experiences, or anxieties about the future (Cook-Cottone, 2017). Can yoga teachers be positive coaches teaching yoga students how to approach discomfort through yoga practices such as breathing through a posture, being with the sensations in a posture, engaging in and deepening a posture, and attending to interoceptive cues and easing out of a posture when that is best? How can this type of prescriptive, targeted approach to yoga instruction be studied? Even more nuanced, can we train yoga teachers to offer instruction in ways that support embodiment and decrease risk, later assessing their effectiveness compared to yoga teachers who do not have this training?

Fifth, where should these studies be conducted? To date, many of the studies have been conducted in settings that are not ideal for rigorous, controlled research such as for-profit treatment centers, yoga studios, and community centers. What are the setting-based factors that contribute to or detract from the influences of yoga on positive embodiment and risk and maintenance of eating disordered behaviors (e.g., the impact of mirrors; see Frayeh & Lewis, 2018). Cook-Cottone and Douglass (2017) propose a host of factors related to the yoga setting that may matter and should be considered for investigation (e.g., content of marketing materials, images on walls, negative or positive body talk, diet talk, fasting and restrictive eating practices, the range of sizes in products sold at studios, and the embodiment of instructors as well as the range of sizes, shapes, and other aspects of diversity embodied by instructors).

Sixth, to date, the concept of dosage has not been adequately addressed (Cook-Cottone, 2013). Is there an optimal dosage of yoga per week that provides a benchmark for achieving therapeutic results including days per week and length of sessions (e.g., 2 to 3 days a week for 60 to 75 minutes per session; Cook-Cottone, 2013)? How long does an individual need to practice yoga before there is sufficient experience to protect or create change (6 months, a year, several years)? Do those who institute a home practice fair better than those who do not (Ross et al., 2012)? Is there a dosage that is too low to make a difference (e.g., <2 times a week) or so high that risk is increased, or pathology is enhanced (e.g., every day for more than 90 minutes a day)?

Seventh, what is the role of contemporary neuroscience? Sullivan et al. (2018) propose a compelling model for the convergence of traditional yoga wisdom and contemporary neuroscience for self-regulation and resilience through yoga practice. They assert that yoga practice integrates bottom-up neurophysiological and top-down neurocognitive mechanisms leading to increased well-being. Further, using the polyvagal theory, they posit that yoga practice can optimally activate the polyvagal system in the promotion of mental health. A recent review of studies examining the effects of yoga practice on brain structures, function, and cerebral blood flow found that collectively these studies demonstrate a positive effect of yoga practice on the structure and/or function of the hippocampus, amygdala, prefrontal cortex, cingulate cortex, and brain networks including the default mode network (Gothe et al., 2019). Disturbances in these areas and processes of the brain are all implicated in the risk and manifestation of eating disorders (Blume et al., 2019; Donnelly et al., 2018; Kot et al., 2020). Accordingly, future research should capitalize on neuroscientific models and techniques to assess the effects of yoga practice among those at risk for and struggling with disordered eating.

Eighth, as clear in the introduction of this special series (Neumark-Stztainer et al., 2020), like us, many researchers studying yoga have a personal practice and have life experience that has led them to study yoga as a prevention and treatment intervention for disordered eating. Intentionally, we began this series explicating our reasons for doing this work taking the first step in minimizing bias – acknowledging it. Now we ask: How can our lines of inquiry, designs, and standards for research provide a stringent and reliable check on our own biases as we explore these questions? Going forward, researchers should strive to reduce bias and increase the opportunity for replication at each step of study development and implementation using registered, RCT designs, blinding participants and instructors to study hypotheses when possible, having naïve research assistants deliver assessments, utilizing sufficient sample sizes, disclosing all measures used, manualizing and sharing the yoga intervention, reporting all outcomes including those that show null or negative effects, providing data for re-analysis, and exploring significant and clinically meaningful outcomes (Ioannidis et al., 2014; Klein & Cook-Cottone, 2013). As editors, we should select critical reviewers and those steeped in knowledge about yoga study designs and shortcomings as well as publish studies with null or negative outcomes.

Moving forward systematically will require challenging, incremental work. It must also balance the rigorous approaches and leave space for innovations and novelty meaning that the need for RCTs must be balanced with space for more pilot studies and creative research. In yoga this is called *sthira and suka*, balancing structure and ease. Much of this research will necessitate measurement development (e.g., broader measures of embodiment), more creative research designs, and using strong theory to inform the research questions we pose. These systematic lines of research will then allow us to continue to refine and build new theories providing better frameworks for the development of yoga interventions to treat and prevent eating disorders. We look forward to the future decades of this work and offer this special issue as a platform for the commencement of the next generation of yoga, embodiment, and eating disorder research.

References

Blume, M., Schmidt, R., & Hilbert, A. (2019). Abnormalities in the EEG power spectrum in bulimia nervosa, binge-eating disorder, and obesity: A systematic review. *European Eating Disorders Review, 27*(2), 124–136. https://doi.org/10.1002/erv.2654

Borden, A., & Cook-Cottone, C. P. (2020). Yoga and eating disorder prevention and treatment: A comprehensive review and meta-analysis. *Eating Disorders: The Journal of Treatment and Prevention, xx*, xx–xx. ((this issue)).

Cook-Cottone, C. P. (2013). Dosage as a critical variable in yoga therapy research. *International Journal of Yoga Therapy, 23*, 11–12.

Cook-Cottone, C. P. (2017). Yoga for the re-embodied self: The therapeutic journey home. *Yoga Therapy Today, Winter, 2016*, 40–42.

Cook-Cottone, C. P. (2020). *Embodiment and the treatment of eating disorders: The body as a resource in recovery*. Norton Books.

Cook-Cottone, C. P., & Douglass, L. L. (2017). Yoga communities and eating disorders: Creating safe space for positive embodiment. *International Journal of Yoga Therapy, 27*(1), 87–93. https://doi.org/10.17761/1531-2054-27.1.87

Cox, A. E., & Tylka, T. L. (2020). A conceptual model describing mechanisms for how yoga practice may support positive embodiment. *Eating Disorders: The Journal of Treatment and Prevention, xx,* xx–xx. ((this issue)).

Cox, A. E., Ullrich-French, S., Cook-Cottone, C., Tylka, T. L., & Neumark-Sztainer, D. (2020). Examining the effects of mindfulness-based yoga instruction on positive embodiment and affective reposes. *Eating Disorders: The Journal of Treatment and Prevention, XX,* XX–XX. ((current issue)).

Donnelly, B., Touyz, S., Hay, P., Burton, A., Russell, J., & Caterson, I. (2018). Neuroimaging in bulimia nervosa and binge eating disorder: A systematic review. *Journal of Eating Disorders, 6*(1), 3. https://doi.org/10.1186/s40337-018-0187-1

Frayeh, A., & Lewis, B. (2018). The effect of mirrors on women's state body image response to yoga. *Psychology of Sport and Exercise, 35,* 47–54. https://doi.org/10.1016/j.psychsport.2017.11.002

Gothe, N. P., Khan, I., Hayes, J., Erlenbach, E., & Damoiseaux, J. S. (2019). Yoga effects on brain health: A systematic review of the current literature. *Brain Plasticity, 5*(1), 105–122. https://doi.org/https://dx.doi.10.3233%2FBPL-190084

Ioannidis, J. P., Munafo, M. R., Fusar-Poli, P., Nosek, B. A., & David, S. P. (2014). Publication and other reporting biases in cognitive sciences: Detection, prevalence, and prevention. *Trends in Cognitive Sciences, 18*(5), 235–241. https://doi.org/10.1016/j.tics.2014.02.010

Klein, J., & Cook-Cottone, C. (2013). The effects of yoga on eating disorder symptoms and correlates: A review. *International Journal of Yoga Therapy, 23*(2), 41–50.

Kot, E., Kucharska, K., Monteleone, A. M., & Monteleone, P. (2020). Structural and functional brain correlates of altered taste processing in anorexia nervosa: A systematic review. *European Eating Disorders Review, 28*(2), 122–140. https://doi.org/10.1002/erv.2713

Neumark-Sztainer, D., Watts, A. W., & Rydell, S. (2018). Yoga and body image: How do young adults practicing yoga describe its impact on their body image. *Body Image, 27,* 156–168. https://doi.org/https://dx.doi.10.1016%2Fj.bodyim.2018.09.001

Perry, I., & Cook-Cottone, C. P. (2020). Eating disorders, embodiment, and yoga: A conceptual overview. *Eating Disorders: The Journal of Treatment and Prevention, xx,* xx–xx. ((this issue)).

Piran, N., & Neumark-Sztainer, D. (2020). Yoga and the experience of embodiment: A discussion and possible links. *Eating Disorders: The Journal of Treatment and Prevention, XX,* XX–XX. ((this issue)).

Ross, A., Friedman, E., Bevans, M., & Thomas, S. (2012). Frequency of yoga practice predicts health: Results from a national survey of yoga practice. *Evidence-based Complementary and Alternative Medicine, 10,* 1–10. https://doi.org/10.1155/2012/983258

Sullivan, M. B., Erb, M., Schmalzl, L., Moonaz, S., Noggle Taylor, J., & Porges, S. W. (2018). Yoga therapy and polyvagal theory: The convergence of traditional wisdom and contemporary neuroscience for self-regulation and resilience. *Frontiers in Human Neuroscience, 12,* 67. https://doi.org/10.3389/fnhum.2018.00067

Webb, J. B., Rogers, C. B., & Thomas, E. V. (2020). Realizing yoga's all-access pass: A social justice critique of Westernized yoga and inclusive embodiment. *Eating Disorders: The Journal of Treatment and Prevention, xx,* xx–xx. ((this issue)).

Index

acceptability 47, 61, 186, 212, 213, 222, 225, 229, 232, 233
advocacy 47, 59–60
affective responses 155, 158–160, 168
age, advancing 56–58
agency 14, 17, 19, 32, 71, 79, 80, 243
Andrew, R. 83
anorexia nervosa (AN) 98
ANOVA 164, 166
Anthis, K. 85
Ariel-Donges, A. H. 98, 124, 194
attitudes toward seeking professional psychological help-short form (ATSPPH-SF) 140
attuned exercise 82–84, 86
attuned self-care 13, 24, 27, 33, 35, 36, 71, 156
attunement 10, 15, 16, 30, 33, 35, 44, 61
awareness 12, 15, 16, 56, 59–60, 76, 78, 99, 100, 175, 178, 184, 185

Ballard, J. 51
baseline body image 183
baseline variables 160, 164
Beck, M. 137
bias 2, 59, 107, 112, 116, 123, 124, 187, 245
Bilger, A. 54
binge eating disorder (BED) 10, 11, 98, 135–139, 146, 148–150
binge eating frequency 135, 137, 138, 143, 146, 150
binge eating scale (BES) 225
bodily desires 13, 14, 27, 35
body appreciation 3, 4, 75–78, 81, 83, 85–87, 157, 159–161, 166, 192–194, 197, 202–204
body awareness 14, 15, 35, 44, 83, 85, 100, 102, 112, 194, 202
body connection 27, 30, 36, 71, 73, 83, 85, 122, 156
body dissatisfaction 98, 99, 112, 191–197, 202, 203, 211, 212, 223
body image 2, 3, 5, 25, 48, 55, 59, 98, 113, 115, 121, 122, 175–178, 183, 185, 187, 233; flexibility 78, 79, 83
Body Mass Index (BMI) 52, 53, 125, 196, 199, 211, 225

body surveillance 74, 75, 77, 83, 87, 112, 117, 157, 159, 161, 167, 192, 193
Boehm, K. 101, 122
Bordo, S. 26
Borenstein, M. 116
bulimia nervosa (BN) 98
bulimia symptoms 107, 112, 119, 121, 122, 126

Calogero, R. M. 84
Carei, T. R. 125
Carmo, C. 122
Clarke, D. P. 137, 146, 148
cognitive behavioral therapy (CBT) 11, 12, 136, 137, 149, 174
Cohen, J. 141
Cole, A. N. 194
competence 14, 19, 44, 79–81, 194; perceptions of 79, 194
comprehensive meta-analysis 116
Conboy, L. A 194
conceptual model 2, 70, 72–74, 87, 88, 99
contemporary yoga scholarship 47, 59
contextual variables 84, 86
control groups 124, 125, 138, 142, 143, 211, 213, 227, 230, 232, 234
Cook-Cottone, C. P. 15, 16, 85, 112, 122, 137, 168
correlational studies 102, 121, 125, 126
Cox, A. E. 77, 78, 87, 193–194, 212
critical theory 26, 27

Dahm, K. A. 148
Dale, L. P. 112
data analyses 164
data collection 2, 116
Daubenmier, J. J. 75, 211
De-Beauvoir, S. 26
Delaney, K. 85
delineating protective experiences 28, 37
demographic questionnaire 196
dependent variables 142, 159, 165, 198, 199, 226, 227
desire 13, 14, 27, 28, 33, 35, 36, 51, 54, 71, 81

developmental theory of embodiment (DTE) 25, 26, 28, 30–32, 34–38, 60, 156, 157, 167
Devlin, M. J. 140
D'Hondt-Taylor, M. 194
dialectic behavioral therapy (DBT) 11, 12, 136, 137, 139
Diers, L. 102
disabilities 37, 55, 56
disordered eating 3, 19, 44–46, 48, 58, 99, 101, 115, 188, 203, 210–212, 242, 244
disrupted embodiment 3, 71
Dittmann, K. A. 102
Domingues, R. B. 122
Douglass, L. L. 85, 168

eating attitudes test 225
eating disorder diagnostic scale (EDDS) 139
eating disorder examination questionnaire (EDE-Q) 140
eating disorders 2, 5, 9, 55, 97, 99, 135–138, 146–150, 156, 174–177, 185–188, 211, 212, 226; treatment of 11, 57, 135, 137, 138, 147, 150, 174–176, 185, 187
education 46, 59–60, 178
effect sizes 101, 116, 117, 119, 121, 141, 166, 200, 226, 232
eight-week Yoga program 138, 141, 148
Eisenberg, M. E. 200
eligibility criteria 102, 115
embodied experiences 12, 13, 74, 241
embodiment 9, 10, 12–17, 19, 25–28, 36, 37, 49, 60, 61, 156, 243; developmental theory of 26; expanding 58; experience of 13, 19, 24, 25, 27, 28, 33, 36, 37, 60, 157; philosophical roots of 12; Piran's developmental theory of 13; positive experiences of 37, 155, 156; psychological theories of 12, 17; research program 27
emotional regulation 11, 107, 136–138, 146–148; difficulties 99, 138, 146, 150
environment 15, 54, 81, 83, 84, 86, 87, 214

Fallon, E. A. 202
feasibility 47, 61, 186, 212, 213, 225, 232–234
Flaherty, M. 194
food 10, 11, 17, 35, 83, 98, 113, 225
forecasted pleasure 157, 159, 161, 163, 165–167
forms of self-criticizing/attacking and self-reassuring scale (FSCRS) 140, 143
Foucault, M. 26
Frankl, V. 13, 16
Frayeh, A. 234
Freedman, M. R. 102
frequent yoga practice 191, 192, 194, 200, 201
functionality 13, 14, 27, 32, 36, 58, 71, 100, 114, 156, 212

Gammage, L. 211
gender non-conforming individuals 45, 51
Gilbert, P. 136, 147
Giles, G. 137
Global eating disorder pathology 119
Goldfein, J. A. 140
Guilamo-Ramos, V. 142

Haddix, M. M. 49
Hall, A. 112
Halliwell, E. 78, 85, 125, 126
Hausenblas, H. A. 202
heterogeneity 116, 117, 176
higher weight 45, 52, 53
Hopkins, L. B. 125
hypothesis testing 165, 233

Impett, E. A. 74
inclusive embodiment 43, 59, 60
individual variables 86
internal consistency 197, 198, 224
internal validity 116, 162
interventions 100, 101, 123, 124, 174–177, 220, 221, 223–225, 232, 233; development 215; interventionists 214; studies 2, 5, 25, 35, 37, 204
intrinsic motivation 80, 81, 87
intuitive eating 44, 60, 61, 83, 86, 107; acceptance model of 60, 83

Jaccard, J. 142
Jopling, D. A. 147
joyful immersion 80, 157

Kamenetz, C. 140
Kane, L. 137
Karlsen, K. E. 125
Klein, J. 122
Kripalani, K. 51
Kripalu Yoga 85, 138
Kwee, J. L. 16

language 32, 34, 36, 85, 156, 162, 177, 212, 215, 218, 221
Launeanu, M. 16
Levine, M. P. 14
Lewis, B. 234
loneliness 99, 211–213, 224
lower socioeconomic status 45, 46

MacLehose, R. F. 107, 200
Mahlo, L. 77
males 45, 50, 126, 149, 201, 202
manipulation check items 162
McGartland, M. 137

McGraw, R. 50
McIver, S. 125, 137, 146
McMahon, A. K. 77, 193, 194, 212
Menzel, J. E. 14, 15
Merleau-Ponty, M. 26
meta-analysis 97, 99–101, 113, 115–117,
    121–124
meta-analytic findings 122
mindfulness 75, 76, 87, 137, 148, 149, 159, 162,
    164, 166, 167, 192, 193, 196, 198, 202, 212, 225;
    condition 164, 166, 167; scale 143; skills 135, 145,
    147, 148, 150
mindfulness-based yoga instruction 155,
    168, 243
mindful self-care 16, 61, 82
Mitchell, K. S. 124
mixed-methods pilot study 173
moderators 72, 73, 84, 85, 87, 195, 242
Multidimensional Body-Self Relations
    Questionnaire (MBSRQ) 197, 223, 224
Murray, S. B. 12

Neff, K. D. 148
negative affect 75, 81, 82, 87, 136, 138, 156, 158,
    211–213, 215, 224
Neumark-Sztainer, D. 85, 107, 200, 233
nonclinical groups 210
non-controlled trials 102, 107, 112
non-randomized studies 107, 112, 126

O'Halloran, P. 137
Ostermann, T. 101, 122
outcome variables 117, 160, 225
overweight 11, 197, 201

Pacanowski, C. R. 200
Park, C. L. 77
participant recruitment 160
Pedrotty, K. N. 84
pilot studies 176, 177, 181, 185, 188, 226, 233, 234, 245
Piran, N. 14, 71, 156
pleasure 14, 19, 34, 80, 81, 155, 157
positive affect 81, 82, 155, 156, 158, 210, 212, 213,
    224, 227, 230, 232, 234
positive embodiment 4, 10, 12, 26, 27, 36, 37,
    71, 72, 84–87, 99, 156, 158, 159, 167, 241, 242;
    variables 86, 159, 167
positive feelings 30–32
potential differential efficacy 126
preliminary analyses 142; manipulation checks 164
primary analyses 143
process evaluation 220
Procter, S. 136, 147
protective factors 26, 28, 30–32, 34–38, 156, 192,
    193, 204, 210

qualitative studies 25, 37, 49, 85, 102, 113, 114, 121,
    185, 186

racial/ethnic minorities 48, 49
randomization 114, 142, 176, 226
randomized controlled trial (RCTs) 101, 102, 113,
    114, 116–119, 121–123, 125, 126, 135, 137, 138,
    158, 176, 242
recruitment 60, 226
Remski, M. 48
restorative yoga 33
retention 226, 233

search strategy 102, 115
self-compassion 76, 77, 83, 85, 87, 137, 138, 141,
    147–150, 197, 204, 212, 224
self-compassion scale-short form (SCS-SF) 140
self-critical individuals 136
self-criticism 99, 135–138, 140, 143, 144, 147,
    148, 150
self-model, embodied 15, 16
self-objectification 10, 15, 58, 61, 74, 75, 80, 107,
    112, 192–194
self-report 117, 150, 187
sexual minorities 45, 54, 55
Sherman, K. J. 124
Siconolfi, D. 54
social action research agenda 61
social justice critique 43
social power 14, 28, 31, 35, 61, 71
Spadola, C. E. 49, 244
stable embodied characteristics 74, 82, 84
state body appreciation 86, 159, 161, 163, 166
state body surveillance 159, 161, 163, 166
state mindfulness 76, 86, 148, 159, 160, 163,
    165–167, 193, 194
statistical analyses 198
study characteristics 102
study selection 116
subgroup analyses 116, 117, 119, 121, 123

theoretical application 60
Tiggemann, M. 77
Toronto mindfulness scale (TMS) 140
transgender non-conforming individuals
    45, 51, 55
treatment research 112
tridimensional ontology 13

Ullrich-French, S. 194

Vogel, H. 101, 122

Watts, A. W. 200
westernized yoga 43, 51

yoga 2, 4, 5, 18, 19, 25, 33, 36, 48, 99, 100, 114, 122, 124, 125, 137, 175, 192, 203, 211; classes 4, 85–87, 126, 141, 142, 159–162, 166, 167, 213, 229; experiences 124, 157, 168, 186, 213; instruction 84, 155, 156, 162, 166, 168, 176, 243; instructors 79–81, 83, 85, 158, 162, 163, 168, 177, 179, 212, 214; knowledge and experience 198; origin basic principles and modern interpretations of 18; participation 55, 56, 75–77, 79–81, 84, 87, 157–159; practice 5, 36–38, 49, 50, 58, 72–74, 79, 81, 113, 191, 193, 194, 241–244; practitioners 31, 35, 37, 44, 45, 47, 57, 58, 74, 75, 78, 79, 83, 86, 156; program 135, 137, 138, 142, 146, 148–150, 176, 177, 180, 181, 187; research on 241; self-efficacy 112, 192, 194–196, 198; series 222, 223, 229, 232, 234; teachers 28, 31, 32, 36, 37, 141, 177, 178, 214, 215, 243

yoga and body image program (YBI) 177, 180, 183–187

yoga-based therapy program 173

For Product Safety Concerns and Information please contact our EU
representative GPSR@taylorandfrancis.com
Taylor & Francis Verlag GmbH, Kaufingerstraße 24, 80331 München, Germany

* 9 7 8 1 0 3 2 0 6 3 2 4 9 *